Bipolar Disorder in Later Life

Bipolar Disorder in Later Life

Edited by

MARTHA SAJATOVIC, M.D.

Professor, Department of Psychiatry
Case Western Reserve University
University Hospitals of Cleveland
Cleveland, Ohio

and

FREDERIC C. BLOW, PH.D.

Professor, Department of Psychiatry
University of Michigan
Director, National Serious Mental Illness
Treatment Research and Evaluation Center
Department of Veterans Affairs
Ann Arbor, Michigan

The Johns Hopkins University Press
Baltimore

© 2007 The Johns Hopkins University Press
All rights reserved. Published 2007
Printed in the United States of America on acid-free paper
2 4 6 8 9 7 5 3 1

The Johns Hopkins University Press
2715 North Charles Street
Baltimore, Maryland 21218-4363
www.press.jhu.edu

Library of Congress Cataloging-in-Publication Data
Bipolar disorder in later life / edited by Martha Sajatovic
and Frederic C. Blow.
p. ; cm.
Includes bibliographical references and index.
ISBN 13: 978-0-8018-8581-5 (hardcover : alk paper)
ISBN 10: 0-8018-8581-7 (hardcover : alk. paper)
1. Manic-depressive illness. 2. Older people — Mental health.
I. Sajatovic, Martha. II. Blow, Frederic C.
[DNLM: 1. Bipolar Disorder. 2. Aged. 3. Middle Aged.
WM 207 B61634 2007]
RC516.B5744 2007
618.97′6895 — dc22   2006026077

A catalog record for this book is available from the British Library.

Contents

Preface

Bipolar disorder is a serious chronic mental illness that is associated with substantial impairments in quality of life and functional outcomes, high rates of suicide, and high financial costs. Although the persistent and chronic nature of bipolar disorder is well known, the unique clinical presentation, health outcomes, and optimal treatments for older adults with bipolar disorder are far less understood. With the changes in demographics in the United States and other industrialized nations and the developing sophistication in the treatment of bipolar illness, there has been a growing awareness of the manifestations of bipolar disorder among older adults. In the past, some clinicians might have been reluctant to make a diagnosis of late-onset bipolar illness in the case of an elderly individual experiencing an apparently new-onset mania. Still persisting is the notion that bipolarity in late life "burns out" or resolves over a period of decades.

The recent resurgence in awareness of and interest in late-life bipolar disorder parallels the growing proportions of elderly persons in the population worldwide. Primarily because of pharmacological advances, the outcomes of geriatric bipolar disorder have improved significantly in the past several decades. Advances in appropriate recognition of bipolar disorder and a rapidly expanding choice of treatments have paved the way for potentially improved care among all individuals with bipolar disorder, including elderly persons. Despite these improvements, geriatric bipolar disorder is still associated with substantial morbidity and mortality, as well as poor psychosocial outcomes. As the chapters in this volume illustrate, bipolar disorder in late life does not "burn out" over time, but rather remains a serious and complex condition that imposes substantial personal and financial burdens on the affected individuals, their families, and society at large.

Clinical research on late-life bipolar disorder has been relatively limited. Clinicians caring for geriatric patients with bipolar illness have few evidence-based guidelines on which to base treatment decisions, and the overwhelming majority of research studies on bipolar disorder involve younger or, at best, mixed-age populations.

The contributors to this volume present the most up-to-date knowledge available, provide frameworks and resoources with which to understand bipolar disorder in late life, and offer guidance to address the paucity of data on this topic.

The chapters are organized into four parts. The first part addresses the epidemiology and assessment of older adults with bipolar disorder, including the use of standardized rating scales and nursing home assessments. Chapter 1 explains changes in diagnosis patterns over the life course, distinctions between early versus later onset of disease, and differences and changes in symptomatology associated with age-related factors. The chapter highlights current research on gender differences, psychiatric comorbidities, patterns of health care utilization, and barriers to care facing this population.

The literature on the application of rating scales to older adults with bipolar disorder is limited. Chapter 2 describes categories of bipolar mood states, explains the characteristics of various mood rating scales and factors that can influence their application in mania, and reviews scales specific to bipolar manic episodes in old age. This chapter provides clinical descriptions of older patients and findings on their psychopathological profiles as measured by rating scales, as well as introducing considerations about assessing manic signs and symptoms in other elderly patient groups.

Little is known about the needs of nursing home residents with serious and persistent mental illness, particularly bipolar disorder. Chapter 3 presents evidence to support the notion that nursing home residents with bipolar disorder are clinically complex individuals who require care in multiple domains, necessitating comprehensive assessments to best determine their overall care needs. This chapter also describes the practical and research applications of the interRAI family of assessment instruments.

Part II is devoted to treatment issues, including treatments for late-onset and secondary mania, pharmacotherapies, psychosocial interventions, and patients' adherence to medication regimens. Chapter 4 concentrates on the epidemiology, etiology, diagnosis, and treatment of secondary mania and late-onset bipolar disorder. This chapter develops the concept of secondary mania and its presentation across the lifespan, details a comprehensive diagnostic workup to identify potential causes of secondary mania, and reviews treatment options.

The pharmacological treatment of bipolar disorder in older adults has been a neglected area of clinical and research focus. Chapter 5 reviews the current state of the evidence on safety, effectiveness, and clinical usage recommendations for specific medications commonly used to treat bipolar disorder in older adults, summarizing the biological treatment options with considerations relevant to older adults.

Data on the appropriateness and effectiveness of psychosocial interventions specifically for older individuals with bipolar disorder are also scarce. Chapter 6 presents recent cross-sectional data from a veteran population with bipolar disorder, and describes the Life Goals Program, a psychoeducational intervention widely used for individuals with bipolar illness. This chapter includes a series of case vignettes of older adults treated with this approach and highlights key themes that emerged from treatment interactions.

Poor adherence to mood-stabilizing medication regimens limits the potential benefits of these medications. Chapter 7 details the determinants of poor adherence to prescribed treatment among patients with bipolar disorder, including older adults. Recent findings on adherence in this population and strategies to improve adherence are presented.

Part III examines complexity and comorbidity, including substance abuse disorders, medical comorbidity, and the issue of culturally aware treatment among those with bipolar disorder in later adulthood. The co-occurrence of a substance use disorder with bipolar disorder raises concerns because of the adverse effects on the course, treatment, and prognoses of both disorders. Chapter 8 reviews the prevalence and correlates of bipolar disorder and substance use disorders in older adults, their co-occurrence in mixed-age samples, and the likely complicating effects of aging on clinical features and outcomes for older adults with co-occurring disorders.

The management and treatment course of late-life bipolar disorder are made more complex by the comorbid medical illnesses commonly found in older adults. Chapter 9 discusses common comorbidities in late-life bipolar disorder, medical disorders related to pharmacological treatment, medication interactions, and the changes in medication dosing and care management made necessary by the co-occurrence of bipolar disorder and medical illnesses.

Culture shapes the ways in which patients, families, and clinicians perceive, communicate about, and address mental illness. Chapter 10 explores how culture affects the experience and meaning of bipolar disorder, including the shaping of symptoms, the management of illness episodes and healing activities, and the management of outcomes. This chapter presents cultural issues that are critical to informing clinical practice in the diagnosis and management of bipolar disorder.

Finally, part IV addresses specialized care delivery, including quality of care, evidenced-based medicine, and legal and ethical issues in bipolar disorder research. The quality of care and subsequent outcomes for older adults with bipolar disorder remain suboptimal, despite pharmacological advances and practice guidelines. Chapter 11 reviews the current knowledge on the quality of psychiatric care and proposes a new paradigm in thinking about quality of care and quality improvement for this population.

Chapter 12 discusses the importance of evidence-based medicine in the treatment of older adults with bipolar disorder, the rationale and methodology for its use in geriatric mental health practices, the evidence supporting the effective treatment of older adults with bipolar disorder, the barriers and approaches to implementing treatment in geriatric mental health care, and the limitations of evidence-based medicine.

Participation in research by elderly adults with bipolar disorder is essential if we are to understand the course of this disease over the lifespan and its cumulative and interactive effects with comorbid conditions. Chapter 13 discusses the significant legal and ethical issues involved in research with participants from this population and how the resolution of these issues may be rendered even more difficult as individuals with bipolar disorder age.

As each of these chapters makes clear, although empirical data have accumulated in recent years, multiple challenges to ensuring optimal outcomes for older adults with bipolar disorder remain. We hope that this book will assist clinicians who are struggling to provide the best possible care for their geriatric patients with bipolar disorder and will add momentum to the growing interest in better understanding later-life bipolar illness.

Contributors

Stephen J. Bartels, M.D., M.S., Professor, Department of Psychiatry, Dartmouth Medical School; Director, Aging Services Research Group, New Hampshire–Dartmouth Psychiatric Research Center, Lebanon, New Hampshire

Mark S. Bauer, M.D., Professor of Psychiatry, Brown University, Department of Veterans Affairs Medical Center, Providence, Rhode Island

Stephen T. Chermack, Ph.D., Assistant Professor, Department of Psychiatry, University of Michigan Addiction Research Center; Chief, Outpatient Mental Health Clinic, and Chief, Substance Abuse Clinic, Ann Arbor Department of Veterans Affairs Healthcare System, Ann Arbor, Michigan

Colin A. Depp, Ph.D., Assistant Professor, Sam and Rose Stein Institute for Research on Aging, Department of Psychiatry, University of California, San Diego, California

Christian R. Dolder, Pharm.D., Assistant Professor, Wingate University School of Pharmacy, Wingate, North Carolina

Brant E. Fries, Ph.D., Professor, Institute of Gerontology and School of Public Health, University of Michigan; Chief, Health Systems Research, Geriatric Research, Education and Clinical Center, Ann Arbor Department of Veterans Affairs Medical Center, Ann Arbor, Michigan

John P. Hirdes, Ph.D., Professor, Department of Health Studies and Gerontology, University of Waterloo; Scientific Director, Homewood Research Institute, Waterloo, Ontario, Canada

Paul E. Holtzheimer III, M.D., Assistant Professor, Fuqua Center for Late-Life Depression, Department of Psychiatry and Behavioral Sciences, Emory University, Atlanta, Georgia

Dilip V. Jeste, M.D., Estelle and Edgar Levi Chair in Aging, Director, Sam and Rose Stein Institute for Research on Aging; Distinguished Professor of Psychiatry and Neurosciences, University of California, San Diego, and San Diego Department of Veterans Affairs Healthcare System, San Diego, California

Helen C. Kales, M.D., Assistant Professor, Department of Psychiatry, University of Michigan; Director, Geriatric Psychiatry Clinic; Affiliated Investigator, Geriatric Research Education and Clinical Center, Ann Arbor Department of Veterans Affairs Healthcare System; Investigator, Department of Veterans Affairs, Health Services Research and Development, Serious Mental Illness Treatment Research and Evaluation Center (SMITREC), Ann Arbor, Michigan

Amy M. Kilbourne, Ph.D., M.P.H., Associate Professor of Psychiatry, University of Michigan and VA Ann Arbor Healthcare System, Serious Mental Illness Treatment Research and Evaluation Center (SMITREC), Ann Arbor, Michigan.

Sana Loue, J.D., Ph.D., M.P.H., Professor, Director, Center for Minority Public Health, School of Medicine, Department of Epidemiology and Biostatistics, Case Western Reserve University, Cleveland, Ohio

Linda McBride, M.S.N., Nurse Clinical Specialist, Mental Health and Behavioral Science Service, Bipolar Disorders Program, Providence Department of Veterans Affairs Medical Center, Providence, Rhode Island

William M. McDonald, M.D., Professor, Fuqua Center for Late-Life Depression, Department of Psychiatry and Behavioral Sciences, Emory University, Atlanta, Georgia

John N. Morris, Ph.D., Co-Director, Institute for Aging Research, Hebrew Senior Life, Boston, Massachusetts

Catherine Peasley-Miklus, Ph.D., Research Associate, Department of Psychiatry, Institute of Geriatric Psychiatry, Weill Medical College of Cornell University and Payne Whitney Westchester, White Plains, New York

Harold A. Pincus, M.D., Vice Chair for Strategic Initiatives, Department of Psychiatry, Columbia University, New York, New York; Director of Quality and Outcomes Research, New York Presbyterian Hospital, New York, New York; RAND Corporation, Pittsburgh, Pennsylvania

Terry Rabinowitz, M.D., Associate Professor of Psychiatry and Family Medicine, University of Vermont College of Medicine; Director, Psychiatric Consultation Service, and Clinical Director, Telemedicine, Fletcher Allen Health Care, Burlington, Vermont

Herbert C. Schulberg, Ph.D., Professor of Psychology in Psychiatry, Department of Psychiatry, Institute of Geriatric Psychiatry, Weill Medical College of Cornell University and Payne Whitney Westchester, White Plains, New York

Marcia Valenstein, M.D., Research Scientist, Department of Veterans Affairs, Health Services Research and Development, Serious Mental Illness Treatment Research and Evaluation Center (SMITREC); Assistant Professor, Department of Psychiatry, University of Michigan, Ann Arbor, Michigan

Aricca D. Van Citters, M.S., Project Coordinator, Aging Services Research Group, New Hampshire–Dartmouth Psychiatric Research Center, Department of Community and Family Medicine, Dartmouth Medical School, Lebanon, New Hampshire

John M. Wryobeck, Ph.D., Assistant Professor, Department of Psychiatry, University of Toledo–Health Sciences Campus, Toledo, Ohio

Robert C. Young, M.D., Professor, Department of Psychiatry, Institute of Geriatric Psychiatry, Weill Medical College of Cornell University and Payne Whitney Westchester, White Plains, New York

Abbreviations

ABS	Aggressive Behavior Scale
ACE	angiotensin-converting enzyme
ADL	activities of daily living
ADRS	Affective Disorder Rating Scale
AIDS	acquired immunodeficiency syndrome
AOI	Awareness of Illness
BMI	body mass index
BPD-SUD	bipolar disorder–substance use disorder
BPRS	Brief Psychiatric Rating Scale
BRMS	Bech-Rafaelson Mania Scale
CBT	cognitive-behavioral therapy
CCC	Complex Continuing Care
CCM	chronic care model
CGI	Clinical Global Impression
CHESS	Changes in Health, End-stage disease and Signs and Symptoms
CIHI	Canadian Institute for Health Information
CMAI	Cohen-Mansfield Agitation Inventory
CMS	Centers for Medicare and Medicaid Services
CNS	clinical nurse specialist
CPS	Cognitive Performance Scale
CYP	cytochrome P450
DBS	deep brain stimulation
DBSA	Depression and Bipolar Support Alliance
DRS	Depression Rating Scale
DSM-III-R	*Diagnostic and Statistical Manual of Mental Disorders*, Third Edition Revised
DSM-IV	*Diagnostic and Statistical Manual of Mental Disorders*, Fourth Edition

DSM-IV-TR	*Diagnostic and Statistical Manual of Mental Disorders,* Fourth Edition Text Revision
EBM	evidence-based medicine
ECT	electroconvulsive therapy
FDA	U.S. Food and Drug Administration
FY	fiscal year
HBQ	Health Belief Questionnaire
HDRS	Hamilton Depression Rating Scale
HIV	human immunodeficiency virus
HRQOL	health-related quality of life
ICD-9	International Classification of Diseases–Ninth Revision
IRB	institutional review board
ISE	Index of Social Engagement
ISS	Internal State Scale
LDL	low-density lipoprotein
MCS	Mental Component Score
MDQ	Mood Disorder Questionnaire
MMSE	Mini Mental State Examination
MMSS	Modified Manic State Scale
MPR	medication possession ratio
MRI	magnetic resonance imaging
NDI	nephrogenic diabetes insipidus
NH	nursing home
NIMH	National Institute of Mental Health
NSAIDs	nonsteroidal anti-inflammatory drugs
OR	odds ratio
PCS	Physical Component Score
PM	participatory management
PTSD	post-traumatic stress disorder
RAI	Resident Assessment Instrument
RAI 2.0	Resident Assessment Instrument 2.0
RAI-MH	Resident Assessment Instrument–Mental Health
RAP	Resident Assessment Protocol
ROMI	Ratings of Medication Influence
RUG-III	Resource Utilization Groups
SD	standard deviation
SIADH	syndrome of inappropriate antidiuretic hormone secretion
SLE	systemic lupus erthythematosus

SMITREC   Serious Mental Illness Treatment Research and Evaluation
              Center
SSRI   selective serotonin reuptake inhibitor
SUD   substance use disorder
TCA   tricyclic antidepressant
UTI   urinary tract infection
VA   U.S. Department of Veterans Affairs
VHA   Veterans Health Administration
WMS-III   Weschler Memory Scale III
YMRS   Young Mania Rating Scale

PART ONE

Epidemiology and Assessment

CHAPTER ONE

Epidemiology of Bipolar Disorder in Later Life

MARTHA SAJATOVIC, M.D.,

AND FREDERIC C. BLOW, PH.D.

Bipolar disorder is a serious and chronic mental illness. It is associated with substantial functional and quality-of-life impairments, increased rates of suicide, and high financial costs. Type I bipolar disorder occurs in 0.4%–1.6% of the U.S. population, affecting between 1 and 3.5 million individuals (Bourdon et al. 1992; Regier et al. 1984). Type II bipolar disorder, characterized by hypomanic episodes and major depressive recurrences, occurs in approximately 0.5% of the U.S. population (Mitchell et al. 2001). These estimates of prevalence are considered conservative (American Psychiatric Association 2002), as bipolar illness is frequently underdiagnosed (Hirschfeld and Vornik 2004). Additionally, illness in some individuals seems to fall within the bipolar spectrum but does not meet the criteria for bipolar I or bipolar II disorder (American Psychiatric Association 2002).

With changes in national demographics and increasing sophistication in the treatment of bipolar illness, there has been a growing awareness of the manifestations of bipolar disorder among older adults. Elderly persons are the fastest-growing segment of the U.S. population: the number of persons aged 65 years and older increased 12% from 1990 to 2000. Over the next three decades, the number of individuals older than 85 years is expected to more than double — to reach an estimated 8.9 million by 2030 (Administration on Aging 2002). This reflects a general aging trend in the population and has important implications for the delivery of health services. By the late 1990s, prevalence rates of bipolar disorder in individuals older than 65 years ranged from 0.1% to 0.4% (Van Gerpen et al. 1999). We can expect the absolute numbers of older adults with bipolar disorder to increase as well.

DIAGNOSIS AND AGE OF ONSET OF BIPOLAR DISORDER IN OLDER ADULTS

Among older adults with bipolar illness, the disorder may first have manifested in young adulthood, persisting into later life, or may be of more recent onset. When studies evaluating age of onset of bipolar disorder in a general population are strati-fied into five-year intervals, the peak age of onset is between 15 and 19 years, closely followed by onset between ages 20 and 24. There is often a period of 5–10 years be-tween the onset of symptoms and first hospitalization or initiation of treatment (Lish et al. 1994; Suppes et al. 2001).

Most research studies define "late-onset" bipolar disorder as onset at age 50 or older, but there is no clear agreement on this definition (Van Gerpen et al. 1999; Wylie et al. 1999). The majority of evidence suggests that the incidence of mania de-clines with age (Depp and Jeste 2004; Loranger and Levine 1978; McDonald 2000; Mendlewicz et al. 1972), although there are contrasting reports of an increased inci-dence of new-onset mania among older adults (Goodwin et al. 1984; Rasanen et al. 1998). Shulman and Post (1980) reported that among geriatric patients with bipolar disorder, only 8% had mania before the age of 40. Hirschfeld and colleagues (2003) reported that 1.6% of individuals aged 55–64 screened positive for bipolar disorder when assessed with the Mood Disorder Questionnaire (MDQ), compared with 0.5% of individuals aged 65 and older.

The proportion of "new" or later-onset cases of bipolar disorder among older in-dividuals with bipolar disorder ranges from 6.1% to 11% (Almeida and Fenner 2002; Cassidy and Carroll 2002; Clayton 1983; Sajatovic et al. 2005a). A recent analysis of a large database from the Veterans Health Administration (VHA) suggests that nearly one-quarter of veterans with bipolar illness are aged 60 or older; of these, approxi-mately 82.5% (n = 13,447) have early-onset illness (Sajatovic et al. 2005a). Almeida and Fenner (2002) reported on an evaluation of a registry of mental health service use involving more than 6,000 individuals whose primary or secondary clinical di-agnosis was bipolar disorder. Most of these patients had an onset of illness between 15 and 45 years of age, but approximately 8% were aged 65 or older at the time of their first contact with mental health services.

Bipolar disorder may first manifest as late as the eighth or ninth decade of life (Sibisi 1990; Spicer et al. 1973). Stone (1989) noted that among patients aged 65 or older, 25% had their first manic episode after the age of 65. Depp and Jeste (2004) identified 13 studies of older patients with bipolar disorder that reported age of onset of any psychiatric disorder and 8 studies that reported age of onset of mania. The sample-weighted mean age of patients in these studies was 68.2 years (SD = 3.9, range 60–72). The weighted mean age of onset of any affective disorder was 48.0 years (SD = 6.4, range 28–65), and age of onset of mania was 56.4 years (SD = 7.3, range 38–70). It seems that, on average, an older adult with bipolar disorder/mania has experienced mood symptoms for approximately 20 years and that older adults have an overall later age of onset than younger populations with bipolar disorder.

Some authors have suggested that late-onset mania is a distinct subtype of bipolar disorder associated with medical and neurological disease (Cassidy and Carroll 2002; Goodwin and Jamison 1990; Moorhead and Young 2003). The term *secondary mania* has been used to describe mania that occurs with identifiable medical or substance use–related etiologies (Krauthammer and Klerman 1978). Goodwin and Jamison (1990) noted that individuals with late-onset bipolar disorder were less likely to have a positive family history of mood disorders and more likely to have concurrent medical and neurological disorders than individuals with early-onset mania. A study by Shulman and Post (1980) found evidence of cerebral organic disease in approximately 24% of elderly patients with bipolar disorder. Cassidy and Carroll (2002) reported that late-onset mania was associated with vascular risks/vascular disorder, including smoking, hypertension, diabetes, coronary artery disease, and atrial fibrillation. New-onset bipolar illness may also be associated with brain changes visible with imaging techniques. Rabins and colleagues (2000) reported that magnetic resonance imaging (MRI) findings among elderly individuals with unipolar and bipolar affective disorders are similar — left sylvian fissure and left and right temporal sulcal enlargement and bilateral cortical atrophy — which differ from the findings in healthy elderly control subjects and elderly individuals with schizophrenia.

A small proportion of older individuals with bipolar disorder (approximately 3%) seem to have had a change in diagnosis over time (Sajatovic et al. 2005b). A typical scenario might involve an older adult with early depressive episodes who has a later-life hypomanic episode. Young and Klerman (1992) noted that individuals with a history of major depression and a family history of bipolar disorder (type V bipolar disorder) may develop type I or type II disorder with age, thus experiencing a "change in polarity" of their mood disorder. In a study comparing new-onset mania in patients older than and younger than 60 years of age, those with late-onset mania had a latency of 17 years between the first depressive episode and the first manic episode, versus 3.5 years for the early-onset mania group (Broadhead and Jacoby 1990).

For cases in which diagnosis is changed from a psychotic illness to bipolar disorder, patients with mania may experience paranoia, agitation, and grandiose delusions. There is substantial symptom overlap with primary psychotic conditions such as schizophrenia; frequently, only a longitudinal symptom assessment allows a clear diagnosis. In the past, individuals with manic psychosis were often misdiagnosed as having schizophrenia. For some elderly patients, a late-life change in diagnosis to bipolar disease may reflect a delayed correction in diagnosis (Young and Klerman 1992).

GENDER DIFFERENCES

Most older individuals with bipolar disorder are women (Almeida and Fenner 2002; Depp and Jeste 2004; Gildengers et al. 2004; Van Gerpen et al. 1999), and this gender disproportion may simply be due to the higher proportion of women in the general geriatric population. Depp and Jeste (2004) reviewed 17 studies of older adults with bipolar disorder in which gender proportion was noted, and reported a weighted mean for proportion of women of 69% (range 45–89).

Some investigators reported no difference in proportions of men and women among older adults with new-onset illness (Cassidy and Carroll 2002; Sajatovic et al. 2005b), whereas others reported a preponderance of women in newer-onset cases, which is due to a later age of illness onset (Shulman and Post 1980). Longitudinal studies of older adults with bipolar disorder found that women have higher suicide rates; however, these reports noted that this disparity does not take into account the twofold higher suicide rates for men in the general population (Angst et al. 2002).

OUTCOMES AND USE OF HEALTH SERVICES

Some research suggests that outcomes of geriatric bipolar disorder have improved significantly in the last several decades, primarily because of pharmacological advances (Van Gerpen et al. 1999). Despite these improvements, geriatric bipolar disorder is still associated with substantial morbidity and mortality. Meeks (1999) found that community-dwelling middle-aged and elderly adults with bipolar disorder have chronic or intermittently cycling manifestations of mood disorder and limited medication treatments. Most are unmarried and impoverished and live alone or with immediate family members. On long-term follow-up (34–38 years), older adults with mood disorders have been reported to have elevated mortality rates, primarily from suicide and circulatory disorders (Angst et al. 2002), and persons older than 65 years who have mania have more psychosocial deficits and poorer outcomes than similarly aged depressed and controlled groups (Berrios and Bakshi 1991). Studies have found that 20%–28.5% of geriatric patients with mania become institutionalized within 3–

10 years of disease onset (Dhingra and Rabins 1991; Shulman et al. 1992; Van Gerpen et al. 1999); concomitant neurological disease may increase the risk of institutionalization (Schulman et al. 1992).

Apart from possible medical and neurological sequelae, health outcomes may be somewhat better for individuals with later-onset bipolar disorder than for those with early-onset illness. Schurhoff and colleagues (2000) noted that compared with individuals with illness onset after age 40, individuals with early-onset bipolar disorder had more severe forms of the illness, with more psychotic features, more mixed episodes, greater comorbidity, and poorer prophylactic lithium response. Sajatovic and colleagues (2005b) reported that among adults aged 60 or older (n = 16,330), those with earlier onset of bipolar disorder were more likely to be divorced or separated, although the risk of becoming homeless was not increased.

Additional research is needed to clarify the prognosis and expected clinical outcomes for geriatric patients with bipolar illness and the way in which these outcomes might differ among late-onset versus early-onset groups. A national consumer and advocacy group, the Depression and Bipolar Support Alliance (DBSA), convened a Consensus Development Panel to review progress made during the past decade on late-life mood disorders and to identify unmet needs in health care delivery and research. The panel was composed of experts in late-life mood disorders, primary care, geriatrics, mental health, and aging policy research and advocacy. This panel concluded that despite the many advances in safe and efficacious treatments, mood disorders remain a significant health care issue for the elderly (Charney et al. 2003). Mood disorders in older adults are associated with disability, reduced functionality, diminished quality of life, substantial caregiver burden, increased use of health services, and increased mortality (Angst et al. 2002; Bartels et al. 2000; Charney et al. 2003). The DBSA panel noted a critical need for improvements in diagnosis, treatment, and delivery of services for older adults with mood disorders. Because the effects of bipolar illness are multidimensional, the suffering and burden related to this illness can be expected to affect not only the older adult with bipolar disorder but also families and society at large.

Bipolar disorder in older adults does not "burn out" over time. The use of health resources by this group continues to be substantial at and beyond the seventh decade of life. Bartels and colleagues (2000) reported that elderly individuals with bipolar disorder have high symptom severity and impaired community-living skills, and that they use almost four times the total mental health services and are four times more likely to be hospitalized compared with older adults with unipolar depression. Similarly, analysis of a large VHA patient database suggested that the use of health resources by older individuals with bipolar disorder increases with advancing age. In this study, middle-aged and older individuals had more hospital admissions than individuals under age 30. Although elderly individuals may be hospitalized at rates similar to or slightly lower than those of middle-aged individuals, they have longer hospital stays, possibly because of the increased medical comorbidity associated with late-life bipolar disorder. Older populations of persons with bipolar disorder also have increased use of outpatient services. Among veterans with bipolar disorder, use of nonpsychiatric outpatient care is markedly greater among older adults, with a mean of 72 visits over a two-year period for individuals aged 60 and older, compared with a mean of 58 visits for individuals aged 30–59 and 24 visits for individuals under the age of 30 (Sajatovic et al. 2004).

Among older adults with bipolar disorder, age of onset seems to be associated with differential use of health services. Older adults with early-onset illness are sicker and use more health services than older adults with a later onset (Meeks 1999; Sajatovic et al. 2005b). Compared with individuals with early-onset illness, individuals with illness of more recent onset have less outpatient care overall ($p < .001$), fewer mental health care visits ($p < .001$), and less medical outpatient care ($p < .001$). Similarly, Meeks (1999) evaluated 86 middle-aged and older adults with bipolar disorder (mean age 53.6 years) and found that earlier age of onset was associated with poorer functioning.

SYMPTOM PRESENTATION

Considerable controversy exists on the question of whether geriatric bipolar symptoms differ from those typically seen in younger populations (Van Gerpen et al. 1999). The available data are limited and somewhat conflicting (Broadhead and Jacoby 1990; Tohen et al. 1994; Yassa et al. 1988). Older adults with bipolar disorder may present with mania, depression, or mixed states (Depp and Jeste 2004; Sajatovic et al. 2004). There may be a tendency toward irritable behavioral characteristics (James 1977), and cognitive symptoms may mimic a dementia. A review of five studies of older adults with bipolar disorder that addressed the prevalence of psychotic symptoms noted that 64% of the patients had psychotic symptoms (range 20%–85%), a proportion similar to that found in mixed-age groups (Goodwin and Jamison 1990). Among community-dwelling adults aged 40–78 years (mean age 53.6) with bipolar disorder, depressive symptoms seemed to predominate and were more predictive of functioning than were manic symptoms (Meeks 1999). Finally, hospitalizations for mania are more common than hospitalizations for depression among older adults with bipolar disorder, regardless of age at onset of illness (Sajatovic et al. 2005b).

Whether bipolar disorder in geriatric patients increases the risk for dementia is not entirely clear, as there are conflicting data reports (Van Gerpen et al. 1999). Burt and colleagues (2002) suggested that patients with bipolar disorder experience greater deterioration in memory functions over the course of their illness than do patients with unipolar disorder. Gildengers and colleagues (2004) recently noted that approximately half of older adults (mean age 68.7 years) score one or more standard deviations below elderly control subjects on standardized cognitive testing (the Mini Mental State Examination and the Mattis Dementia Rating Scale). The rates of cognitive impairment do not seem to differ between geriatric patients with mania and those with depression (Young and Klerman 1992).

In elderly populations, delirium and adverse drug effects may also profoundly affect symptom presentation. Delirious mania is a condition in which the signs and symptoms of delirium manifest in the context of a manic episode (Bond 1980). Weintraub and Lippmann (2001) suggested that elderly individuals with a history of bipolar disorder who become delirious may present with symptoms consistent with their underlying mood disorder.

COMORBIDITY

A substantial factor that leads to treatment complications and cost inflation for individuals with bipolar disorder is psychiatric comorbidity. Sixty-five percent of individuals with bipolar disorder meet *Diagnostic and Statistical Manual*, Fourth Edition (DSM-IV) criteria for at least one comorbid lifetime axis I disorder (American Psychiatric Association 1994), with comorbid substance abuse and anxiety disorders being particularly problematic and common among individuals with bipolar disorder (McElroy et al. 2001). Bauer and colleagues (2005) recently noted that nearly 30% of patients treated for bipolar disorder in public sector care have multiple current comorbidities. Few reports have specifically focused on comorbidity in late-life bipolar disorder. Among younger populations with bipolar disorder, comorbidity is associated with greater functional impairment, higher health care costs, and worse health outcomes (Kleinman et al. 2003; Singh et al. 2005; Tondo and Ghiani 2003).

In one of the few studies specific to older adults, a large VHA study of patients aged 60 or older with bipolar disorder (n = 16,330) found that 28.6% had a co-occurring disorder (Sajatovic et al. 2006). Comorbid conditions among older veterans with bipolar disorder included the following: substance abuse in 8.9%; posttraumatic stress disorder (PTSD), 5.4%; other anxiety disorders, 9.7%; and dementia, 4.5%. Individuals with substance abuse in this population were more likely to be younger, unmarried, homeless, and of a minority racial/ethnic group compared with elderly persons with bipolar disorder and anxiety disorders or dementia. Older veterans with bipolar disorder without comorbidities had fewer hospital stays and out-patient visits than veterans with bipolar disorder and comorbid PTSD, substance abuse, anxiety, or dementia. Use of inpatient care was greater among geriatric veterans with bipolar disorder and dementia than among veterans with bipolar disorder and other comorbid conditions. Geriatric patients with comorbid PTSD had the greatest overall use of outpatient services. In summary, this study indicated that clinical characteristics, use of health resources, and health care costs differ among groups of geriatric patients with bipolar disorder, depending on the type of comorbidity.

Comorbid substance use is of particular concern among individuals with bipolar disorder (Bauer et al. 2005; McElroy et al. 2001). Rates of substance use disorders are as high as 50% in individuals with bipolar disorder (Sonne and Brady 1999; Weiss et al. 1999) and are associated with a variety of negative sequelae, including reduced response to treatment (Goldberg et al. 1999) and increased interpersonal difficulties (Bauer et al. 2005). For example, individuals with bipolar disorder and substance abuse are generally less responsive to lithium than individuals with bipolar disorder and no substance abuse (McElroy et al. 2001; Post et al. 1996). The research on the impact of low-level substance use on the course of psychiatric symptoms/disorders in older adulthood is limited. Given the evidence among younger individuals, however, it is highly likely that even relatively low levels of substance use can complicate the clinical course of bipolar disorder among older adults. The effect of moderate or at-risk substance use on bipolar disorder has important implications for both the course and the treatment of this disorder in older adults. Substance use in the presence of psychiatric illness is associated with more severe symptoms, increased suicidality, poor compliance with medication regimens and treatment interventions, and adverse mental health outcomes (Hasegawa et al. 1990; Schuckit et al. 1997; Tsuang et al. 1995). It is reasonable to expect that these problems are magnified in older adults with a diagnosis of bipolar disorder (see chapter 8 for a more thorough discussion).

BARRIERS TO CARE

Highet and colleagues (2004) recently summarized the barriers to optimal health care identified by individuals with bipolar disorder. These include delayed or inaccurate diagnosis of bipolar disorder, unmet needs in primary care, unmet needs in specialist mental health care, adverse experiences with hospitalizations, unsatisfactory interactions with health professionals, fragmented medical and psychological care, inadequate community-based crisis management, and exclusion of caregivers and families from management decisions. Such problems are likely to be compounded for older adults with bipolar disorder.

Patients, families, and providers unfamiliar with mental diagnoses may not accurately identify new-onset mania in elderly persons. McDonald and Nemeroff (1996) noted that late-onset mania may be associated with poor recognition of mood symptoms by providers, resulting in increased caregiver burden, premature placement of the patient in a nursing home, and a more rapid functional decline. Older individuals receiving psychotropic medications are likely to be receiving concomitant nonpsychotropic pharmacological treatments for medical conditions such as hypertension and diabetes, thus increasing the risk of drug-related adverse events, relapse, and hospitalization. Cognitive impairment may adversely affect an older person's ability to communicate with family and care providers. Older individuals on fixed incomes may experience difficulty in paying for prescriptions or medical care. Finally, societal barriers such as stigma may limit care and optimal health outcomes. Public awareness campaigns to destigmatize mental illness over the past decade have been helpful, but they may have had less impact on attitudes toward such illness in older individuals.

TREATMENT

There is no consensus on the best treatments for late-life bipolar disorder. Current treatment guidelines are fairly cursory (American Psychiatric Association 2002; Keck et al. 2004). No randomized controlled treatment trials specific to geriatric bipolar disorder have been published on which one could make evidence-based recommendations. Information on psychosocial treatments is also extremely limited. And most data on medication treatments are based on uncontrolled studies, mixed-age samples, or retrospective analyses.

In younger adults, lithium is a first-line treatment for bipolar mania (American Psychiatric Association 2002; Goldberg 2000), with more than 50% of individuals in mixed-age samples receiving lithium (Ahmed and Anderson 2001; Levine et al. 2000). However, for older adults with bipolar disorder, lithium is often poorly tolerated and possibly less efficacious than for younger adults (McDonald 2000; Tueth et al. 1998).

The introduction of novel anticonvulsants and the atypical antipsychotics for treating bipolar disorder has substantially broadened the available treatment options for all adult age groups. Some novel treatments may be more effective and better tolerated among older adults, but their efficacy in comparison to lithium for this geriatric populations is not known. In spite of the dearth of data on the efficacy and tolerability of these medications, clinicians are widely prescribing novel treatments for older patients with bipolar disorder (Sajatovic et al. 2004; Shulman et al. 2003). An analysis from the Ontario (Canada) Drug Benefit Program from 1993 to 2001 demonstrated that the number of new valproic acid (valproate) users surpassed new lithium users in 1997, with a steady decline in new lithium users and a steady increase in new valproic acid users between 1993 and 2000 (Shulman et al. 2003). The authors questioned the relatively rapid shift in prescription patterns in the absence of evidence-based data and suggested that before the use of lithium is abandoned, clinicians need adequate evidence that valproic acid offers a comparable or superior efficacy, effectiveness, and safety profile.

In 2001, just over 40% of individuals with bipolar disorder received some type of antipsychotic agent, largely atypical compounds. Patterns of use for each atypical antipsychotic seemed to be similar across the age spectrum (Sajatovic et al. 2004). Meeks (1999) reported on a sample of older adults with bipolar disorder in which use of maintenance neuroleptics was as high as 49%.

Again, despite widespread use of novel medication treatments for bipolar disorder among older adults, it is not clear whether treatments known to be efficacious and well tolerated in younger populations will work equally well in geriatric populations. Long-term outcome analyses of older adults with bipolar disorder suggest that those who receive medication tend to live longer and have a 2.5-fold lower suicide rate than those with untreated bipolar disorder (suicides in 5.2% treated vs. 13.1% untreated individuals) (Angst et al. 2002). Thus, although treatment may be helpful, in the absence of controlled studies focused on the pharmacological treatment of geriatric bipolar disorder, "first-line" treatments for bipolar disorder in elderly persons remain to be established.

CONCLUSIONS

Older adults with bipolar disorder represent a growing population of individuals with serious mental illness and significant treatment needs. Despite substantial gains in our understanding of the prevalence, presentation, and outcomes of bipolar disorder in recent years, there are still gaps in our knowledge that prevent the optimal delivery of care to this vulnerable population. Prospective studies with appropriate sampling could provide an accurate determination of the prevalence and characteristics of this illness, as well as a more standardized definition of late-onset illness. Controlled treatment studies for this patient population are almost entirely lacking, and there is an urgent need for both medication and psychosocial intervention trials that could be used to assist clinicians in determining best treatments and best practices. Finally, effectiveness studies are needed to evaluate the characteristics of older adults with bipolar disorder in "real world" settings, including populations with medical and psychiatric comorbidity, individuals receiving care in primary care practices, and populations of varying ethnicity and culture.

REFERENCES

Administration on Aging. 2002. A profile of older Americans: 2001. www.aoa.dhhs.gov/aoa/ STATS/profile/2001/highlights.html

Ahmed, Z., and Anderson, I. M. 2001. Treatment of bipolar affective disorder in clinical practice. *J Psychopharmacol* 15:55–57.

Almeida, O. P., and Fenner, S. 2002. Bipolar disorder: similarities and differences between patients with illness onset before and after 65 years of age. *Int Psychogeriatr* 14:311–322.

American Psychiatric Association. 1994. *Diagnostic and statistical manual of mental disorders* (4th ed.). Washington, DC: American Psychiatric Association Press.

American Psychiatric Association. 2002. Practice guideline for the treatment of patients with bipolar disorder (revision). *Am J Psychiatry* 159(4 suppl.):1–50.

Angst, F., Stassen, H. H., Clayton, P. J., et al. 2002. Mortality of patients with mood disorders: follow-up over 34–38 years. *J Affect Disord* 68(2–3):167–181.

Bartels, S. J., Forester, B., Miles, K. M., et al. 2000. Mental health service use by elderly patients with bipolar disorder and unipolar major depression. *Am J Geriatr Psychiatry* 8:160–166.

Bauer, M. S., Altshuler, L., Evans, D. R., et al. 2005. Prevalence and distinct correlates of anxiety, substance, and combined comorbidity in a multi-site public sector sample with bipolar disorder. *J Affect Disord* 85:301–315.

Berrios, G. E., and Bakshi, N. 1991. Manic and depressive symptoms in the elderly: their relationships to treatment outcome, cognition, and motor symptoms. *Psychopathology* 24:31–38.

Bond, T. C. 1980. Recognition of acute delirious mania. *Arch Gen Psychiatry* 37:553–554.

Bourdon, K. H., Rae, D. S., Locke, B. Z., et al. 1992. Estimating the prevalence of mental disorders in US adults from the Epidemiologic Catchment Area Survey. *Public Health Rep* 107:663–668.

Broadhead, J., and Jacoby, R. 1990. Mania in old age: a first prospective study. *Int J Geriatr Psychiatry* 5:215–222.

Burt, T., Prudic, J., Peyser, S., et al. 2002. Learning and memory in bipolar and unipolar major depression: effects of aging. *Neuropsychiatry Neuropsychol Behav Neurol* 13:246–253.

Cassidy, F., and Carroll, B. J. 2002. Vascular risk factors in late-onset mania. *Psychol Med* 32:359–362.

Charney, D. S., Reynolds, C. F. 3rd, Lebowitz, B. L., et al. 2003. Depression and Bipolar Support Alliance consensus statement on the unmet needs in diagnosis and treatment of mood disorders in late life. *Arch Gen Psychiatry* 60:664–672.

Clayton, P. J. 1983. The prevalence and course of the affective disorders. In Davis, J. M., and

Maas, J. W. (eds.), *The affective disorders* (pp. 93–201). Washington, DC: American Psychiatric Association Press.

Depp, C., and Jeste, D. V. 2004. Bipolar disorder in older adults: a critical review. *Bipolar Disord* 6:343–367.

Dhingra, U., and Rabins, P. V. 1991. Mania in the elderly: a 5–7 year follow-up. *J Am Geriatr Soc* 39:581–583.

Gildengers, A. G., Butters, M. A., Seligman, K., et al. 2004. Cognitive functioning in late-life bipolar disorder. *Am J Psychiatry* 161:736–738.

Goldberg, J. F. 2000. Treatment guidelines: current and future management of bipolar disorder. *J Clin Psychiatry* 61(suppl. 13):12–18.

Goldberg, J. F., Garno, J. L., Leon, A. C., et al. 1999. A history of substance abuse complicates remission from acute mania in bipolar disorder. *J Clin Psychiatry* 60:733–740.

Goodwin, F. K., and Jamison, K. R. 1990. *Manic depressive illness.* Oxford: Oxford University Press.

Goodwin, F. K., Jamison, K. R., Post, R. M., et al. (eds.). 1984. *The natural course of manic-depressive illness: neurobiology of mood disorders.* Baltimore: Williams and Wilkins.

Hasegawa, K., Mukasa, H., Nakazawa, Y., et al. 1990. Primary and secondary depression in alcoholism — clinical features and family history. *Drug Alcohol Depend* 27:275–281.

Highet, N. J., McNair, B. G., Thompson, M., et al. 2004. Experience with treatment services for people with bipolar disorder. *Med J Aust* 181:S47–S51.

Hirschfeld, R., Calabrese, J., Weisman, M., et al. 2003. Screening for bipolar disorder in the community. *J Clin Psychiatry* 64:53–59.

Hirschfeld, R. M., and Vornik, L. A. 2004. Recognition and diagnosis of bipolar disorder. *J Clin Psychiatry* 65(suppl. 15):5–9.

James, N. M. 1977. Early and late-onset bipolar affective disorder. *Arch Gen Psychiatry* 34:511–518.

Keck, P. E., Perlis, R. H., Otto, M. W., et al. 2004. The Expert Consensus Guideline Series: treatment of bipolar disorder 2004. *Postgrad Med Spec Rep*, Dec., 1–120.

Kleinman, L., Lowin, A., and Flood, E. 2003. Costs of bipolar disorder. *Pharmacoeconomics* 21:601–622.

Krauthammer, C., and Klerman, L. G. 1978. Secondary mania. *Arch Gen Psychiatry* 35:1333–1339.

Levine, J., Chengappa, K. N., Brar, J. S., et al. 2000. Psychotropic drug prescription patterns among patients with bipolar I disorder. *Bipolar Disord* 2:120–130.

Lish, J. D., Dime-Meenan, S., Whybrow, P. C., et al. 1994. The National Depressive and Manic-Depressive Association (DMDA) survey of bipolar members. *J Affect Disord* 31:281–294.

Loranger, A. W., and Levine, P. M. 1978. Age of onset of bipolar affective illness. *Arch Gen Psychiatry* 35:1345–1348.

McDonald, W. M. 2000. Epidemiology, etiology, and treatment of geriatric mania. *J Clin Psychiatry* 61:3–11.

McDonald, W. M., and Nemeroff, C. B. 1996. The diagnosis and treatment of mania in the elderly. *Bull Menninger Clin* 60:175–196.

McElroy, S. L., Altshuler, L. L., Suppes, T., et al. 2001. Axis I psychiatric comorbidity and its relationship to historical illness variables in 288 patients with bipolar disorder. *Am J Psychiatry* 158:420–426.

Meeks, S. 1999. Bipolar disorder in the latter half of life: symptom presentation, global functioning and age of onset. *J Affect Disord* 52:161–167.

Mendlewicz, J., Fieve, R. R., Rainer, J. D., et al. 1972. Manic-depressive illness: a comparative study of patients with and without family history. *Br J Psychiatry* 120:523–530.

Mitchell, P. B., Wilhelm, K., Parker, G., et al. 2001. The clinical features of bipolar depression: a comparison with matched major depressive disorder patients. *J Clin Psychiatry* 62:212–216.

Moorhead, S. R., and Young, A. H. 2003. Evidence for a late onset bipolar-I disorder sub-group from 50 years. *J Affect Disord* 73:271–277.

Post, R. M., Ketter, T. A., Denicoff, K., et al. 1996. The place of anticonvulsant therapy in bipolar illness. *Psychopharmacology (Berl)* 128:115–129.

Rabins, P. V., Aylward, E., Holroyd, S., et al. 2000. MRI findings differentiate between late-onset schizophrenia and late-life mood disorder. *Int J Geriatr Psychiatry* 15:954–960.

Rasanen, P., Tiihonen, J., and Hakko, H. 1998. The incidence and onset-age of hospitalized bipolar affective disorder in Finland. *J Affect Disord* 48:63–68.

Regier, D. A., Myers, J. K., Kramer, M., et al. 1984. The NIMH Epidemiologic Catchment Area program: historical context, major objectives, and study population characteristics. *Arch Gen Psychiatry* 41:934–941.

Sajatovic, M., Bingham, C. R., Campbell, E., et al. 2005a. Bipolar disorder in older adult inpatients. *J Nerv Ment Dis* 193:417–419.

Sajatovic, M., Blow, F. C., Ignacio, R. V., et al. 2004. Bipolar disorder in the Veterans Health Administration: age-related modifiers of clinical presentation and health services use. *Psychiatr Serv* 55:1014–1021.

Sajatovic, M., Blow, F. C., Ignacio, R. V., et al. 2005b. New-onset bipolar disorder in later life. *Am J Geriatr Psychiatry* 13:282–289.

Sajatovic, M., Blow, F. C., and Ignacio, R. V. 2006. Psychiatric comorbidity in older adults with bipolar disorder. *Int J Geriatr Psychiatry* 21:1–6.

Schuckit, M. A., Tipp, J. E., Bergman, M., et al. 1997. Comparison of induced and independent major depression disorders in 2,945 alcoholics. *Am J Psychiatry* 154:948–957.

Schurhoff, F., Bellivier, F., Jouvent, R., et al. 2000. Early and late onset bipolar disorders: two different forms of manic-depressive illness? *J Affect Disord* 58:215–221.

Shulman, K., and Post, F. 1980. Bipolar affective disorder in old age. *Br J Psychiatry* 186:26–32.

Shulman, K. I., Tohen, M., Satlin, A., et al. 1992. Mania compared with unipolar depression in old age. *Am J Psychiatry* 149:341–345.

Shulman, K. I., Rochon, P., Suykora, K., et al. 2003. Changing prescription patterns for lithium and valproic acid in old age: shifting practice without evidence. *BMJ* 326:960–961.

Sibisi, C. D. T. 1990. Sex differences in the age of onset of bipolar affective illness. *Br J Psychiatry* 156:842–845.

Singh, J., Mattoo, S. K., Sharan, P., et al. 2005. Quality of life and its correlates in patients with dual diagnosis of bipolar affective disorder and substance dependence. *Bipolar Disord* 7:187–191.

Sonne, S. C., and Brady, K. T. 1999. Substance abuse and bipolar comorbidity. *Psychiatr Clin North Am* 22:609–627.

Spicer, C. C., Hare, E. J., and Slater, D. 1973. Neurotic and psychotic forms of depressive illness: evidence from age-incidence in a national sample. *Br J Psychiatry* 123:535–541.

Stone, K. 1989. Mania in the elderly. *Br J Psychiatry* 155:220–224.

Suppes, T., Leverich, G. S., Keck, P. E., et al. 2001. The Stanley Foundation Bipolar Treatment Outcome Network. II: Demographics and illness characteristics of the first 261 patients. *J Affect Disord* 67(1–3):45–59.

Tohen, M., Shulman, K. I., and Satlin, A. 1994. First-episode mania in late life. *Am J Psychiatry* 151:130–132.

Tondo, L., and Ghiani, C. 2003. Psychiatric comorbidity in bipolar disorder. *Bipolar Disord* 5(suppl. 1):13–26.

Tsuang, D., Cowley, D., Ries, R., et al. 1995. The effects of substance use disorder on the clinical presentation of anxiety and depression in an outpatient psychiatric clinic. *J Clin Psychiatry* 56:549–555.

Tueth, M. J., Murphy, T. K., and Evans, D. L. 1998. Special considerations: use of lithium in children, adolescents, and elderly populations. *J Clin Psychiatry* 590(suppl. 6):66–73.

Van Gerpen, M. W., Johnson, J. E., and Winstead, D. K. 1999. Mania in the geriatric patient population: a review of the literature. *Am J Geriatr Psychiatry* 7:188–202.

Weintraub, D., and Lippmann, S. 2001. Delirious mania in the elderly. *Int J Geriatr Psychiatry* 16:374–377.

Weiss, R. D., Najavits, L. M., and Greenfield, S. F. 1999. A relapse prevention group for patients with bipolar and substance use disorder. *J Subst Abuse Treat* 16:47–54.

Wylie, M. E., Mulsant, B. H., Pollack, B. G., et al. 1999. Age at onset in geriatric bipolar disorder: effects on clinical presentation and treatment outcomes in an inpatient sample. *Am J Geriatr Psychiatry* 7:77–83.

Yassa, R., Nair, N. P. V., and Iskandar, H. 1988. Late-onset bipolar disorder. *Psychiatr Clin North Am* 11:117–131.

Young, R. C., and Klerman, G. L. 1992. Mania in late life: focus on age at onset. *Am J Psychiatry* 149:867–876.

CHAPTER TWO

Mood Rating Scales and the Psychopathology of Mania in Old Age

Selected Applications and Findings

ROBERT C. YOUNG, M.D.,

CATHERINE PEASLEY-MIKLUS, PH.D.,

AND HEBERT C. SCHULBERG, PH.D.

Clinical research on bipolar disorder in later life has been relatively limited. However, increasing professional and lay recognition of the clinical challenges and public health importance of bipolar disorder in elderly persons has markedly raised the priority and resources assigned to such research, including controlled treatment trials. Appropriate psychometrically validated assessment instruments are essential to progress in this area. Several instruments for rating affective psychopathology in bipolar mania and related disorders are available, but the clinical evidence base derived from the use of these instruments for older persons remains sparse.

In this chapter, we review the categories of bipolar mood states, the characteristics of various mood rating scales and the factors that can influence their application in mania, and the scales that have been applied specifically in studies of bipolar manic episodes in old age. We present clinical descriptions of elderly patients and what rating scales reveal about their psychopathological profiles, and consider the assessment of manic signs and symptoms in other elderly patient groups. This discussion is illustrative and is not intended to be comprehensive.

CATEGORIES OF BIPOLAR EPISODES

Mania and hypomania. According to the *Diagnostic and Statistical Manual of Mental Disorders,* Fourth Edition (DSM-IV), the predominant affective signs and symptoms of mania are acceleration and/or excesses of behavior, mental activity, and elated or irritable mood (American Psychiatric Association 1994). Manic episodes are the most studied aspect of bipolar disorder in the geriatrics literature (Young 2004). *Hypomania* refers to syndromes with fewer, milder signs and symptoms. Such episodes can occur in type I bipolar disorder and are characteristic of type II bipolar disorder. Hypomania has received less study than mania in later-life bipolar disorder.

Mixed manic states. Depressive features can occur in the context of bipolar manic states, and these states are referred to as mixed mania (e.g., DSM-IV [American Psychiatric Association 1994]) or dysphoric mania (Swann 1995). The literature on these states in later life is sparse.

Bipolar depression. Episodes of major depression occur in persons with bipolar disorder, including older persons. Bipolar depression has received minimal description in the case of older patients, however, and we will only briefly discuss ratings of depressive symptoms in elderly persons with mania.

USES OF MOOD RATING SCALES IN MANIA
AND BIPOLAR DISORDER

Rating scales for mood symptoms can be used in research and in clinical practice; their application is more limited in the latter circumstance. An important application of mood rating scales in research is in the definition or classification of patient groups. In treatment studies, in particular, minimum baseline severity scores often serve as key inclusion criteria to increase the homogeneity of the study sample (Baldessarini 2002).

Rating scale scores are also used to assess the outcomes of controlled treatment or naturalistic management. For patients with bipolar disorder, total scores have been used to define categorical outcomes such as treatment "response," "euthymia," and "remission" (Chengappa et al. 2003). An example of this application of rating scale scores in elderly persons with bipolar disorder is provided in a recent report by Gildengers and colleagues (2005).

Another research use for information derived from rating scales is in testing associations between overall severity (total score) or individual item scores, or item-score profiles (e.g., factors), of a manic episode and other demographic, clinical, or laboratory variables. For example, the potential relation of the presenting symptoms to outcomes of pharmacotherapies has been an ongoing focus of investigation in young patients with bipolar mania (Swann et al. 2002).

Clinicians can administer self-report scales to patients to screen for psychiatric symptoms in nonpsychiatric settings such as primary medical clinics. Only relatively recently, however, has attention turned to detecting bipolar disorder in primary care practices (Das et al. 2005).

TYPES OF MOOD RATING SCALES USED TO ASSESS PATIENTS WITH BIPOLAR DISORDER

Mood rating scales used in the assessment of manic psychopathology can be categorized by their structure and by the source of information.

Structure. The two main types of rating scale are *multi-item* and *global* scales. The Young Mania Rating Scale (YMRS), developed by Young and colleagues (1978), and the Modified Manic State Scale (MMSS; Blackburn et al. 1977) are examples of multi-item scales. From a psychometric perspective, it is easier to achieve adequate inter-rater reliability with multi-item scales than with global ones. Multi-item scales can also provide a range of specific information that can be used, or "reduced," analytically. The Clinical Global Impression (CGI) scale (Guy 1976; Meaden et al. 2000) is an example of a global instrument and is simpler to score. This type of scale generates an overall assessment based on information considered relevant, but without assigning specified weights to its multiple components. When retrospective information is being used to derive a clinical assessment, global scales are probably more feasible than multi-item scales.

Type of rater. There are three main types of information source. *Interviewer-rated scales* are designed for completion by trained interviewers, who generate a score after considering both the patient's observed behavior and the content of his or her responses to questions. This assessment procedure is consistent with performing a mental status examination. While some rating scales distinguish subjective from observed information, other instruments, such as the Hamilton Depression Rating Scale (HDRS; Hamilton 1960), combine the data sources in constructing an item severity score. *Observer-rated scales* are designed for administration by caregivers or other observers, without an interview-based elicitation of a patient's subjective report. An example of this type of instrument is the Affective Disorder Rating Scale (ADRS; Murphy et al. 1974); no data have been reported on the use of this instrument specifically for elderly persons. Observer-rated scales are particularly valuable in situations where a patient's self-report may be unreliable because of severe illness or cognitive impairment. *Self-report scales* have been administered to young ambulatory patients with bipolar disorder; an example is the Internal State Scale (ISS; Bauer et al. 1991). However, the validity of self-report scales is of concern when patients have severe symptoms or substantial cognitive impairments.

MOOD RATING SCALES USED FOR ELDERLY PERSONS
WITH BIPOLAR MANIA

As noted above, there are relatively few published reports on the application of mood rating scales for elderly persons with bipolar disorder. Examples are listed in table 2.1. Many studies of mood state have used global assessments, which sometimes are based on global instruments with unknown psychometric properties; examples are the global scales applied by van der Velde (1970) and by Himmelhoch and colleagues (1980). Other investigators have used the CGI. The CGI has recently been modified for use in research on bipolar disorder (Meaden et al. 2000; Spearing et al. 1997), with separate items pertaining to overall psychopathology, depressive features, and manic features.

Several studies have presented data generated by multi-item, interviewer-rated mood scales. Some of these scales were explicitly designed for patients with mania. These include the MMSS (Blackburn et al. 1977), the Bech-Rafaelson Mania Scale (BRMS; Bech et al. 1978), and the YMRS (Young et al. 1978).

Other scales have also been used in studies of bipolar mania in older persons. The Brief Psychiatric Rating Scale (BPRS; Overall and Gorham 1962) is a well-known

TABLE 2.1

Rating scales used in assessing manic states in older persons: examples of studies

Scale focus	Scale	Acronym	Scale reference	Studies using the scale
Manic features	Young Mania Rating Scale	YMRS	Young et al. 1978	Gildengers et al. 2005; Young and Falk 1989; Young et al. 2004
	Modified Manic State Scale	MMSS	Blackburn et al. 1977	Broadhead and Jacoby 1990
	Bech-Rafaelson Mania Scale	BRMS	Bech et al. 1978	Tariot et al. 2001
Depressive features	Hamilton Depression Rating Scale	HDRS	Hamilton 1990	Gildengers et al. 2005
Other psycho-pathology	Brief Psychiatric Rating Scale	BPRS	Overall and Gorham 1962	Puryear et al. 1995; Tariot et al. 2001
	Cohen Mansfield Agitation Inventory	CMAI	Cohen-Mansfield et al. 1989	Puryear et al. 1995; Tariot et al. 2001
Global	Clinical Global Impression	CGI	Guy 1976	Chen et al 1999; Noagiul et al. 1998
	Other		None	Himmelhoch et al. 1980; Van der Velde 1970

interviewer-rated scale, which has been used in studies of young patients with bipolar disorder (Shopsin et al. 1975). Another scale that has been applied in research on bipolar mania in older persons is the Cohen-Mansfield Agitation Inventory (CMAI; Cohen-Mansfield et al. 1989), which is a caregiver/observer-rated scale. A recent study of elderly persons with mood states that included mania used information obtained with the HDRS (Gildengers et al. 2005).

CLINICAL DESCRIPTIONS AND RATING SCALE FINDINGS FOR ELDERLY PERSONS WITH BIPOLAR DISORDER

We outline here some perspectives on manic psychopathology, mixed features, and psychotic features in later-life bipolar disorder, from clinically derived descriptions and from studies using rating scales. Where the evidence permits, we comment on the effects of age and of age at onset of illness on psychopathology, given the association of late onset versus early onset of mania and bipolar illness with different etiologies and pathophysiologies (Shulman and Post 1980).

Manic Psychopathology

Clinical Description Observers have suggested that older patients with bipolar mania may have an attenuation of overall severity, and an accentuation or attenuation of particular clinical features, compared with younger patients. Thus, Slater and Roth (1977) proposed that many cases of late-life mania are "relatively mild." In elderly patients, they suggested, euphoria often is not "infectious," but "hostility and resentment" may be prominent. Slater and Roth described elderly patients with mania as manifesting speech and thought that lack "sparkle and versatility" and as commonly exhibiting ideation that is "threadbare and repetitious." Post (1965) similarly proposed that elderly persons with mania seldom display the flight of ideas typifying this syndrome. There has been little comment in the literature about differences in psychopathology in older patients with mania with late versus early onset of illness (Glasser and Rabins 1984).

Findings with Rating Scales Several studies have used rating scales to compare the manic psychopathology of elderly and younger patients — that is, to examine age effects. Both total scores and individual item scores have been examined for this analytical purpose. On overall severity, Young and Falk (1989) found no significant association between age and total YMRS score. In a subsequent study of bipolar mania across the age spectrum, Young and colleagues (2004) again found no significant correlation between age and total YMRS score. Broadhead and Jacoby (1990), by contrast, found that total scores on the MMSS administered on hospital admission to elderly patients with mania were lower than those of a younger adult comparison group. On examining individual YMRS item scores, Young and colleagues (2004) observed that in keeping with an earlier observation (Young and Falk 1989), age was weakly but significantly associated with lower scores on the sexual interest item. On the other hand, age was associated with higher scores on an item measuring rate and amount of speech. In their study of elderly patients with mania, Broadhead and Jacoby (1990) found lower scores on the "religiosity" item of the MMSS, but other items did not differentiate older and young patients.

Comparing elderly persons with mania of early versus late onset, Broadhead and Jacoby (1990) detected no differences in severity but did find higher average item ratings for "happiness" and "cheerfulness" on the MMSS for the patients with late-onset illness.

Mixed Features

Clinical Description On the basis of clinical impressions, Post (1965) suggested that older patients with mania exhibit concomitant depressive features more often than do younger patients.

Findings with Rating Scales In the study by Broadhead and Jacoby (1990), depression item scores did not differ between patients in the two age groups. The investigators also found no difference in depression item scores based on age at onset of illness for hospitalized elderly patients with mania.

Psychotic Features

Clinical Description Psychotic symptoms — that is, delusions and hallucinations — can occur in bipolar mania. Post (1965) suggested that the frequency of non-mood-congruent persecutory delusions is greater in older than in younger patients.

In a study by Wylie and colleagues (1999), 58% of the symptomatic geriatric patients with bipolar disorder in manic or depressed states were psychotic; these investigators did not include a younger patient comparison group. Benazzi (1999) observed in his private practice that among aged, as well as younger, patients with depression, those who had psychotic features more often had bipolar disorder than did those without these features. Wylie and colleagues (1999) observed an association between late age at onset and psychosis in a sample of elderly patients with bipolar disorder in manic and depressed states. Tohen and coauthors (1994) reported delusions in 45% of their patients with late-onset mania. However, Broadhead and Jacoby (1990) detected no difference in rates of delusion between early-onset and late-onset mania in elderly persons.

Findings with Rating Scales A prospective assessment of a mixed-age sample of inpatients with mania found no association between age and the presence of hallucinations and/or delusions (Young et al. 1983). An evaluation of geriatric patients with mania similarly revealed no difference in ratings of psychotic features compared with younger patients (Broadhead and Jacoby 1990).

MOOD RATINGS: OTHER SPECIAL SITUATIONS IN ELDERLY PERSONS

"Bipolarity" in later life covers a heterogeneous and complex group of patients. Thus, a discussion of assessment of manic mood symptoms in elderly persons should include mention of the possible implications of comorbid medical conditions and dementias as well as conditions in other poorly studied subgroups, such as older persons with schizoaffective bipolar disorder.

Signs and symptoms of mania in patients with comorbid medical conditions have received little study in elderly persons. Black and colleagues (1988) reported that global "severity" scores overlapped in populations of mixed-age patients with and without comorbid conditions. Berrios and Bakshi (1991) determined that YMRS scores in elderly persons in manic states, but not those in depressed states, were positively associated with Hachinski scale score (Hachinski et al. 1975), an index of vascular brain disease.

Partial and complete manic syndromes can occur in patients with dementia (Young 2004). Thus, the BRMS (Bech et al. 1978) was administered in early studies of patients with dementia (Tariot et al. 2001). Information obtained from caregivers/observers may be particularly useful in assessing these patients; the Neuropsychiatric Inventory (Cummings 1997) and the Dementia Signs and Symptoms Scale (Loreck et al. 1994) use this strategy and include items pertinent in such cases.

ASSESSMENT OF OTHER CLINICAL DOMAINS

Our focus here has been on rating scale assessments of mood psychopathology in elderly persons with bipolar disorder, but we should mention that instruments are also available for assessing other broad clinical domains that may be pertinent to research and clinical practice in this patient population. One such domain is cognitive performance, for which the Mini Mental State Examination (MMSE; Folstein et al. 1975) has been applied in research (Gildengers et al. 2004) and in clinical care. The limitations of the MMSE for research include its low sensitivity. Medication side effects, behavioral function/quality of life, and caregiver burden are other clinically important domains that warrant assessment. There are challenges and complexities in assessing each of these domains, and the age-specific literature on these topics is very limited. Discussion of these domains exceeds the scope of this chapter, but we should note that measures related to these clinical domains can be better understood when the patient's mood state is taken into account.

CONCLUSIONS

Geropsychiatrists and investigators studying bipolar disorder in elderly persons can make meaningful use of mood rating scales whose validity and utility have been established in younger patients. The (limited) available evidence derived from rating scales suggests that age alone has minimal effects on manic symptoms. The literature on the application of rating scales for elderly persons with bipolar disorder is generally sparse.

REFERENCES

American Psychiatric Association. 1994. *Diagnostic and statistical manual of mental disorders* (4th ed.). Washington, DC: American Psychiatric Association Press.

Baldessarini, R. J. 2002. Treatment research in bipolar disorder: issues and recommendations. *CNS Drugs* 16:721–729.

Bauer, M. S., Crits-Christoph, P., Ball, W. A., et al. 1991. Independent assessment of manic and depressive symptoms by self-rating. *Arch Gen Psychiatry* 48:807–812.

Bech, P., Rafaelsen, O. J., Kramp, P., et al. 1978. The Mania Rating Scale: scale construction and interobserver agreement. *Neuropsychopharmacology* 17:430–431.

Benazzi, F. 1999. Psychotic late-life depression: a 376-case study. *Int Psychogeriatr* 11:325–332.

Berrios, G. E., and Bakshi, N. 1991. Manic and depressive symptoms in the elderly: their relationships to treatment outcome, cognition and motor symptoms. *Psychopathology* 24:31–38.

Black, D. W., Winokur, G., Bell, S., et al. 1988. Complicated mania. *Arch Gen Psychiatry* 45:232–236.

Blackburn, J., Loudon, J., and Ashworth, C. 1977. A new scale for measuring mania. *Psychol Med* 7:453–458.

Broadhead, J., and Jacoby, R. 1990. Mania in old age: a first prospective study. *Int J Geriatr Psychiatry* 5:215–222.

Chen, S. T., Altshuler, L. L., Melnyk, K. A., et al. 1999. Efficacy of lithium vs valproate in the treatment of manna in the elderly: a retrospective study. *J Clin Psychiatry* 60:181–185.

Chengappa, K. N. R., Baker, R. W., Shao, L., et al. 2003. Rates of response, euthymia and remission in two placebo-controlled olanzapine trials for bipolar mania. *Bipolar Disord* 5: 1–5.

Cohen-Mansfield, J., Marx, M. S., and Rosenthal, A. S. 1989. A description of agitation in a nursing home. *J Gerontol* 44:M77–M84.

Cummings, J. L. 1997. The Neuropsychiatric Inventory. *Neurology* 48:S10–S16.

Das, A. K., Olfson, M., Gameroff, M. J., et al. 2005. Screening for bipolar disorder in primary care practice. *JAMA* 293:956–963.

Folstein, M. F., Folstein, S. E., and McHugh, P. R. 1975. Mini-Mental State: a practical method for grading the cognitive state of patients for the clinician. *J Psychiatr Res* 12:189–198.

Gildengers, A. G., Butters, M. A., Seligman, K., et al. 2004. Cognitive impairment in late life bipolar disorder. *Am J Psychiatry* 161:736–738.

Gildengers, A. G., Mulsant, B. H., Begley, A. E., et al. 2005. A pilot study of standardized treatment in geriatric bipolar disorder. *Am J Geriatr Psychiatry* 13:319–323.

Glasser, M., and Rabins, P. 1984. Mania in the elderly. *Age Aging* 13:210–213.

Guy, W. 1976. *ECDEU assessment manual for psychopharmacology* (rev. ed.). Rockville, MD: U.S. Department of Health, Education and Welfare.

Hachinski, V. C., Illiff, L. D., Dihlka, E., et al. 1975. Cerebral blood flow in dementia. *Arch Neurol* 32:632–637.

Hamilton, M. 1960. A rating scale for depression. *J Neurol Neurosurg Psychiatry* 23:56–62.

Himmelhoch, J., Neil, J. R., Ray, S. J., et al. 1980. Age, dementia, dyskinesias, and lithium response. *Am J Psychiatry* 137:941–945.

Loreck, D. J., Bylsma, F. W., and Folstein, M. F. 1994. The Dementia Signs and Symptoms Scale. *Am J Geriatr Psychiatry* 2:60–74.

Meaden, P. M., Daniel, R. E., and Zajecka, J. 2000. Construct validity of life chart functioning scales for use in naturalistic studies of bipolar disorder. *J Psychiatr Res* 34:187–192.

Murphy, D. L., Biegel, A., Weingartner, H., et al. 1974. The quantitation of manic behavior. In Pichot, P. (ed.), *Psychological measurements in psychopharmacology*, Modern Problems in Pharmacopsychiatry (pp. 203–220). Paris: Karger.

Noagiul, S., Narayan, M., and Nelson, C. J. 1998. Divalproex treatment of mania in elderly patients. *Am J Geriatr Psychiatry* 6:257–262.

Overall, J. E., and Gorham, D. R. 1962. The Brief Psychiatric Rating Scale. *Psychol Rep* 10:799–812.

Post, F. 1965. *The clinical psychiatry of late life.* Oxford: Pergamon Press.

Puryear, L. J., Kunik, M. E., and Workman, R. 1995. Tolerability of divalproex sodium in elderly psychiatric patients with mixed diagnoses. *J Geriatr Psychiatry Neurol* 8:234–237.

Shopsin, B., Gershon, S., Thompson, H., et al. 1975. Psychoactive drugs in mania. *Arch Gen Psychiatry* 32:34–42.

Shulman, K., and Post, F. 1980. Bipolar affective disorders in old age. *Br J Psychiatry* 136:26–32.

Slater, E., and Roth, M. 1977. *Mayer-Gross, Slater, and Roth's clinical psychiatry* (3rd ed.). London: Bailliere, Tindall and Cassell.

Spearing, M. K., Post, R. M., Leverich, G. S., et al. 1997. Modification of the Clinical Global Impressions (CGI) scale for use in bipolar illness (CGI-BP). *Psychiatr Res* 73:159–171.

Swann, A. C. 1995. Mixed or dysphoric manic states: psychopathology and treatment. *J Clin Psychiatry* 56(suppl. 3):6–10.

Swann, A. C., Bowden, C. L., Calabrese, J. R., et al. 2002. Pattern of response to divalproex, lithium, or placebo in four naturalistic subtypes of mania. *Neuropsychopharmacology* 26:530–536.

Tariot, P. N., Schneider, L. S., Mintzer, J. E., et al. 2001. Safety and tolerability of divalproex sodium in the treatment of signs and symptoms of mania in elderly patients with dementia: results of a double-blind, placebo-controlled trial. *Curr Ther Res* 62:51–67.

Tohen, M., Shulman, K. I., and Satlin, A. 1994. First-episode mania in late life. *Am J Psychiatry* 151:30–132.

van der Velde, C. D. 1970. Effectiveness of lithium carbonate in the treatment of manic-depressive illness. *Am J Psychiatry* 123:345:351.

Wylie, M. E., Mulsant, B. H., Pollock, B., et al. 1999. Age at onset in geriatric bipolar disorder. *Am J Geriatr Psychiatry* 7:77–83.

Young, R. C. 2004. Bipolar disorders. In Roose, S. P., and Sackeim, H. A. (eds.), *Late-life depression* (pp. 34–48). New York: Oxford University Press.

Young, R. C., and Falk, J. R. 1989. Age, manic psychopathology and treatment response. *Int J Geriatr Psychiatry* 4:73–78.

Young, R. C., Biggs, J. T., Ziegler, V. E., et al. 1978. A rating scale for mania: reliability, validity, and sensitivity. *Br J Psychiatry* 133:429–435.

Young, R. C., Schreiber, M. T., and Nysewander, R. W. 1983. Psychotic mania. *Biol Psychiatry* 18:1167–1173.

Young, R. C., Kiosses, D., Murphy, C. F., et al. 2004. Age and ratings of manic psychopathology. *American Association for Geriatric Psychiatry 2004 annual meeting poster abstracts* (no. 1). Bethesda, MD: American Association for Geriatric Psychiatry.

CHAPTER THREE

Comprehensive Assessment of Persons with Bipolar Disorder in Long-Term Care Settings

The Potential of the interRAI Family of Instruments

JOHN P. HIRDES, PH.D., BRANT E. FRIES, PH.D.,
TERRY RABINOWITZ, M.D., AND JOHN N. MORRIS, PH.D.

Following the trend to de-institutionalize patients in psychiatric hospitals, which began in the 1950s and continued through the mid-1970s, nursing homes (NHs) began to take over the care of increasing numbers of persons with severe and persistent mental illness. The number of elderly people living in psychiatric hospitals in the United States decreased 40%, while the number of individuals with mental illness living in NHs increased more than 100% (Mechanic and McAlpine 2000). One estimate indicates that two of every three NH residents meet established criteria for at least one mental disorder, including dementia and depression, and more than a quarter have depressive symptoms (Colenda et al. 1999). Another study estimated the prevalence of mental illness among NH residents at 80%–91%. About 80% of residents have dementia, 25%–50% have psychotic symptoms, and behavioral disturbances are relatively common (Snowdon 2001).

It follows that NHs need to address not only those mental disorders that are expected and highly prevalent among NH residents (e.g., Alzheimer disease) but also depression, anxiety, schizophrenia, and other mental illnesses. An estimated 50%–60% of NH residents have a history of a psychiatric disturbance, most often related to depression. Psychotic disorders are also quite common (Meeks et al. 1990). NH placement is likely for large numbers of elderly persons with severe and persistent mental illness, especially for those who have little social support or whose illness adversely affects their functional abilities (Bartels et al. 1997).

While considerable attention has been paid to Alzheimer disease, other dementias, and depression among NH residents, much less is known about the needs of residents with severe and persistent mental illness. This is particularly true for bipolar disorder. In a comprehensive review of the literature on bipolar disorder in older adults, Depp and Jeste (2004) found only two studies of bipolar disorder in NH residents. In part, this dearth of information may be a consequence of the lower prevalence of bipolar disorder than other mental disorders in long-term care settings. Tariot and colleagues (1993) reported a prevalence of bipolar disorder of 3% in a sample of 80 NH residents. Depp and Jeste (2004) estimated a prevalence of bipolar disorder among community-dwelling elderly persons of about 0.1%, in contrast to 8%–10% among psychiatry inpatients; the prevalence seemed to decline among older residents. Despite speculation in earlier literature that individuals with bipolar disorder become less symptomatic over time (Winokur et al. 1969), more recent studies argue that aging is associated with a worsening of bipolar symptoms (Post et al. 1986). These contradictions in the literature led Depp and Jeste (2004) to conclude that "many clinical observations about bipolar disorder remain empirically unconfirmed" (344).

Although older persons with bipolar disorder make up a small proportion of residents in long-term care settings, it is important to gain a clearer understanding of the strengths, preferences, and needs of NH residents with this condition. With regard to patterns of service use and clinical characteristics, older persons with bipolar disorder have been described as an intermediate group between individuals with schizophrenia and those with unipolar depression (Depp and Jeste 2004).

THE INTERRAI FAMILY OF ASSESSMENT INSTRUMENTS

It is reasonable to hypothesize that symptoms of bipolar disorder in nursing home residents add substantially to the overall level of complexity of residents' care needs. The best test of this hypothesis at the individual level is through a comprehensive geriatric assessment that includes a review of psychiatric symptoms, with the understanding that these assessments, if performed at regular intervals, can identify changes over time. Moreover, when such assessments are performed as part of a standardized approach to care for the *entire* long-term care population, they provide a large database within which the needs of smaller subgroups (e.g., those with bipolar disorder) can be compared.

One such comprehensive geriatric assessment is provided by interRAI, an international research collaborative (www.interrai.org). The interRAI family of assessment instruments provides a unique opportunity to examine the characteristics and responses of persons with various medical conditions (including psychiatric disor-

ders) across multiple sectors of the health care system (Hirdes et al. 1999). These instruments were designed to function as an integrated health information system
through the use of a common assessment methodology that allows direct comparisons of similar individuals in different care settings. The interRAI instruments include assessments designed for use in long-term care, home care, inpatient and community mental health, assisted living, palliative care, acute care, and rehabilitation
settings. Each instrument measures domain areas such as cognition, mood, behavior, functional ability, social function, service utilization, treatments and procedures,
medical and psychiatric diagnoses, and psychiatric and health symptoms. While the
specific item set of each instrument is tailored to the specific sector for which it was
designed, all instruments share a core set of data elements.

The most established and widely used instrument in the interRAI family is the
Resident Assessment Instrument 2.0 (RAI 2.0; Morris et al. 1997). The RAI 2.0 was
originally created after the Omnibus Budget Reconciliation Act of 1987 mandated
that the U.S. Health Care Financing Administration (now the Centers for Medicare
and Medicaid Services [CMS]) develop and implement a nationwide uniform instrument that could provide a comprehensive functional assessment and guide the
development of an individualized plan of care for each NH resident (Hawes et al.
1997b; Morris et al. 1990). Earlier studies had found that comprehensive geriatric assessment has positive effects on the health and well-being of elderly persons (Applegate et al. 1990; Hendriksen et al. 1984). Similar results were obtained in evaluations of the effect of implementing the Resident Assessment Instrument (RAI) in the
United States (Fries et al. 1997a; Hawes et al. 1997a; Mor et al. 1997; Phillips et al.
1997a, 1997b).

The RAI is mandated for use in all U.S. nursing homes that receive federal fund-
ing under Medicare or Medicaid. Assessments are performed on admission of new
residents and at least annually thereafter, with a shorter version performed at quarterly intervals. The RAI was implemented in 1991 as a paper-based instrument; in
1998, a new mandate required all nursing homes to regularly report RAI data to the
CMS.

Through interRAI, research using the RAI 2.0 has been performed in more than
20 countries (e.g., Fries et al. 1997b; Fries and Fahey 2003; Sgadari et al. 1997), and
the RAI 2.0 is now used in several countries, states, and provinces, including seven
Canadian provinces/territories (Hirdes et al. 2003b; Morris et al. 1990). Data from
these efforts may provide the best opportunity so far to study the characteristics of
persons with bipolar disorder in long-term care settings. In addition, a second inter-
RAI instrument — the RAI–Mental Health (RAI-MH; Hirdes et al. 2001, 2002) — became the mandatory assessment system for all adult psychiatry inpatients in Ontario,

Canada, effective October 2005. With these two data sources, it will soon be possible to make direct comparisons of older persons with bipolar disorder in the two major non–community care settings where they receive services (Complex Continuing Care units and psychiatric hospitals, and NHs in the near future).

Each of the interRAI instruments is designed to support at least four major applications: (1) care planning, (2) resource allocation, (3) quality measurement, and (4) outcome evaluation (Hirdes et al. 1999). The nursing home RAI 2.0 includes 18 Resident Assessment Protocols (RAPs) that are designed to trigger the production of care plans that address a broad range of clinical conditions or situations, including, for example, depression, cognition, behavioral disturbance, use of psychotropic medication, use of restraints, and activities of daily living (ADL) rehabilitation (Hawes et al. 1997a; Morris et al. 1990). These RAPs are one of the important features that differentiate the interRAI assessment methodology from other approaches.

Each RAP includes (1) a summary of the underlying clinical problem; (2) a set of "triggers" in the form of a coding algorithm that uses items from the assessment form to signal when the condition of interest is present or at imminent risk of emerging; and (3) a set of guidelines that suggest (a) clinical issues to consider should the RAP be triggered, (b) additional conditions to assess so as to differentiate potential false positives from true positives for that clinical problem, and (c) treatment options to consider.

The Resource Utilization Groups (RUG-III) case mix system (Fries et al. 1994), which is calculated from 100 or so individual-level clinical variables in the Minimum Data Set form of the RAI 2.0, is an algorithm that predicts the relative resource intensity of NH residents. RUG-III forms the basis for the federal payment systems in all U.S. and Icelandic NHs, as well as for Ontario Complex Continuing Care (CCC) hospitals/units. A variety of quality indicators that use RAI 2.0 data elements have also been developed to measure the process and outcomes of care in NH settings (Morris et al. 2004; Phillips et al. 1997c; Zimmerman et al. 1995). These quality indicators are employed on the CMS "NH Compare" website (www.medicare.gov/NHcompare) and in the annual Ontario hospital report for CCC hospitals/units (www.hospitalreport.ca/HospitalReport2003CCCReport.html).

All interRAI instruments include a series of embedded scales that can track individual outcomes and provide a multidimensional profile of individuals or groups (Morris et al. 2000). The scales in the RAI 2.0 include the following:

— Cognitive Performance Scale (CPS; Morris et al. 1994): a 7-point scale with values ranging from 0 (cognitively intact) to 6 (severely cognitively impaired).

The CPS has a correlation of −.91 with the Mini Mental State Examination (MMSE).

— Depression Rating Scale (DRS; Burrows et al. 2000): a 15-point scale that has been validated against the Hamilton and Cornell Depression Scales.

— ADL Hierarchy Scale (Morris et al. 1999): a 7-point scale that combines four ADL measures to describe disability, with values ranging from 0 (independent) to 6 (severely impaired in late-loss ADLs).

— Index of Social Engagement (ISE; Mor et al. 1995): a 6-point scale measuring involvement in social activities in long-term care settings; this has been validated against recreation activity times.

— Changes in Health, End-stage disease and Signs and Symptoms (CHESS) scale (Hirdes et al. 2003a): a 6-point scale measuring medical complexity and instability of health that is highly predictive of mortality and acute medical procedures.

— Pain Scale (Fries et al. 2001): a 4-point scale that combines the frequency and severity of pain; this has been validated against the Visual Analogue Scale.

— Aggressive Behavior Scale (ABS): a scale that summarizes verbal abuse, physical abuse, resistance to care, and socially inappropriate behavior; it has a high correlation (.85) with the Cohen-Mansfield Agitation Inventory (CMAI) aggression subscale.

In addition, the RAI 2.0 contains more than 400 individual data elements that can be used on their own or in other combinations to track longitudinal changes in a host of domain areas.

USE OF THE RAI 2.0 TO DESCRIBE OLDER ADULTS WITH BIPOLAR DISORDER IN LONG-TERM CARE

Here and in the following sections we present RAI 2.0 data to compare the characteristics of persons with bipolar disorder, schizophrenia, and other psychiatric conditions in Ontario CCC hospitals/units. These facilities provide post-acute care to frail elderly individuals with complex health needs, similar to the care provided to residents of skilled nursing facilities in the United States (Price Waterhouse Coopers 2001). The RAI 2.0 was first mandated for use in Ontario CCC hospitals/units in 1996, and "de-identified" data are made available to interRAI annually for research purposes.

The current RAI 2.0 database for Ontario CCC hospitals/units contains almost

TABLE 3.1

Clinical and sociodemographic profile of Complex Continuing Care hospital/unit residents with bipolar disorder, schizophrenia, and other diagnoses

	New admissions			Established residents		
	Bipolar disorder (n = 760)	Schizophrenia (n = 845)	Other diagnoses (n = 83,873)	Bipolar disorder (n = 146)	Schizophrenia (n = 156)	Other diagnoses (n = 9,600)
Age and scale scores (mean [95% confidence limits])						
Age (years)	70.7 (69.8–71.6)	68.2 (67.3–69.1)	77.0 (77.0–77.1)	69.6 (67.3–71.9)	66.1 (63.8–68.5)	73.8 (73.5–74.1)
Depression Rating Scale (DRS)	2.8 (2.6–3.0)	2.3 (2.1–2.5)	1.5 (1.5–1.5)	3.2 (2.6–3.7)	3.1 (2.5–3.6)	2.0 (1.9–2.0)
Cognitive Performance Scale (CPS)	2.6 (2.5–2.8)	3.0 (2.9–3.1)	2.2 (2.2–2.3)	3.3 (3.0–3.7)	3.7 (3.4–3.9)	3.3 (3.2–3.3)
Index of Social Engagement (ISE)	2.0 (1.9–2.2)	1.6 (1.5–1.7)	2.3 (2.2–2.3)	1.8 (1.5–2.2)	1.4 (1.1–1.6)	1.9 (1.8–1.9)
ADL Hierarchy Scale	3.3 (3.1–3.4)	3.14 (3.3–3.6)	3.7 (3.7–3.7)	4.2 (3.9–4.5)	4.1 (3.8–4.3)	4.4 (4.3–4.4)
Aggressive Behavior Scale (ABS)	1.8 (1.6–2.0)	1.8 (1.6–2.0)	0.8 (0.7–0.8)	2.5 (2.0–3.1)	2.8 (2.3–3.4)	1.5 (1.5–1.6)
Pain Scale	1.1 (1.0–1.2)	1.0 (1.0–1.1)	1.3 (1.3–1.3)	1.0 (1.8–1.1)	0.9 (0.7–1.0)	1.1 (1.0–1.1)
CHESS Scale	1.7 (1.6–1.8)	1.6 (1.5–1.7)	1.9 (1.8–1.9)	1.1 (0.9–1.3)	0.9 (0.8–1.1)	1.0 (1.0–1.0)
Resident characteristics (%)						
Male	36.5	36.5	42.3	34.9	48.7	47.7
Marital status						
Married	35.0	24.5	40.2	29.5	11.5	38.9
Never married	10.5	32.8	8.4	17.8	43.0	13.7
Separated/divorced	16.4	13.5	6.1	14.4	16.7	9.3
Widowed	32.9	22.5	41.2	34.9	22.4	35.9
Mental health service use						
Prior psychiatric admissions	10.8	15.9	0.7	NA	NA	NA
Mental health history	46.5	61.7	3.9	NA	NA	NA
Admitted from psychiatric hospital unit	2.5	5.1	0.3	5.5	10.3	1.0

*All chi-square values were significant at $p < .0001$, except for percentage male in existing patients, which was significant at $p < .01$

Abbreviations: ADL, activities of daily living; CHESS, Changes in Health, End-stage disease and Signs and Symptoms.

300,000 assessments of about 85,000 persons assessed from July 1996 through March 2004. Our analyses are based on all individuals in that database who had an admission assessment. In addition, we use the first annual assessment for individuals who remained in the facility for at least one year. Note that the majority of CCC residents were discharged to other care settings (or died) within 90 days of admission, so those remaining for a year or more represent a distinct subgroup of residents. All RAI 2.0 assessments were performed by trained professionals (usually registered nurses) who completed each assessment as part of routine practice. CCC hospitals/units submit the results to the Canadian Institute for Health Information (CIHI), which applies error-checking protocols to increase the quality of the data. All data provided to interRAI have been encrypted to protect individuals' privacy, according to Canadian privacy laws.

Data on persons with bipolar disorder, schizophrenia, and other conditions are examined in two main stages. We first provide a general descriptive overview based on sociodemographic variables and the various interRAI scales described above, then perform a series of thematic analyses to illustrate how RAI 2.0 data can enhance knowledge of the psychiatric, social, medical, and service-use issues for these populations.

All comparisons among the three types of residents — those with "bipolar disorder," "schizophrenia," and "other diagnoses" — were tested for differences with the chi-squared test. Given the large sample sizes, most results were statistically significant; therefore, the discussion here focuses on substantiality.

A PRELIMINARY SNAPSHOT OF COMPLEX CONTINUING CARE RESIDENTS WITH BIPOLAR DISORDER

Table 3.1 (and subsequent tables and figures) compares, on a variety of dimensions, CCC residents with bipolar disorder and their counterparts with schizophrenia and with other diagnoses. In addition, all persons newly admitted ("new admissions") to CCC hospitals/units are compared with the subset of established residents who have been in the facility for at least one year. As noted previously, the large majority of new admissions to CCC are discharged within several months, so residents who have been there for a year probably represent distinctive subgroups of each of the three types compared here.

Demographic Descriptors

Residents with bipolar disorder are distinct from the general CCC population in a number of important domains. For example, they tend to be younger, somewhat less physically disabled, and in less pain than residents with diagnoses other than schizophrenia or bipolar disorder. On the other hand, their mean scores on the DRS and the ABS are almost double those of residents in the other-diagnoses category. They are also more cognitively impaired than those with other diagnoses, but less cognitively impaired than those in the schizophrenia group. As noted elsewhere (Bartels et al. 1997), residents with bipolar disorder have some similarities to those with schizophrenia. The residents with bipolar disorder are more depressed, slightly older, and somewhat more engaged in the activities of the facility; however, they are not significantly different from residents with schizophrenia with respect to ADL impairment, aggressive behavior, pain, or medical complexity (based on the CHESS scale).

It is noteworthy that many of the group differences in clinical characteristics seen on admission are less pronounced in established residents. The two main exceptions to this are DRS scores and aggressive behavior, which continue to be substantially higher in the bipolar disorder group. Equally important, established residents with bipolar disorder have higher scores on cognitive impairment, ADL impairment, and aggressive behavior than the admission cohort. On the other hand, the level of medical complexity indicated by the CHESS score seems to be lower in the established residents. These patterns are also evident for residents with schizophrenia in the new admission and established resident cohorts.

There are potentially important differences in the patterns of interpersonal relationships for the three groups of CCC residents. Those with neither bipolar nor schizophrenic disorders are most likely to be married or to have been married and their marital relationship ended by death of a male spouse. Residents with bipolar disorder are more likely to be married than are persons with schizophrenia, but about as likely as the schizophrenia group to have their marital relationship end in separation or divorce. In contrast, the schizophrenia group is most likely to have never been married.

The three groups also differ markedly in the patterns of use of mental health services. Both the bipolar disorder and the schizophrenia groups are much more likely (1) to have a history of psychiatric admissions, (2) to have a psychiatric history noted on their medical records, and (3) to have been admitted to the CCC hospital/unit from a psychiatric hospital. However, in each instance, the rate for the bipolar disorder group is intermediate between those for the schizophrenia and other-diagnoses groups. While a history of psychiatric problems is noted for almost two-thirds of the schizophrenia group, this is true for less than half of the bipolar disorder group.

The RAI 2.0 can also be used to better understand group differences in more narrowly focused areas that are likely to affect residents' quality of life and quality of care.

Mental Health Indicators

Table 3.2 and figure 3.1 present a variety of mental health indicators, including indicators of delirium, psychosis, negative symptoms, sleep, and behavioral disturbance. The delirium, or "periodic disordered thinking," indicators are based only on behaviors or symptoms that are of recent onset (i.e., different from the resident's baseline status). Among the new admissions, residents with bipolar disorder and schizophrenia are similar on all six indicators, and they tend to have higher rates than the other-diagnoses group (table 3.2). On the other hand, among established residents, delirium indicator rates are lower in the schizophrenia group, while rates for the bipolar group remain higher. Residents with bipolar disorder are most likely to experience, among the indicators examined, changes in level of cognitive function over the course of the day (14.1%), periods of restlessness (12.8%), and episodes of being easily distracted (12.0%). An important clinical question to be resolved for each individual presenting with these indicators is whether the symptoms are due to bipolar disorder itself (e.g., mania/hypomania) or are indicative of delirium. Incorrect diagnosis or incorrect medication management can have serious consequences. For example, if delirium is mistaken for mania or hypomania, the addition of or increase in dose or frequency of either lithium or antipsychotics might lead to increased confusion, more pronounced extrapyramidal symptoms, or anticholinergic overload (Rabinowitz 2002; Rabinowitz et al. 2003).

Not surprisingly, established residents with bipolar disorder are more likely to show new-onset cognitive indicators than other residents who have been in the facility for a year. Given the cyclical nature of the symptoms of bipolar disorder, those affected are more likely to be in a *state of change* than are the other resident groups. However, even for residents with a reliable history of bipolar disorder, a diagnosis of mania or hypomania should be delayed until an exhaustive "rule-out" of other causes of symptoms is completed.

Table 3.2 also shows that a substantial proportion of residents with bipolar disorder have psychotic symptoms, at a rate between the schizophrenia and other-diagnoses groups. The rate of delusions in the bipolar disorder group is more than three times higher than, and the rate of hallucinations is more than double, that in the other-diagnoses group, both at admission and among established residents. On the other hand, while delusions are almost as prevalent in the bipolar disorder group as in the schizophrenia group, the rates of hallucinations are slightly more than half that noted among residents with schizophrenia.

In contrast, residents with bipolar disorder and with schizophrenia are about

TABLE 3.2

Percentage of Complex Continuing Care hospital/unit residents with indicators of delirium, psychosis, negative symptoms, or sleep disturbance, by diagnostic group

	New admissions			Established residents		
	Bipolar disorder	Schizophrenia	Other diagnoses	Bipolar disorder	Schizophrenia	Other diagnoses
Indicators of delirium or periodic disordered thinking (new onset of symptom)						
Easily distracted	12.0	11.5	7.5	8.9	5.1	4.4
Periods of altered perception or awareness of surroundings	9.9	8.6	6.6	8.2	5.1	3.7
Episodes of disorganized speech	10.9	9.1	6.6	11.0	4.50	4.0
Periods of restlessness	12.8	13.0	8.5	9.6	5.8	5.2
Periods of lethargy	9.0	10.4	8.7	8.9	5.1	4.8
Mental function varies over the course of the day	14.1	14.1	10.8	14.4	8.3	5.7
Any indicator	20.0	21.3	16.1	19.2	9.6	10.0
Indicators of psychosis						
Delusions	13.8	16.8	3.7	15.1	21.2	4.5
Hallucinations	7.2	12.1	3.3	10.3	18.6	3.5
Negative symptoms						
Withdrawal from activities of interest	33.8	36.7	23.7	38.4	35.9	23.3
Reduced social interaction	39.3	44.1	29.2	43.8	42.1	28.5
Sleep disturbance						
Insomnia or change in usual sleep pattern	30.7	27.7	20.9	21.9	25.6	16.3

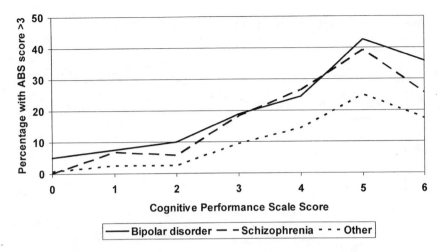

Fig. 3.1. Percentage of residents in Ontario Complex Continuing Care hospitals/units with an Aggressive Behavior Scale score of 3 or more, by cognitive performance (Cognitive Performance Scale score) and resident type.

equally likely to show negative symptoms (withdrawal from activities of interest, reduced social interaction), and both groups are more likely to have negative symptoms than the group with other diagnoses. For those with bipolar disorder, this may be a reflection of anhedonia associated with depression, which occurs at a higher rate and with greater severity in this group, as indicated by the DRS scores reported above. In addition, when compared with residents with other diagnoses at admission, new admissions with bipolar disorder are more likely to have insomnia or changes in sleep patterns noted on admission, but this difference is less pronounced in the established residents group.

Figure 3.1 illustrates the relations among aggressive behavior (verbal abuse, physical abuse, and socially inappropriate behavior such as spitting, throwing objects, and resisting care), cognitive impairment, and resident type. Among all three resident subgroups, the mean score on the ABS increases markedly with more severe cognitive impairment, but tapers off in the highest CPS category, which represents the most severely cognitively impaired (e.g., those with end-stage dementia). However, there is also clear evidence of an interactive effect of bipolar disorder and schizophrenia with cognitive impairment. That is, at moderate or worse levels of cognitive impairment, substantially more pronounced behavioral disturbance occurs in the bipolar disorder and schizophrenia groups than in the group with other diagnoses. Illustrated in figure 3.2 is the interesting companion finding that this type of inter-

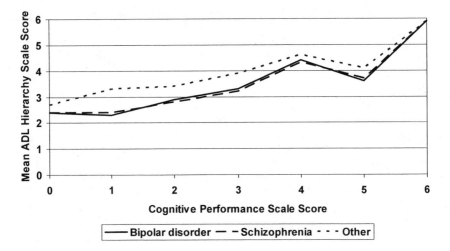

Fig. 3.2. Mean ADL (Activities of Daily Living) Hierarchy Scale score among residents in Ontario Complex Continuing Care hospitals/units, by cognitive performance (Cognitive Performance Scale score) and resident type.

action is *not* present for ADL impairment. In fact, at lower levels of cognitive impairment, the bipolar disorder and schizophrenia groups have slightly lower mean scores than other residents on the ADL Hierarchy Scale.

Social Relationships

There are some striking differences in social conflict and social isolation for residents with bipolar disorder compared with other residents (table 3.3). Particularly among new admissions, conflict with others is more pervasive among those with bipolar disorder. These individuals are about twice as likely as residents with other diagnoses at admission to have been in conflict with or critical of staff, family, or friends. They are about three times more likely to show daily signs of persistent anger with themselves or others and to be unhappy with other residents. For most of these indicators of conflict, the rates for residents with schizophrenia are similar to those for the bipolar disorder group, and all rates tend to be higher among established residents than new admissions.

No significant differences among groups are apparent in the proportion of residents who have little involvement in activities at the CCC facility, but differences in the rate of absence of personal contact with family or friends are especially striking. A quarter (26.3%) of residents newly admitted with schizophrenia have no contact with friends or family members. The rate among those with bipolar disorder is

TABLE 3.3
Percentage of Complex Continuing Care with indicators of conflict and social isolation, by diagnostic group

	New admissions			Established residents		
	Bipolar disorder	Schizophrenia	Other diagnoses	Bipolar disorder	Schizophrenia	Other diagnoses
Indicators of conflict						
Conflict/criticism of staff	11.6	9.4	5.6	18.5	11.5	10.2
Conflict/anger with family/friends	15.7	11.0	7.7	15.6	15.4	11.2
Unhappy with roommate	6.6	7.5	4.5	9.6	9.6	7.4
Unhappy with residents	8.0	8.2	2.5	12.3	17.3	6.8
Persistent anger with self or others (daily)	14.2	11.5	5.4	19.2	21.8	10.4
Indicators of social isolation						
Absence of personal contact with family or friends	12.2	26.3	7.2	22.6	31.4	9.5
Little involvement in activities in facility	49.2	54.9	51.7	50.1	55.1	53.1

TABLE 3·4
Percentage of Complex Continuing Care hospital/unit residents receiving psychotropic medications and mental health interventions, by diagnostic group

	New admissions			Established residents		
	Bipolar disorder	Schizophrenia	Other diagnoses	Bipolar disorder	Schizophrenia	Other diagnoses
Psychotropic medications						
Antidepressants	50.3	28.2	22.2	54.1	29.5	29.2
Antipsychotics	54.1	67.7	14.8	60.3	77.6	18.4
Anxiolytics	43.4	36.8	31.9	42.5	43.6	28.7
Sedatives	17.5	15.5	12.4	16.4	16.0	10.5
No psychotropics	14.6	15.3	42.5	13.7	10.9	41.7
Three or more types of psychotropics	20.7	13.0	3.7	21.9	19.9	5.5
Mental health interventions						
Behavioral symptom evaluation	11.2	10.7	2.9	14.4	12.8	3.8
Licensed mental health professional visit in past 90 days	34.5	29.1	7.5	25.3	21.2	5.3
Group therapy	4.1	3.4	2.2	4.8	8.3	4.2
Reorientation (e.g., cueing)	38.4	41.0	28.8	37.0	43.6	27.2

half that of the schizophrenia group, but roughly double the rate for new admissions with other diagnoses. In contrast, among the established residents, the rates for those with schizophrenia and those with other diagnoses climb modestly, but absence of personal contact with family or friends almost doubles for the bipolar disorder group. This suggests that while other residents tend to have fairly stable patterns of contact with informal networks (i.e., the schizophrenia group remains consistently high and the other-diagnoses group stays consistently low), residents with bipolar disorder may be at increased risk of having a major decline in informal contact over the course of their residential care. This may be, at least in part, a reflection of the patterns of conflict and behavioral disturbance in this group, as well as the observed differences in marital history.

Treatments and Interventions

Given the findings for mental health indicators, behavioral disturbance, and patterns of conflict with others, it is not surprising to find that CCC residents with bipolar disorder are much more likely to receive psychotropic medications and mental health interventions than are residents with other diagnoses (table 3.4). In fact, the profile of residents with bipolar disorder is in many ways similar to that of residents with schizophrenia. Of the three resident groups analyzed, those with bipolar disorder are the most likely to receive antidepressants. Most residents with bipolar disorder also receive antipsychotic medications, and this rate of antipsychotics use is highest among established residents. The bipolar disorder group is about three times more likely than the other-diagnoses group to receive some type of psychotropic medication and is the most likely to receive three or more classes of psychotropics.

With respect to mental health services, residents with bipolar disorder and those with schizophrenia are more likely than residents in the other-diagnoses group to have (1) undergone evaluation of behavioral symptoms, (2) seen a licensed mental health professional, and (3) received reorientation from staff. Only minor differences are evident in access to group therapy, which was rarely used with any group of residents.

Medication Side Effects: The Resident Assessment Protocols on Psychotropic Drug Use

Potential medication-related side effects include hypotension, gait disturbance, and physical discomfort (e.g., constipation). The "trigger items" used to identify the need for care planning in the psychotropic drug use RAP are listed in table 3.5, and

TABLE 3.5
Indicators of potential drug-related hypotension, gait disturbance, or discomfort in the RAI 2.0 Resident Assessment Protocol (RAP) for psychotropic drug use

Potential drug-related hypotension or gait disturbance	Potential drug-related discomfort
Repetitive physical movement	Constipation
Balance while sitting	Fecal impaction
Hypotension	Lung aspiration
Dizziness/vertigo	
Syncope	
Unsteady gait	
Fall in past 30 days	
Fall in past 31–180 days	
Hip fracture	
Swallowing problem	

analyses of how these triggers relate to resident type are shown in table 3.6. The residents in the bipolar disorder and the schizophrenia groups are equally likely to trigger the items related to discomfort and hypotension or gait disturbance. Both groups have significantly higher rates of these side effects than the other-diagnoses group. In fact, about three-quarters of the residents with bipolar disorder or schizophrenia have hypotension or gait disturbance, conditions that place an older person at increased risk of injury (e.g., falls) and subsequent increased morbidity. One of the more prevalent medication-related side effects is repetitive physical movements (e.g., pacing, hand wringing, restlessness, fidgeting, picking). These symptoms occurred daily in about 20% of newly admitted or established residents with bipolar disorder. No doubt some of these symptoms are related to bipolar disorder itself rather than a medication side effect, but it is also safe to infer that a significant proportion are related to medications.

Figure 3.3 illustrates the relation among resident type, antipsychotic use, and daily repetitive movements. When no antipsychotics are used, daily repetitive movements are significantly more common among residents with bipolar disorder and schizophrenia than among those with other diagnoses (about 15% vs. 8%, respectively). However, for all three resident groups, the rate of daily repetitive movements increases to about 25% for those receiving antipsychotics: this rate is significantly higher for those taking antipsychotics than for those not receiving this medication class. Although interRAI recommends that RAI 2.0 assessments include a detailed summary of the specific medications taken, this section was *not* part of the mandate in Ontario (or in the United States). Therefore, it is not possible with this dataset to differentiate between residents who received conventional versus atypical antipsychotics.

TABLE 3.6

Percentage of Complex Continuing Care hospital/unit residents with potential drug-related hypotension, gait disturbance, or discomfort, by diagnostic group

	New admissions			Established residents		
	Bipolar disorder	Schizophrenia	Other diagnoses	Bipolar disorder	Schizophrenia	Other diagnoses
Potential drug-related discomfort: one or more indicators present (see table 3.5)	24.7	25.3	16.7	28.1	26.9	15.9
Potential drug-related hypotension or gait disturbance: one or more indicators present (see table 3.5)	72.6	72.3	45.6	76.0	77.6	49.7
Repetitive physical movements						
Not present	65.9	65.3	81.4	60.3	62.2	73.7
Less than daily	14.5	14.1	9.7	16.4	16.7	11.6
Daily	19.6	20.6	8.9	23.3	21.2	14.7

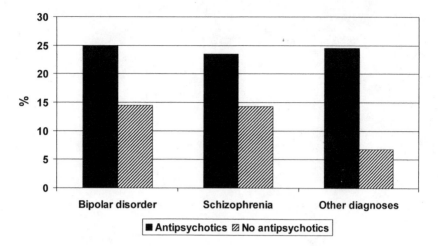

Fig. 3.3. Percentage of residents in Ontario Complex Continuing Care hospitals/units with daily repetitive physical movements, by use/nonuse of antipsychotic medication and resident type.

CLINICAL AND POLICY IMPLICATIONS

Given the paucity of data on the characteristics of persons with bipolar disorder in long-term care settings, the findings presented here raise some ideas about clinical practice and policy for this population. The evidence clearly supports the notion that nursing home residents with bipolar disorder comprise a unique subpopulation with special needs. They are clinically complex individuals who require care in multiple domains. For example, although persons with bipolar disorder seem to have levels of medical instability and functional impairment comparable to those of other residents in long-term care, in bipolar disorder these conditions are further influenced by psychiatric, behavioral, and social problems that may adversely affect individuals' quality of life. The most direct clinical implication of this finding is that persons with bipolar disorder in long-term care require comprehensive assessment to determine their overall care needs. The interRAI instruments seem well-suited for providing a broad, resident-focused assessment suitable for use with this population.

As mentioned earlier in the chapter, some reports suggest that elderly persons with bipolar disorder comprise an intermediate group between those with schizophrenia and the general population of older adults (Depp and Jeste 2004). While some aspects of this assertion are borne out by the evidence presented here, such a characterization is simplistic and implies that bipolar symptoms are less disabling than symptoms of schizophrenia. The findings show, for example, that the bipolar disorder and schizophrenia groups have a similar prevalence rate of behavioral disturbance, and that the association between behavioral disturbance and cognition is more pronounced in the bipolar disorder group. On the other hand, the rate and severity of depressive symptoms are considerably higher in the bipolar disorder group than in the schizophrenia group. Given that the lifetime risk of suicide among persons with bipolar disorder may be as high as 15% (Perlis et al. 2004), and that this is comparable to the risk for persons with schizophrenia (Henderson et al. 2004), the importance of both disorders should not be underestimated.

Our analysis also reveals two subgroups among NH residents with bipolar disorder. Newly admitted persons differ in several ways from those who have been in the facility for at least a year. Established residents have more severe overall impairments, are more difficult to treat, and have fewer social resources, making them harder to discharge or place in less-intensive care settings. The preliminary evidence that institutional placement is associated with a severance of informal ties is especially important, because this may have profound effects on discharge potential, advocacy, quality of care, and quality of life for persons with bipolar disorder.

Understanding the combined effects of depression and behavioral disturbance in NH residents with bipolar disorder may facilitate the development of an appropriate, comprehensive intervention strategy for these individuals. Conflict and social isolation seem to be pervasive in their lives. Persons with bipolar disorder are much more likely than the general long-term care population to receive mental health interventions, but the relatively high rate of use of antipsychotic medications may be a disproportionate response to disturbed behavior in this cohort. There is evidence of potential adverse drug reactions associated with at least some of these medications. In summary, persons with bipolar disorder seem to be affected by a complex array of interconnected clinical problems that are difficult to address if the treatment strategies are overly narrow in focus.

Individuals with bipolar disorder in long-term care are more likely than the general NH population to have been in contact with the mental health system. For these individuals, interRAI assessment instruments may be a particularly useful mechanism for improving communication and continuity of care among different sectors of the health care system. For example, effective October 2005, the RAI-MH became the mandatory admission and discharge assessment instrument for all adult psychiatric inpatients in Ontario, including inpatients in acute, long-term, forensic, and geriatric psychiatry. Therefore, all persons now discharged from a psychiatric facility in this province have been assessed with the RAI-MH; data from these assessments are seamlessly compatible with the RAI 2.0 assessment used in the long-term care setting. Thus, clinicians in Ontario now have information that will allow smoother transitions across sectors and more appropriate clinical responses for persons with bipolar disorder earlier in their long-term care.

The results reported here suggest that research based on the interRAI family of assessment instruments can substantially contribute to knowledge about bipolar disorder in older adults. One can begin addressing the dearth of research on this population by using the substantial data resources already in hand. In addition, as the use of these assessment instruments increases across sectors of the health care system, and increases internationally, new opportunities will arise to study this population in different care settings and in different cultures. The results we present are derived from data on residents in Ontario's Complex Continuing Care hospitals/units. Although these facilities are similar to U.S. skilled nursing facilities, one cannot be certain that the findings generalize to lighter-care NHs that serve a less clinically complex population. Further analyses of older persons with bipolar disorder in other care settings and other countries would be most useful.

CONCLUSIONS

The findings presented in this chapter are based on cross-sectional analyses aimed at exploring, at a basic level, a broad range of issues affecting individuals with bipolar disorder in institutional settings. The results suggest that many research questions can be addressed with analyses of interRAI data. Future research should include more detailed multivariate analyses to determine what specific factors have the most important effect on the lives of nursing home residents with bipolar disorder. In addition, longitudinal models are needed to determine the temporal ordering of variables (e.g., behavioral disturbance and disruption of social ties).

The interRAI data also provide at least two unique opportunities for better understanding the needs of this population: cross-national and cross-sectoral comparisons. That is, it would be helpful to determine whether the results reported here are unique to Canadian facilities or to more-intensive care settings such as CCC hospitals/units. Linking the records of persons with bipolar disorder as they move through different sectors of the health care system (e.g., inpatient psychiatry, home care, long-term care) would be especially informative. This type of analysis could yield information on the factors that precipitate the long-term care placement of persons with bipolar disorder, and it could shed light on potential interventions that would support the integration of these individuals into the community.

REFERENCES

Applegate, W. B., Blass, J. P., and Williams, T. F. 1990. Instruments for the functional assessment of older patients. *N Engl J Med* 322:1207–1214.

Bartels, S. J., Mueser, K. T., and Miles, K. M. 1997. A comparative study of elderly patients with schizophrenia and bipolar disorder in nursing homes and the community. *Schizophr Res* 27:181–190.

Burrows, A. B., Morris, J. N., Simon, S. E., et al. 2000. Development of a RAI-based Depression Rating Scale for use in nursing homes. *Age Ageing* 29:165–172.

Colenda, C. C., Streim, J., Greene, J. A., et al. 1999. The impact of OBRA 87 on psychiatric services in nursing homes. Joint testimony of the American Psychiatric Association and the American Association for Geriatric Psychiatry. *Am J Geriatr Psychiatry* 7:12–17.

Depp, C. A., and Jeste, D. V. 2004. Bipolar disorder in older adults: a critical review. *Bipolar Disord* 6:343–367.

Fries, B. E., and Fahey, C. 2003. Introduction: lessons learned from eight countries. In Fries, B. E., and Fahey, C. (eds.), *Implementing the Resident Assessment Instrument: case studies of policymaking for long-term care in eight countries* (pp. 5–8). New York: Milbank Memorial Fund.

Fries, B. E., Schneider, D. P., Foley, W. J., et al. 1994. Refining a case-mix measure for nursing homes: Resource Utilization Groups (RUG-III). *Med Care* 32:668–685.

Fries, B. E., Hawes, C., Morris, J. N., et al. 1997a. Effect of the national Resident Assessment Instrument on selected health conditions and problems. *J Am Geriatr Soc* 45:994–1001.

Fries, B. E., Schroll, M., Hawes, C., et al. 1997b. Approaching cross-national comparisons of nursing home residents. *Age Ageing* 26(suppl. 2):13–18.

Fries, B. E., Simon, S. E., Morris, J. N., et al. 2001. Pain in US nursing homes: validating a pain scale for the Resident Assessment Instrument. *Gerontologist* 41:173–179.

Hawes, C., Mor, V., Phillips, C. D., et al. 1997a. The OBRA-87 nursing home regulations and implementation of the Resident Assessment Instrument: effects on process quality. *J Am Geriatr Soc* 45:977–985.

Hawes, C., Morris, J., Phillips, C. D., et al. 1997b. Development of the nursing home Resident Assessment Instrument in the USA. *Age Ageing* 26(suppl. 2):19–25.

Henderson, D. C., Kunkel, L., and Goff, D. C. 2004. Psychosis and schizophrenia. In Stern, T. A., and Herman, J. B. (eds.), *Massachusetts General Hospital psychiatry update and board preparation* (pp. 97–102). New York: McGraw-Hill Medical Publishing.

Hendriksen, C., Lund, E., and Stromgard, E. 1984. Consequences of assessment and intervention among elderly people: a three-year randomized controlled trial. *BMJ* 289:1522–1524.

Hirdes, J. P., Fries, B. E., Morris, J. N., et al. 1999. Integrated health information systems based on the RAI/MDS series of instruments. *Healthcare Manage Forum* 12:30–40.

Hirdes, J. P., Marhaba, M., Smith, T. F., et al. 2001. Development of the Resident Assessment Instrument–Mental Health (RAI-MH). *Hosp Q* 4:44–51.

Hirdes, J. P., Smith, T. F., Rabinowitz, T., et al. 2002. The Resident Assessment Instrument–

Mental Health (RAI-MH)(c): inter-rater reliability and convergent validity. *J Behav Health Serv Res* 29:419–432.

Hirdes, J. P., Frijters, D. H., and Teare, G. F. 2003a. The MDS-CHESS scale: a new measure to predict mortality in the institutionalized elderly. *J Am Geriatr Soc* 51:96–100.

Hirdes, J. P., Sinclair, D., King, J., et al. 2003b. From anecdotes to evidence: Complex Continuing Care at the dawn of the information age in Ontario. In Fries, B. E., and Fahey, C. (eds.), *Implementing the Resident Assessment Instrument: case studies of policymaking for long-term care in eight countries* (pp. 44–63). New York: Milbank Memorial Fund.

Mechanic, D., and McAlpine, D. D. 2000. Use of nursing homes in the care of persons with severe mental illness: 1985 to 1995. *Psychiatr Serv* 51:354–358.

Meeks, S., Carstensen, L. L., Stafford, P. B., et al. 1990. Mental health needs of the chronically mentally ill elderly. *Psychol Aging* 5:163–171.

Mor, V., Branco, K., Fleishman, J., et al. 1995. The structure of social engagement among nursing home residents. *J Gerontol B Psychol Sci* 50:P1–P8.

Mor, V., Intrator, O., Hiris, J., et al. 1997. Impact of the MDS on changes in nursing home discharge rates and destinations. *J Am Geriatr Soc* 45:1002–1010.

Morris, J., Hawes, C., Fries, B. E., et al. 1990. Designing the national Resident Assessment Instrument for nursing homes. *Gerontologist* 30:293–307.

Morris, J. N., Fries, B. E., Mehr, D. R., et al. 1994. MDS Cognitive Performance Scale. *J Gerontol Med Sci* 49:M174–M182.

Morris, J., Nonemaker, S., Murphy, K., et al. 1997. A commitment to change: revision of HCFA's RAI. *J Am Geriatr Soc* 45:1011–1016.

Morris, J. N., Fries, B. E., and Morris, S. A. 1999. Scaling ADLs within the MDS. *J Gerontol A Med Sci* 54:M546–M553.

Morris, J., Carpenter, G. I., Berg, K., et al. 2000. Outcome measures for use with home care clients. *Can J Aging* 19(suppl. 2):87–105.

Morris, J. N., Jones, R. N., Fries, B. E., et al. 2004. Convergent validity of MDS-based performance quality indicators in post-acute care settings. *Am J Med Qual* 19:242–247.

Perlis, R. H., and Ghaemi, S. N. 2004. Bipolar disorder. In Stern, T. A., and Herman, J. B. (eds.), *Massachusetts General Hospital psychiatry update and board preparation* (pp. 113–120). New York: McGraw-Hill Medical Publishing.

Phillips, C. D., Hawes, C., Mor, V., et al. 1997a. Geriatric assessment in nursing homes in the United States: impact of a national program. *Generations* 21:15–20.

Phillips, C. D., Morris, J. N., Hawes, C., et al. 1997b. The impact of the RAI on ADLs, continence, communication, cognition, and psychosocial well-being. *J Am Geriatr Soc* 45:986–993.

Phillips, C. D., Zimmerman, D., Bernabei, R., et al. 1997c. Using the Resident Assessment Instrument for quality enhancement in nursing homes. *Age Ageing* 26(suppl. 2):77–81.

Post, R., Rubinow, D., and Ballenger, J. 1986. Conditioning and sensitization in the longitudinal course of affective illness. *Br J Psychiatry* 149:191–201.

Price Waterhouse Coopers. 2001. *Report of a study to review levels of service and responses to need in a sample of Ontario long term care facilities and selected comparators.* Prepared for the Ontario Long Term Care Association and the Ontario Association of Non-Profit Homes and Services for Seniors. Toronto: Price Waterhouse Coopers.

Rabinowitz, T. 2002. Delirium: an important (but often unrecognized) clinical syndrome. *Curr Psychiatry Rep* 4:202–208.

Rabinowitz, T., Murphy, K. M., Nagle, K. J., et al. 2003. Delirium: pathophysiology, recognition, prevention and treatment. *Expert Rev. Neurotherapeutics* 3:89–101.

Sgadari, A., Topinkova, E., Bjornson, J., et al. 1997. Urinary incontinence in nursing home residents: a cross-national comparison. *Age Ageing* 27(suppl. 2):49–54.

Snowdon, J. 2001. Psychiatric care in nursing homes: more must be done. *Psychiatry Old Age* 9:108–112.

Tariot, P. N., Podgorski, C. A., Blazina, L., et al. 1993. Mental disorders in the nursing home: another perspective. *Am J Psychiatry* 150:1063–1069.

Winokur, G., Clayton, P., and Reich, T. 1969. *Manic-depressive illness*. St. Louis, MO: Mosby.

Zimmerman, D. R., Karon, S. L., Arling, G., et al. 1995. Development and testing of nursing home quality indicators. *Health Care Financ Rev* 16:104–127.

PART TWO

Treatment

CHAPTER FOUR

Late-Onset Bipolar Disorder and Secondary Mania

PAUL E. HOLTZHEIMER III, M.D.,

AND WILLIAM M. MCDONALD, M.D.

Mood disorders, including bipolar disorder, are underdiagnosed in elderly persons (Charney et al. 2003). While some older persons with mania may have a history of early-onset bipolar disorder, others may have developed mania for the first time in late life. Those with late-onset mania may have idiopathic late-onset bipolar disorder or "secondary mania," that is, mania resulting from an underlying medical condition. This chapter focuses on the epidemiology, etiology, diagnosis, and treatment of secondary mania and late-onset bipolar disorder.

EPIDEMIOLOGY
Definitions of Secondary Mania and Its Presentation across the Lifespan

Krauthammer and Klerman (1978) originally noted that manic symptomatology could develop in people with no history of mood disorder who develop certain medical illnesses (e.g., epilepsy, cancer, metabolic abnormalities), and these authors used the term *secondary mania* to describe this condition. Secondary mania was formally defined as a disorder, lasting at least one week, occurring in association with some medical or pharmacological disturbance and characterized by an elated or irritable mood and at least two of the following behavioral symptoms: hyperactivity, grandiosity, flight of ideas, pressured speech, distractibility, decreased sleep, and lack of judgment. Additionally, for a condition to be classified as secondary mania, the patient should have no history of primary mood disorder and no evidence of delirium (e.g., disorientation or clouding of consciousness). Stasiek and Zetin (1985) confirmed this definition through the presentation and summary of several cases of secondary mania associated with various medications, metabolic disturbances, and neurological conditions. The primary significance of defining secondary mania was to alert clinicians to the possibility that an underlying medical condition or drug treatment could potentially induce a manic syndrome practically identical to that seen in patients with "idiopathic" bipolar disorder or manic-depressive illness. It was therefore suggested that the proper workup for a patient presenting with manic symptoms should include careful consideration of, and examination for, potential medical causes of those symptoms before a diagnosis of idiopathic bipolar disorder was made.

Secondary mania was recognized as a condition that could occur at any point across the lifespan, and the diagnosis is not restricted to use in older adults. Most medical conditions and treatments associated with secondary mania (described in more detail below and listed in table 4.1) can occur in people of any age. The literature describing cases of secondary mania shows a clear overlap in age of onset for secondary mania and idiopathic bipolar disorder (i.e., late teen years to mid-thirties). Therefore, the possibility of secondary mania should be considered in *any* patient presenting with manic symptoms, especially if associated with an underlying medical or pharmacological-related condition. That said, secondary mania is indeed more common in older than in younger patients. This is reasonable, given the higher prevalence of potentially causative medical conditions and treatments in older adults (Krauthammer and Klerman 1978; Stasiek and Zetin 1985).

Incidence and Prevalence of Late-Onset "Idiopathic" Mania

Idiopathic bipolar disorder refers to a mood disorder consisting of manic, hypomanic, depressive, and/or mixed episodes in cases where secondary mania has been ruled out. The average age of onset for idiopathic bipolar disorder is about 20 years (American Psychiatric Association 2000). The incidence and prevalence of late-onset idiopathic bipolar disorder are uncertain (see chapter 1), but onset after 40 years of age is unusual and incidence is believed to decrease significantly with age. For example, in a community sample in Western Australia, the prevalence of bipolar disorder was 0.4%, with only 1 in 12 subjects presenting with manic symptoms for the first time after age 65 years (Almeida and Fenner 2002). In a sample of 1,157 patients at an urban primary care clinic, 7.6% of those aged 55–70 years screened positive for bipolar disorder (Das et al. 2005). In a second sample, consist-

TABLE 4.1
Causes of secondary mania

Neurological
  Basal ganglia disease (e.g., Parkinson disease)
  Brain tumors (primary or metastatic)
  Cerebrovascular disease
  Dementia
  Epilepsy
  HIV encephalopathy/AIDS dementia
  Infectious encephalitis
  Multiple sclerosis
  Neurosyphilis
  Traumatic brain injury
Medical/systemic
  Cushing syndrome
  Paraneoplastic syndromes
  Systemic infections
  Systemic lupus erythematosus
  Thyroid abnormalities (especially hyperthyroidism)
  Uremia
Iatrogenic
  Medications
    Antidepressants
    Benzodiazepine (use and/or withdrawal)
    Corticosteroids
    Dopamine agonists
    Thyroid replacement
  Surgical treatments for Parkinson disease
    Deep brain stimulation of subthalamic nucleus
    Pallidotomy
Other
  Circadian rhythm changes
  Substance intoxication/withdrawal

ing of 246 patients who presented to their primary care physician for first treatment of mania, only 9% were older than 55 years. Among patients with late-onset mania, eight (3%) were between 56 and 65 years old, nine (4%) were between 66 and 75, and six (2%) were older than 75 (Kennedy et al. 2005). Finally, a sample from a bipolar disorder clinic found that 6.3% of 366 clinic patients had late onset of illness; however, this was defined as onset after 47 years of age (Cassidy and Carroll 2002).

Among patients with late-onset mania due to idiopathic bipolar disorder, about half have no clear history of a mood disorder, while half have a history of depression (Stone 1989). Up to 17 years may elapse between the first depressive episode and first manic episode in late-onset bipolar disorder (Broadhead and Jacoby 1990; Shulman et al. 1992; Snowdon 2001; Stone 1989). Mania can occur at any age, with de novo manic symptoms described in patients in their eighth and ninth decades (Kellner and Neher 1991; Summers 1983; Walter-Ryan 1983). Some investigators have shown that men, but not women, have an increased incidence of mania in late life, especially in their eighth and ninth decades (Eagles and Whalley 1985; Sibisi 1990; Spicer et al. 1973). However, other studies have demonstrated that the risk for developing mania in late life is at least equal among men and women, and possibly greater for women (Almeida and Fenner 2002; Kennedy et al. 2005). Individuals with late-onset mania are less likely to have family members with mood disorders, suggesting that genetic factors may be less important in the etiology of late- versus early-onset mania (Depp and Jeste 2004; Engstrom et al. 2003; Hays et al. 1998; Moorhead and Young 2003; Schurhoff et al. 2000; Snowdon 1991; R. C. Young 1992).

Summary of Epidemiology

Secondary mania refers to a manic syndrome resulting from an associated medical or pharmacological disturbance in a person with no history of mood disorder and no evidence of delirium. Secondary mania can occur at any age but is more common in older adults. Conversely, idiopathic bipolar disorder is less likely to present de novo in older adults, and secondary mania probably accounts for more cases of late-onset mania in older adults than does idiopathic illness (while the reverse is probably true for younger patients). Definitive studies of the epidemiology of late-onset idiopathic bipolar disorder are lacking, and the available data must be interpreted cautiously. Based on the data, 7%–9% of individuals with idiopathic bipolar disorder have new onset of mania in later life. The relative incidence of late-onset mania in men versus women is unclear. Genetic factors may be less relevant to the etiology of idiopathic bipolar disorder in late-onset versus early-onset mania.

ETIOLOGY
Secondary Mania

As discussed above, secondary mania has been associated with a range of medical, neurological, and iatrogenic (including pharmacological) causes (table 4.1). Stroke is an established cause of secondary mania (Celik et al. 2004; Cummings and Mendez 1984; Fenn and George 1999; Kulisevsky et al. 1993; Robinson and Starkstein 1989; Starkstein et al. 1988; Starkstein and Robinson 1989), with right-sided strokes showing a stronger association than left-sided strokes (Robinson 1997; Shulman 1997). Similarly, focal traumatic brain injury may result in new-onset mania (Jorge et al. 1993; Shukla et al. 1987; Starkstein et al. 1988, 1990). Patients with complex partial seizures and other forms of epilepsy may present with manic symptoms either ictally or post-ictally (Barczak et al. 1988; Chakrabarti et al. 1999; Gillig et al. 1988; Guillem et al. 2000; Pascualy et al. 1997). Other neurological conditions associated with secondary mania include dementia, such as Alzheimer disease, Pick disease, and vascular dementia (Assal and Cummings 2002; Levy et al. 1996; McDonald and Thompson 2001; Migliorelli et al. 1995; Nilsson et al. 2002; Shulman 1997); Parkinson disease and related basal ganglia disorders (Kim et al. 1994; Lauterbach 2004; Lauterbach et al. 1998; Rosenblatt and Leroi 2000); multiple sclerosis (Feinstein 2004; Heila et al. 1995; Kwentus et al. 1986; Mapelli and Ramelli 1981; Peselow et al. 1981); human immunodeficiency virus (HIV) encephalopathy and acquired immunodeficiency syndrome (AIDS) dementia (el-Mallakh 1991; Kieburtz et al. 1991; Lyketsos et al. 1993, 1997; McGowan et al. 1991; Rosenbaum 1992; Schmidt and Miller 1988); neurosyphilis (Galindo Menendez 1996; Hoffman 1982; Rosenbaum 1992); infectious encephalitis (Lendvai et al. 1999); and central nervous system neoplasms (Binder 1983; Filley and Kleinschmidt-DeMasters 1995; Greenberg and Brown 1985; Mazure et al. 1999; Salazar-Calderon Perriggo et al. 1993; Starkstein et al. 1988).

Systemic medical conditions and metabolic disturbances associated with the development of late-onset mania include cortisol abnormalities, such as Cushing syndrome (Kelly 1996; Reed et al. 1983); thyroid abnormalities, especially hyperthyroidism (Krauthammer and Klerman 1979; Nath and Sagar 2001); systemic lupus erthythematosus (SLE) (Khan et al. 2000); vitamin deficiencies (e.g., B_{12} [Goggans 1984; Lindenbaum et al. 1988; Scott et al. 2004] and niacin [Rudin 1981]); paraneoplastic syndromes (Collins and Oakley-Browne 1988); systemic infections (e.g., influenza [Maurizi 1985; Steinberg et al. 1972]); and uremia (el-Mallakh et al. 1987; Thomas and Neale 1991).

Many iatrogenic causes have also been attributed to the development of mania. Presenting an exhaustive list of medications associated with new-onset mania is not possible here. Some common associations include corticosteroids (Brown and Suppes 1998; Ganzini et al. 1993; Sultzer and Cummings 1989); thyroid replacement therapy (Evans et al. 1986; Ganzini et al. 1993; Josephson and Mackenzie 1980); pharmacotherapies for Parkinson disease, especially dopamine agonist medications (Cummings 1991; Harsch et al. 1985; Kurlan and Dimitsopulos 1992; Ryback and Schwab 1971; B. K. Young et al. 1997); and benzodiazepine use (Burke 1987; Dorevitch 1991; Goodman and Charney 1987; Reddy et al. 1996) and withdrawal (Lapierre and Labelle 1987; Rigby et al. 1989; Turkington and Gill 1989). As in younger patients, antidepressant medications may precipitate mania in older adults, with tricyclic antidepressants posing the greatest risk (R. C. Young et al. 2003).

Other somatic treatments have been associated with late-onset mania. Electroconvulsive therapy (ECT) has induced mania (Sanders and Deshpande 1990; Serby 2001), although it can also be an effective treatment for mania (McDonald and

Thompson 2001; Mukherjee et al. 1994; Tsao et al. 2004). Surgical treatments for Parkinson disease have been associated with new-onset mania, including pallidotomy (Okun et al. 2003) and deep brain stimulation (DBS) of the subthalamic nucleus (Herzog et al. 2003; Kulisevsky et al. 2002; Romito et al. 2002a, 2000b) and the internal globus pallidus (Anderson and Mullins 2003; Miyawaki et al. 2000).

Other conditions may potentially induce mania. Substance intoxication or withdrawal may mimic or cause manic symptoms, especially in older adults; common substances include alcohol, cocaine, methamphetamine, and opiates. Caffeine intoxication (Machado-Vieira et al. 2001; Ogawa and Ueki 2003) and nicotine withdrawal (Benazzi 1989; Cohen 1990) have been associated with mania. Linton and Warner (2000) described three elderly patients with "travel-induced psychosis"; however, two of the three patients had a clear history of bipolar disorder, and the third had a history of recurrent severe depression.

Idiopathic Late-Onset Bipolar Disorder

The etiology of idiopathic bipolar disorder (at any age of onset) remains poorly understood. However, the relative lack of family history for mood disorders in patients with late-onset bipolar disorder suggests that late-onset mania may result, at least in part, from different pathophysiological processes from those associated with the early-onset form of the illness.

A growing database suggests that vascular disease may play an important role in the development of late-onset mood disorders. As noted above, strokes have been clearly linked with the development of secondary mania as well as depression (Robinson 2003), and subclinical vascular disease, especially in subcortical white matter, has been linked with late-onset depression (Alexopoulos et al. 1997; Krishnan et al. 1997; McDonald and Krishnan 1992). Increased cerebrovascular disease risk factors and evidence of ischemic damage to white matter have also been found in patients with late-onset mania (Broadhead and Jacoby 1990; Cassidy and Carroll 2002; McDonald et al. 1991; Shulman and Post 1980; Wylie et al. 1999). Other brain changes found in late-onset bipolar disease include decreased right caudate volume compared with healthy older controls (Beyer et al. 2004), decreased total brain volume compared with patients with early-onset bipolar illness (Beyer et al. 2004), greater cortical atrophy compared with matched patients with schizophrenia (Rabins et al. 2000), and a greater prevalence of patients with silent cerebral infarction compared with those with early-onset illness and late-onset depression (Fujikawa et al. 1995). Thus, it is likely that late-life mood disorders in general, including late-onset mania, can result from vascular-ischemic-related changes in the brain that are associated with aging. Longitudinal studies on the relation between risk factors for vascular disease, neuroimaging findings, and development of bipolar disorder are needed to further clarify this relationship.

Summary of Etiology

Before making a diagnosis of idiopathic bipolar disorder, the clinician should consider the potential causes of secondary mania (table 4.1). The etiology of late-onset idiopathic bipolar disorder, like that of the early-onset illness, is poorly understood. However, a growing database suggests that vascular damage plays a significant etiological role in late-onset versus early-onset bipolar illness.

DIAGNOSIS AND ASSESSMENT
Clinical Presentation

Symptoms of mania include elevated or irritable mood, mood lability, distractibility, decreased need for sleep, increased talkativeness, racing thoughts, impulsivity, grandiosity, increased goal-directed activity, and excessive engagement in risky behavior (American Psychiatric Association 1994); mania may present with or without psychosis. Elderly persons with new-onset mania often have the same symptoms as younger persons. One small study suggested that patients with late-onset mania have less psychopathology than those with early-onset illness (Depp et al. 2004). However, another study found that patients with late-onset mania had more psychosis than those with early onset, although the response to inpatient treatment was the same in the two groups (Wylie et al. 1999).

Mania in the older adult should be clearly differentiated from delirium or dementia with agitated behavior. Older persons with mania may present with pseudo-dementia, consisting of confusion, memory impairment, mild disorientation, and distractibility (Casey and Fitzgerald 1988; Kellner and Neher 1991; Koenigsberg 1984; Liptzin 1992). Significant cognitive disturbance and disorientation should raise the possibility of dementia or delirium — and delirium should be considered especially if there is an associated clouding of consciousness. Recognizing mania in the context of dementia may be difficult, because individuals are less able to express subjective changes in mood and thought content; also, the patient may already demonstrate impulsivity and/or agitation related to the underlying dementia. In attempting to clarify the diagnosis, the clinician should keep in mind that mania is primarily characterized by significant *mood* changes (either elevated or irritable), whereas dementia and delirium typically are not. Considering the time course may also assist in distinguishing among these conditions: mania tends to develop over days to weeks; dementia, and behavioral disturbances associated with dementia, typically evolve over months to years; and delirium generally develops within hours to days.

Diagnostic Workup

The most important aspect of the diagnostic workup for late-onset mania is to identify potential causes of secondary mania. A careful history and physical examination, appropriate laboratory tests, and neuroimaging (when indicated) should be performed. The clinical history should focus on changes in mood and behavior, changes in neurovegetative signs (sleep, appetite, activity level, energy), changes in medications or new medical diagnoses, associated physical signs and symptoms (especially neurological symptoms such as syncope, seizures, and tremor), and observations reported by family members and other caregivers. The development of mania in younger persons is often clinically obvious as a clear change from baseline, but in older persons, physical disability from other illnesses may limit the expression of manic symptoms. Thus, careful attention should be paid to *any* new behavior that may indicate mania, such as hypersexuality, physical aggression, or impulsivity. The mental status examination should emphasize tests of cognitive function (including attention, concentration, and executive function). Physical examination should be performed to identify evidence of medical illnesses. Careful attention to the neurological examination is crucial. Table 4.2 provides a suggested workup for late-onset mania.

The laboratory workup should include a complete blood count, basic chemistries, renal function tests, hepatic function tests, thyroid function tests, B_{12}/folate level, urinalysis, and urine toxicology. An electrocardiogram (EKG) will help identify any new or newly unstable cardiac illness. When indicated by the clinical history and examination, measures of serum levels of medications and/or lumbar puncture are appropriate. In most cases of new-onset mania in elderly persons, screening imaging of the head (typically a noncontrast computed tomography scan) is indicated. However, magnetic resonance imaging should be considered only if the differential diagnosis (based on other elements in the clinical history) includes neoplasm, encephalitis, multiple sclerosis, or vasculitis. An electroencephalogram may be useful to evaluate for seizure disorder or delirium.

Summary of Diagnosis and Assessment

The presentation of mania in an older adult may be complicated by symptoms of pseudodementia and the presence of comorbid medical conditions. During as-

TABLE 4.2
Suggested workup for late-onset mania

Clinical history
    Current physical/neurological symptoms
    Family history of mood disorder
    History of mood disorder
    Neurovegetative changes (e.g., sleep, appetite, energy)
    Past medical history
    Recent medication changes
    Recent mood and behavioral changes
Physical examination, including careful neurological exam
Mental status examination, including tests of cognitive function
Laboratory tests
    B_{12}, folate
    Complete blood count
    Electrolytes, including calcium
    Kidney function
    Liver function
    Lumbar puncture (if indicated)
    Serum medication levels (if indicated)
    Thyroid function
    Urinalysis
    Urine toxicology
Electrocardiogram
Neuroimaging
    Electroencephalogram (if indicated)
    Noncontrast head computed tomography (screening only)
    Magnetic resonance imaging (if indicated)

sessment of the older patient with possible mania, careful attention should be paid to *any* changes in mood, behavior, physical signs and symptoms, medical illnesses, and medications. Any observations by family and other caregivers are important in clarifying the presentation. The diagnostic workup should focus on identifying medical conditions that may be causing or contributing to symptoms.

TREATMENT BASICS

Treatment of mania in the older adult is addressed in detail elsewhere (see chapters 5–7), and we present here just some basic aspects of treating late-onset mania (including secondary mania). The first step is to adequately treat underlying medical conditions that may be causing or contributing to symptoms. This would include correcting thyroid function or other metabolic abnormalities, treating any contributing medical illness (such as epilepsy or Parkinson disease), stopping (if possible) the use of corticosteroids or other medications that may be exacerbating or causing symptoms, and carefully assessing for substance use, intoxication, and/or withdrawal.

The use of mood-stabilizing, antipsychotic, and sedating medications can be helpful in achieving mood and behavioral stability in an older person with mania, even if he or she clearly has secondary mania. Indeed, treatment with one or more of these medications may be necessary to ensure the safety of the patient and others while the secondary mania is being treated. Lithium — a first-line agent in the management of mania and bipolar disorder in younger patients — has been used successfully in older patients with mania, but may have significantly more side effects in older patients and in those with underlying neurological disease (Himmelhoch et al. 1980; Kemperman et al. 1989; Roose et al. 1979; Smith and Helms 1982). These side effects can include tremor, gastrointestinal complaints, increased thirst, muscle weakness, and fatigue. Cardiac side effects of lithium use may be more problematic in older than in younger patients. Neurological side effects of lithium may also be greater in patients with underlying neurological disease. Finally, given the narrow therapeutic window for lithium, this drug may be difficult to use appropriately for older adults, for several reasons: poor medication compliance (due to memory problems and confusion), decreased renal clearance, and concomitant medications, some of which (e.g., thiazide diuretics) may result in clinically significant interactions.

Certain anticonvulsant medications have clear efficacy for treating mania in younger individuals, and a growing database suggests good efficacy and tolerability in older adults as well. Additionally, patients with mania who have a primary neurological illness may respond better to anticonvulsants than to lithium (McCoy et al. 1993; McElroy et al. 1992; Stoll et al. 1994). That said, the use of some anticonvulsant medications (such as valproic acid [valproate] or carbamazepine) may be limited by the tolerability of side effects, drug-drug interactions (especially with carbamazepine), and other adverse reactions (such as thrombocytopenia associated with valproic acid). The short-term use of benzodiazepines can be considered in cases of extreme agitation associated with late-onset mania; however, at lower doses these medications may be associated with paradoxical increases in agitation and behavioral disturbance caused by cortical disinhibition, and patients may become overly sedated, hypotensive, or hypocapneic when taking higher doses.

Several atypical antipsychotic medications have shown efficacy in treating acute mania and in treating agitation in persons with dementia (Alexopoulos et al. 2004; Yatham 2002). The use of atypical antipsychotics in the treatment of late-onset and secondary mania is generally accepted by experts (Alexopoulos et al. 2004), but this requires further investigation. A developing concern about the use of atypical antipsychotics by older patients is the possible increased mortality associated with use by patients with dementia and agitation (see www.fda.gov/cder/drug/advisory/ antipsychotics.htm).

In the treatment of the older patient with mania, particular attention should be paid to the risk-benefit ratio of specific treatments. Certain medications may have the potential to cause severe side effects (e.g., lithium or valproic acid), but the consequences of untreated mania can be significant and just as detrimental to the patient's overall health and well-being. Despite the difficulty associated with benzodiazepine use in older patients (especially those with underlying neurological problems), short-term use of these medications may be necessary to prevent harm to the individual or others resulting from severe agitation or behavioral dyscontrol. Discontinuing current antidepressant medications should be considered, especially in severe mania (Alexopoulos et al. 2004); however, discontinuing antidepressants may increase the risk of a depressive episode in patients with bipolar disorder (Altshuler et al. 2001). ECT can be a particularly safe, rapid, and effective treatment for mania, especially when the use of mood-stabilizing medications raises concerns about side effects, adverse events, or drug-drug interactions. Patients should be carefully screened, however, for intracranial and cardiac contraindications before instituting ECT treatment, and it should be noted that ECT may temporarily worsen cognitive impairments and confusion.

If the individual with mania cannot be effectively and safely cared for in the home environment, hospitalization will be necessary; hospitalization may also facilitate the diagnostic workup needed to clarify causative and contributing factors. In addition to providing a safe environment for treating the patient with mania, the hospital can also provide a low level of environmental stimulation that may have a calming effect. Light-dark and sleep-wake cycles should be normalized if possible. Caregivers should be educated and supported in caring for the older person with bipolar disorder, especially in the proper use of scheduled and as-needed medications, potential triggers for mood episodes, and early symptoms of relapse. Even more so than younger patients, older patients with bipolar disorder are likely to be cared for in complex health care settings that include a primary caregiver (spouse or other close relative), other caregivers, long-term care facilities, and multiple health care providers. Adequate communication and cooperation among these various entities is mandatory for the optimal diagnosis and treatment of older persons with mania.

In summary, the first step in treating mania in the older adult is to treat any underlying medical conditions that may be causing or contributing to symptoms. Medications with proven efficacy in treating mania in younger adults may also be used for older adults, although they may not be as well tolerated. Electroconvulsive therapy is a generally safe and effective treatment option for mania in the older person. Optimal treatment of the geriatric patient with mania often necessitates a high level of communication and cooperation across various systems, including the patient, the patient's family, other caregivers, multiple medical providers, hospitals, and residential/long-term care facilities.

REFERENCES

Alexopoulos, G. S., Meyers, B. S., Young, R. C., et al. 1997. "Vascular depression" hypothesis. *Arch Gen Psychiatry* 54:915–922.

Alexopoulos, G. S., Streim, J., Carpenter, D., et al. 2004. Using antipsychotic agents in older patients. *J Clin Psychiatry* 65(suppl. 2):5–99.

Almeida, O. P., and Fenner, S. 2002. Bipolar disorder: similarities and differences between patients with illness onset before and after 65 years of age. *Int Psychogeriatr* 14:311–322.

Altshuler, L., Kiriakos, L., Calcagno, J., et al. 2001. The impact of antidepressant discontinuation versus antidepressant continuation on 1-year risk for relapse of bipolar depression: a retrospective chart review. *J Clin Psychiatry* 62:612–616.

American Psychiatric Association. 1994. *Diagnostic and statistical manual of mental disorders* (4th ed.). Washington, DC: American Psychiatric Association Press.

American Psychiatric Association. 2000. *Diagnostic and statistical manual of mental disorders* (4th ed.). Washington, DC: American Psychiatric Association Press.

Anderson, K. E., and Mullins, J. 2003. Behavioral changes associated with deep brain stimulation surgery for Parkinson's disease. *Curr Neurol Neurosci Rep* 3:306–313.

Assal, F., and Cummings, J. L. 2002. Neuropsychiatric symptoms in the dementias. *Curr Opin Neurol* 15:445–450.

Barczak, P., Edmunds, E., and Betts, T. 1988. Hypomania following complex partial seizures: a report of three cases. *Br J Psychiatry* 152:137–139.

Benazzi, F. 1989. Severe mania following abrupt nicotine withdrawal. *Am J Psychiatry* 146:1641.

Beyer, J. L., Kuchibhatla, M., Payne, M., et al. 2004. Caudate volume measurement in older adults with bipolar disorder. *Int J Geriatr Psychiatry* 19:109–114.

Binder, R. L. 1983. Neurologically silent brain tumors in psychiatric hospital admissions: three cases and a review. *J Clin Psychiatry* 44:94–97.

Broadhead, J., and Jacoby, R. 1990. Mania in old age: a first prospective study. *Int J Geriatr Psychiatry* 5:215–222.

Brown, E. S., and Suppes, T. 1998. Mood symptoms during corticosteroid therapy: a review. *Harv Rev Psychiatry* 5:239–246.

Burke, W. J. 1987. Benzodiazepine-induced hypomania? *J Clin Psychopharmacol* 7:356–357.

Casey, D. A., and Fitzgerald, B. A. 1988. Mania and pseudodementia. *J Clin Psychiatry* 49:73–74.

Cassidy, F., and Carroll, B. J. 2002. Vascular risk factors in late onset mania. *Psychol Med* 32:359–362.

Celik, Y., Erdogan, E., Tuglu, C., et al. 2004. Post-stroke mania in late life due to right temporoparietal infarction. *Psychiatry Clin Neurosci* 58:446–447.

Chakrabarti, S., Aga, V. M., and Singh, R. 1999. Postictal mania following primary generalized seizures. *Neurol India* 47:332–333.

Charney, D. S., Reynolds, C. F. 3rd, Lewis, L., et al. 2003. Depression and Bipolar Support Alliance consensus statement on the unmet needs in diagnosis and treatment of mood disorders in late life. *Arch Gen Psychiatry* 60:664–672.

Cohen, S. B. 1990. Mania after nicotine withdrawal. *Am J Psychiatry* 147:1254–1255.

Collins, C., and Oakley-Browne, M. 1988. Mania associated with small cell carcinoma of the lung. *Aust N Z J Psychiatry* 22:207–209.

Cummings, J. L. 1991. Behavioral complications of drug treatment of Parkinson's disease. *J Am Geriatr Soc* 39:708–716.

Cummings, J. L., and Mendez, M. F. 1984. Secondary mania with focal cerebrovascular lesions. *Am J Psychiatry* 141:1084–1087.

Das, A. K., Olfson, M., Gameroff, M. J., et al. 2005. Screening for bipolar disorder in a primary care practice. *JAMA* 293:956–963.

Depp, C. A., and Jeste, D. V. 2004. Bipolar disorder in older adults: a critical review. *Bipolar Disord* 6:343–367.

Depp, C. A., Jin, H., Mohamed, S., et al. 2004. Bipolar disorder in middle-aged and elderly adults: is age of onset important? *J Nerv Ment Dis* 192:796–799.

Dorevitch, A. 1991. Mania associated with clonazepam. *DICP: Ann Pharmacother* 25:938–939.

Eagles, J. M., and Whalley, L. J. 1985. Ageing and affective disorders: the age at first onset of affective disorders in Scotland, 1969–1978. *Br J Psychiatry* 147:180–187.

el-Mallakh, R. S. 1991. Mania and paranoid psychosis in AIDS. *Psychosomatics* 32:362.

el-Mallakh, R. S., Shrader, S. A., and Widger, E. 1987. Mania as a manifestation of end-stage renal disease. *J Nerv Ment Dis* 175:243–245.

Engstrom, C., Brandstrom, S., Sigvardsson, S., et al. 2003. Bipolar disorder: II. Personality and age of onset. *Bipolar Disord* 5:340–348.

Evans, D. L., Strawn, S. K., Haggerty, J. J. Jr., et al. 1986. Appearance of mania in drug-resistant bipolar depressed patients after treatment with L-triiodothyronine. *J Clin Psychiatry* 47:521–522.

Feinstein, A. 2004. The neuropsychiatry of multiple sclerosis. *Can J Psychiatry* 49:157–163.

Fenn, D., and George, K. 1999. Post-stroke mania late in life involving the left hemisphere. *Aust N Z J Psychiatry* 33:598–600.

Filley, C. M., and Kleinschmidt-DeMasters, B. K. 1995. Neurobehavioral presentations of brain neoplasms. *West J Med* 163:19–25.

Fujikawa, T., Yamawaki, S., and Touhouda, Y. 1995. Silent cerebral infarctions in patients with late-onset mania. *Stroke* 26:946–949.

Galindo Menendez, A. 1996. [Parenchymal neurosyphilis: insidious onset (dementia) and acute onset (manic type) forms]. *Actas Luso Esp Neurol Psiquiatr Cienc Afines* 24:261–267.

Ganzini, L., Millar, S. B., and Walsh, J. R. 1993. Drug-induced mania in the elderly. *Drugs Aging* 3:428–435.

Gillig, P., Sackellares, J. C., and Greenberg, H. S. 1988. Right hemisphere partial complex seizures: mania, hallucinations, and speech disturbances during ictal events. *Epilepsia* 29:26–29.

Goggans, F. C. 1984. A case of mania secondary to vitamin B_{12} deficiency. *Am J Psychiatry* 141:300–301.

Goodman, W. K., and Charney, D. S. 1987. A case of alprazolam, but not lorazepam, inducing manic symptoms. *J Clin Psychiatry* 48:117–118.

Greenberg, D. B., and Brown, G. L. 1985. Mania resulting from brain stem tumor. *J Nerv Ment Dis* 173:434–436.

Guillem, E., Plas, J., Musa, C., et al. 2000. Ictal mania: a case report. *Can J Psychiatry* 45:493–494.

Harsch, H. H., Miller, M., and Young, L. D. 1985. Induction of mania by L-dopa in a non-bipolar patient. *J Clin Psychopharmacol* 5:338–339.

Hays, J. C., Krishnan, K. R., George, L. K., et al. 1998. Age of first onset of bipolar disorder: demographic, family history, and psychosocial correlates. *Depress Anxiety* 7:76–82.

Heila, H., Turpeinen, P., and Erkinjuntti, T. 1995. Case study: mania associated with multiple sclerosis. *J Am Acad Child Adolesc Psychiatry* 34:1591–1595.

Herzog, J., Reiff, J., Krack, P., et al. 2003. Manic episode with psychotic symptoms induced by subthalamic nucleus stimulation in a patient with Parkinson's disease. *Mov Disord* 18:1382–1384.

Himmelhoch, J. M., Neil, J. F., May, S. J., et al. 1980. Age, dementia, dyskinesias, and lithium response. *Am J Psychiatry* 137:941–945.

Hoffman, B. F. 1982. Reversible neurosyphilis presenting as chronic mania. *J Clin Psychiatry* 43:338–339.

Jorge, R. E., Robinson, R. G., Starkstein, S. E., et al. 1993. Secondary mania following traumatic brain injury. *Am J Psychiatry* 150:916–921.

Josephson, A. M., and Mackenzie, T. B. 1980. Thyroid-induced mania in hypothyroid patients. *Br J Psychiatry* 137:222–228.

Kellner, M. B., and Neher, F. 1991. A first episode of mania after age 80. *Can J Psychiatry* 36:607–608.

Kelly, W. F. 1996. Psychiatric aspects of Cushing's syndrome. *QJM* 89(7):543–551.

Kemperman, C. J., Gerdes, J. H., De Rooij, J., et al. 1989. Reversible lithium neurotoxicity at normal serum level may refer to intracranial pathology. *J Neurol Neurosurg Psychiatry* 52:679–680.

Kennedy, N., Boydell, J., Kalidindi, S., et al. 2005. Gender differences in incidence and age at onset of mania and bipolar disorder over a 35-year period in Camberwell, England. *Am J Psychiatry* 162:257–262.

Khan, S., Haddad, P., Montague, L., et al. 2000. Systemic lupus erythematosus presenting as mania. *Acta Psychiatr Scand* 101:406–408; discussion 408.

Kieburtz, K., Zettelmaier, A. E., Ketonen, L., et al. 1991. Manic syndrome in AIDS. *Am J Psychiatry* 148:1068–1070.

Kim, E., Zwil, A. S., McAllister, T. W., et al. 1994. Treatment of organic bipolar mood disorders in Parkinson's disease. *J Neuropsychiatry Clin Neurosci* 6:181–184.

Koenigsberg, H. W. 1984. Manic pseudodementia: case report. *J Clin Psychiatry* 45:132–134.

Krauthammer, C., and Klerman, G. L. 1978. Secondary mania: manic syndromes associated with antecedent physical illness or drugs. *Arch Gen Psychiatry* 35:1333–1339.

Krauthammer, C., and Klerman, G. L. 1979. Mania secondary to thyroid disease. *Lancet* 1:827–828.

Krishnan, K. R., Hays, J. C., and Blazer, D. G. 1997. MRI-defined vascular depression. *Am J Psychiatry* 154:497–501.

Kulisevsky, J., Berthier, M. L., and Pujol, J. 1993. Hemiballismus and secondary mania following a right thalamic infarction. *Neurology* 43:1422–1424.

Kulisevsky, J., Berthier, M. L., Gironell, A., et al. 2002. Mania following deep brain stimulation for Parkinson's disease. *Neurology* 59:1421–1424.

Kurlan, R., and Dimitsopulos, T. 1992. Selegiline and manic behavior in Parkinson's disease. *Arch Neurol* 49:1231.

Kwentus, J. A., Hart, R. P., Calabrese, V., et al. 1986. Mania as a symptom of multiple sclerosis. *Psychosomatics* 27:729–731.

Lapierre, Y. D., and Labelle, A. 1987. Manic-like reaction induced by lorazepam withdrawal. *Can J Psychiatry* 32:697–698.

Lauterbach, E. C. 2004. The neuropsychiatry of Parkinson's disease and related disorders. *Psychiatr Clin North Am* 27:801–825.

Lauterbach, E. C., Cummings, J. L., Duffy, J., et al. 1998. Neuropsychiatric correlates and treatment of lenticulostriatal diseases: a review of the literature and overview of research opportunities in Huntington's, Wilson's, and Fahr's diseases. A report of the ANPA Committee on Research, American Neuropsychiatric Association. *J Neuropsychiatry Clin Neurosci* 10:249–266.

Lendvai, I., Saravay, S. M., and Steinberg, M. D. 1999. Creutzfeldt-Jakob disease presenting as secondary mania. *Psychosomatics* 40:524–525.

Levy, M. L., Miller, B. L., Cummings, J. L., et al. 1996. Alzheimer disease and frontotemporal dementias: behavioral distinctions. *Arch Neurol* 53:687–690.

Lindenbaum, J., Healton, E. B., Savage, D. G., et al. 1988. Neuropsychiatric disorders caused by cobalamin deficiency in the absence of anemia or macrocytosis. *N Engl J Med* 318:1720–1728.

Linton, C., and Warner, N. J. 2000. Travel-induced psychosis in the elderly. *Int J Geriatr Psychiatry* 15:1070–1072.

Liptzin, B. 1992. Treatment of mania. In C. Salzman (ed.), *Clinical Geriatric Psychopharmacology* (2nd ed., pp. 177–190.). Baltimore: Williams and Wilkins.

Lyketsos, C. G., Hanson, A. L., Fishman, M., et al. 1993. Manic syndrome early and late in the course of HIV. *Am J Psychiatry* 150:326–327.

Lyketsos, C. G., Schwartz, J., Fishman, M., et al. 1997. AIDS mania. *J Neuropsychiatry Clin Neurosci* 9:277–279.

Machado-Vieira, R., Viale, C. I., and Kapczinski, F. 2001. Mania associated with an energy drink: the possible role of caffeine, taurine, and inositol. *Can J Psychiatry* 46:454–455.

Mapelli, G., and Ramelli, E. 1981. Manic syndrome associated with multiple sclerosis: secondary mania? *Acta Psychiatr Belg* 81:337–349.

Maurizi, C. P. 1985. Influenza and mania: a possible connection with the locus ceruleus. *South Med J* 78:207–209.

Mazure, C. M., Leibowitz, K., and Bowers, M. B., Jr. 1999. Drug-responsive mania in a man with a brain tumor. *J Neuropsychiatry Clin Neurosci* 11:114–115.

McCoy, L., Votolato, N. A., Schwarzkopf, S. B., et al. 1993. Clinical correlates of valproate augmentation in refractory bipolar disorder. *Ann Clin Psychiatry* 5:29–33.

McDonald, W. M., Husain, M., Doraiswamy, P. M., et al. 1991. A magnetic resonance image study of age-related changes in human putamen nuclei. *Neuroreport* 2:57–60.

McDonald, W. M., and Krishnan, K. R. 1992. Magnetic resonance in patients with affective illness. *Eur Arch Psychiatry Clin Neurosci* 241:283–290.

McDonald, W. M., and Thompson, T. R. 2001. Treatment of mania in dementia with electroconvulsive therapy. *Psychopharmacol Bull* 35:72–82.

McElroy, S. L., Keck, P. E. Jr., Pope, H. G. Jr., et al. 1992. Valproate in the treatment of bipolar disorder: literature review and clinical guidelines. *J Clin Psychopharmacol* 12(1 suppl.):42S–52S.

McGowan, I., Potter, M., George, R. J., et al. 1991. HIV encephalopathy presenting as hypomania. *Genitourin Med* 67:420–424.

Migliorelli, R., Petracca, G., Teson, A., et al. 1995. Neuropsychiatric and neuropsychological correlates of delusions in Alzheimer's disease. *Psychol Med* 25:505–513.

Miyawaki, E., Perlmutter, J. S., Troster, A. I., et al. 2000. The behavioral complications of pallidal stimulation: a case report. *Brain Cogn* 42:417–434.

Moorhead, S. R., and Young, A. H. 2003. Evidence for a late onset bipolar-I disorder sub-group from 50 years. *J Affect Disord* 73:271–277.

Mukherjee, S., Sackeim, H. A., and Schnur, D. B. 1994. Electroconvulsive therapy of acute manic episodes: a review of 50 years' experience. *Am J Psychiatry* 151:169–176.

Nath, J., and Sagar, R. 2001. Late-onset bipolar disorder due to hyperthyroidism. *Acta Psychiatr Scand* 104:72–73; discussion 74–75.

Nilsson, F. M., Kessing, L. V., Sorensen, T. M., et al. 2002. Enduring increased risk of developing depression and mania in patients with dementia. *J Neurol Neurosurg Psychiatry* 73:40–44.

Ogawa, N., and Ueki, H. 2003. Secondary mania caused by caffeine. *Gen Hosp Psychiatry* 25:138–139.

Okun, M. S., Bakay, R. A., DeLong, M. R., et al. 2003. Transient manic behavior after pallidotomy. *Brain Cogn* 52:281–283.

Pascualy, M., Tsuang, D., Shores, M., et al. 1997. Frontal-complex partial status epilepticus misdiagnosed as bipolar affective disorder in a 75-year-old man. *J Geriatr Psychiatry Neurol* 10:158–160.

Peselow, E. D., Fieve, R. R., Deutsch, S. I., et al. 1981. Coexistent manic symptoms and multiple sclerosis. *Psychosomatics* 22:824–825.

Rabins, P. V., Aylward, E., Holroyd, S., et al. 2000. MRI findings differentiate between late-onset schizophrenia and late-life mood disorder. *Int J Geriatr Psychiatry* 15:954–960.

Reddy, J., Khanna, S., Anand, U., et al. 1996. Alprazolam-induced hypomania. *Aust N Z J Psychiatry* 30:550–552.

Reed, K., Watkins, M., and Dobson, H. 1983. Mania in Cushing's syndrome: case report. *J Clin Psychiatry* 44:460–462.

Rigby, J., Harvey, M., and Davies, D. R. 1989. Mania precipitated by benzodiazepine withdrawal. *Acta Psychiatr Scand* 79:406–407.

Robinson, R. G. 1997. Mood disorders secondary to stroke. *Semin Clin Neuropsychiatry* 2:244–251.

Robinson, R. G. 2003. Poststroke depression: prevalence, diagnosis, treatment, and disease progression. *Biol Psychiatry* 54:376–387.

Robinson, R. G., and Starkstein, S. E. 1989. Mood disorders following stroke: new findings and future directions. *J Geriatr Psychiatry* 22:1–15.

Romito, L. M., Raja, M., Daniele, A., et al. 2002a. Transient mania with hypersexuality after surgery for high frequency stimulation of the subthalamic nucleus in Parkinson's disease. *Mov Disord* 17:1371–1374.

Romito, L. M., Scerrati, M., Contarino, M. F., et al. 2002b. Long-term follow up of subthalamic nucleus stimulation in Parkinson's disease. *Neurology* 58:1546–1550.

Roose, S. P., Bone, S., Haidorfer, C., et al. 1979. Lithium treatment in older patients. *Am J Psychiatry* 136:843–844.

Rosenbaum, M. 1992. Mania in AIDS and syphilis (paresis). *Am J Psychiatry* 149:416.

Rosenblatt, A., and Leroi, I. 2000. Neuropsychiatry of Huntington's disease and other basal ganglia disorders. *Psychosomatics* 41:24–30.

Rudin, D. O. 1981. The major psychoses and neuroses as omega-3 essential fatty acid deficiency syndrome: substrate pellagra. *Biol Psychiatry* 16:837–850.

Ryback, R. S., and Schwab, R. S. 1971. Manic response to levodopa therapy: report of a case. *N Engl J Med* 285:788–789.

Salazar-Calderon Perriggo, V. H., Oommen, K. J., and Sobonya, R. E. 1993. Silent solitary right parietal chondroma resulting in secondary mania. *Clin Neuropathol* 12:325–329.

Sanders, R. D., and Deshpande, A. S. 1990. Mania complicating ECT. *Br J Psychiatry* 157:153–154.

Schmidt, U., and Miller, D. 1988. Two cases of hypomania in AIDS. *Br J Psychiatry* 152:839–842.

Schurhoff, F., Bellivier, F., Jouvent, R., et al. 2000. Early and late onset bipolar disorders: two different forms of manic-depressive illness? *J Affect Disord* 58:215–221.

Scott, T. M., Tucker, K. L., Bhadelia, A., et al. 2004. Homocysteine and B vitamins relate to brain volume and white-matter changes in geriatric patients with psychiatric disorders. *Am J Geriatr Psychiatry* 12:631–638.

Serby, M. 2001. Manic reactions to ECT. *Am J Geriatr Psychiatry* 9:180.

Shukla, S., Cook, B. L., Mukherjee, S., et al. 1987. Mania following head trauma. *Am J Psychiatry* 144:93–96.

Shulman, K. I. 1997. Disinhibition syndromes, secondary mania and bipolar disorder in old age. *J Affect Disord* 46:175–182.

Shulman, K., and Post, F. 1980. Bipolar affective disorder in old age. *Br J Psychiatry* 136:26–32.

Shulman, K. I., Tohen, M., Satlin, A., et al. 1992. Mania compared with unipolar depression in old age. *Am J Psychiatry* 149:341–345.

Sibisi, C. D. 1990. Sex differences in the age of onset of bipolar affective illness. *Br J Psychiatry* 156:842–845.

Smith, R. E., and Helms, P. M. 1982. Adverse effects of lithium therapy in the acutely ill elderly patient. *J Clin Psychiatry* 43:94–99.

Snowdon, J. 1991. A retrospective case-note study of bipolar disorder in old age. *Br J Psychiatry* 158:485–490.

Snowdon, J. 2001. Prevalence of depression in old age. *Br J Psychiatry* 178:476–477.

Spicer, C. C., Hare, E. H., and Slater, E. 1973. Neurotic and psychotic forms of depressive illness: evidence from age-incidence in a national sample. *Br J Psychiatry* 123:535–541.

Starkstein, S. E., Boston, J. D., and Robinson, R. G. 1988. Mechanisms of mania after brain injury: 12 case reports and review of the literature. *J Nerv Ment Dis* 176:87–100.

Starkstein, S. E., Mayberg, H. S., Berthier, M. L., et al. 1990. Mania after brain injury: neuroradiological and metabolic findings. *Ann Neurol* 27:652–659.

Starkstein, S. E., and Robinson, R. G. 1989. Affective disorders and cerebral vascular disease. *Br J Psychiatry* 154:170–182.

Stasiek, C., and Zetin, M. 1985. Organic manic disorders. *Psychosomatics* 26:394–396, 399, 402.

Steinberg, D., Hirsch, S. R., Marston, S. D., et al. 1972. Influenza infection causing manic psychosis. *Br J Psychiatry* 120:531–535.

Stoll, A. L., Banov, M., Kolbrener, M., et al. 1994. Neurologic factors predict a favorable valproate response in bipolar and schizoaffective disorders. *J Clin Psychopharmacol* 14:311–313.

Stone, K. 1989. Mania in the elderly. *Br J Psychiatry* 155:220–224.

Sultzer, D. L., and Cummings, J. L. 1989. Drug-induced mania — causative agents, clinical characteristics and management: a retrospective analysis of the literature. *Med Toxicol Adverse Drug Exp* 4:127–143.

Summers, W. K. 1983. Mania with onset in the eighth decade: two cases and a review. *J Clin Psychiatry* 44:141–143.

Thomas, C. S., and Neale, T. J. 1991. Organic manic syndrome associated with advanced uraemia due to polycystic kidney disease. *Br J Psychiatry* 158:119–121.

Tsao, C. I., Jain, S., Gibson, R. H., et al. 2004. Maintenance ECT for recurrent medication-refractory mania. *J ECT* 20:118–119.

Turkington, D., and Gill, P. 1989. Mania induced by lorazepam withdrawal: a report of two cases. *J Affect Disord* 17:93–95.

Walter-Ryan, W. G. 1983. Mania with onset in the ninth decade. *J Clin Psychiatry* 44:430–431.

Wylie, M. E., Mulsant, B. H., Pollock, B. G., et al. 1999. Age at onset in geriatric bipolar disorder: effects on clinical presentation and treatment outcomes in an inpatient sample. *Am J Geriatr Psychiatry* 7:77–83.

Yatham, L. N. 2002. The role of novel antipsychotics in bipolar disorders. *J Clin Psychiatry* 63(suppl. 3):10–14.

Young, B. K., Camicioli, R., and Ganzini, L. 1997. Neuropsychiatric adverse effects of antiparkinsonian drugs: characteristics, evaluation and treatment. *Drugs Aging* 10:367–383.

Young, R. C. 1992. Geriatric mania. *Clin Geriatr Med* 8:387–399.

Young, R. C., Jain, H., Kiosses, D. N., et al. 2003. Antidepressant-associated mania in late life. *Int J Geriatr Psychiatry* 18:421–424.

CHAPTER FIVE

Biological Treatments of Bipolar Disorder in Later Life

CHRISTIAN R. DOLDER, PHARM.D.,

COLIN A. DEPP, PH.D., AND DILIP V. JESTE, M.D.

The pharmacological treatment of bipolar disorder in older adults has been a ne-glected area of clinical and research focus. Current treatment guidelines for bipolar disorder do not provide specific recommendations for adapting treatment to older adults (Snowdon 2000). The recent consensus statement of the Depression and Bipolar Support Alliance on unmet needs in the diagnosis and treatment of mood disorders in later life noted that the treatment of late-life bipolar disorder is especially understudied, in part because of the absence of a placebo-controlled trial of any med-ication for this group of patients (Charney et al. 2003).

Among younger adults, pharmacological treatment of bipolar disorder is com-plex, employing monotherapy or combination therapy with mood stabilizers, an-tipsychotics, antidepressants, sedatives, and/or electroconvulsive therapy (ECT). Adding to the challenges of treating bipolar disorder for any age group are special considerations germane to geriatric pharmacology, including factors such as de-creased tolerance to medications, medical comorbidity, and cognitive impairment (see chapter 9 for a more thorough discussion of these topics). In this chapter, we re-view the current evidence on the safety, effectiveness, and clinical usage recom-mendations for specific medications commonly used to treat bipolar disorder in older adults. Table 5.1 provides a summary of biological treatment options, with con-siderations relevant to older adults.

TABLE 5.1
Considerations in treating bipolar disorder in older adults

Medication	Treatment of mania		Treatment of bipolar depression		Side effects and other considerations
	Younger adults	Older adults	Younger adults	Older adults	
Lithium	++	+	++	+	Cognitive impairment, sedation, cardiovascular effects, thyroid effects, polyuria; narrow therapeutic index
Anticonvulsants					
Carbamazepine	++	+/−	+/−	+/−	Cognitive impairment, sedation, neurological impairment, hematological alterations, dermatological effects, gastrointestinal effects
Gabapentin	−	+	+/−	+/−	
Lamotrigine	+/−	+/−	++	+	
Oxcarbazepine	+/−	+/−	+/−	+/−	
Topiramate	+/−	+/−	+/−	+/−	
Valproate	++	+	+	+/−	
Antipsychotics					
Conventional	++	+			Anticholinergic effects (sedation, orthostasis, constipation, urinary retention), and motor side effects
Atypical					Glucose abnormalities, weight gain, lipid abnormalities, sedation, orthostasis (quetiapine, clozapine), stroke (olanzapine, risperidone)
Aripiprazole	++	+/−			
Clozapine	+	+/−			
Olanzapine	++	+	+		
Quetiapine	++	+	++		
Risperidone	++	+			
Ziprasidone	++	+/−			
Antidepressants					
Selective serotonin reuptake inhibitors			++	+	Sexual dysfunction, gastrointestinal effects, sleep disturbances, induction of mania, withdrawal symptoms
Tricyclics			++	+	Anticholinergic effects (sedation, orthostasis, constipation, urinary retention); overdose precautions
Benzodiazepines	+	+/−			Cognitive impairment, dependence, withdrawal symptoms
Electroconvulsive therapy	++	+/−	++	+	Cognitive impairment (anterograde/retrograde amnesia)

++ efficacy supported by controlled trials; + efficacy supported primarily by open studies or retrospective studies; +/− mixed findings or lack of data; − efficacy not supported by controlled trials.

GENERAL CONSIDERATIONS IN THE TREATMENT
OF BIPOLAR DISORDER

Before we describe the specific medications used for treatment of bipolar disorder, it is important to consider several questions.

1. Which symptoms will be targeted? As pointed out by M. S. Bauer and Mitchner (2004), the ideal medication for bipolar disorder would reduce acute mania as well as acute depression and also prevent future episodes of depression or mania. This is a lofty standard for a single medication and accounts, in part, for the common use of combination strategies. Many of the existing outcome data concern the treatment of acute mania, with fewer studies on bipolar depression and even less available information on the prevention of either mania or depression.

2. For which patient subgroup? Bipolar disorder is extremely heterogeneous, perhaps even more so among elderly individuals. Features of bipolar disorder in a particular patient, such as the presence of psychosis or mixed symptoms, may dictate decisions about treatment, as does the presence of psychiatric comorbidity (e.g., substance abuse, anxiety disorders). Among older adults with bipolar disorder, medical and neurological comorbidity are common (Depp and Jeste 2004), emphasizing the need to monitor toxic or cognitive effects.

3. Is the person likely to adhere to treatment? In an analysis of the pharmacy records of 1,500 individuals, the median duration of continuous use of lithium after it was prescribed was only 76 days (Johnson and McFarland 1996). Nonadherence to medication regimens occurs in roughly 40% of patients with bipolar disorder at any given time. Predictors of nonadherence include comorbid substance abuse and attitudinal factors, such as denial of the need for medications (Scott and Pope 2002). Nonadherence by elderly patients may also result from other factors, such as forgetfulness, polypharmacy, and/or cost of medications or other barriers to treatment access.

4. How should treatment choices be adapted for aging persons? As described in more detail elsewhere in this volume, the challenge of effectively treating bipolar disorder in elderly persons may increase as a result of the physiological changes related to aging. In general, older adults are more susceptible to medication-induced side effects. This increased susceptibility is most often explained by pharmacokinetic and pharmacodynamic changes associated with aging: reduced renal elimination of drugs, resulting from diminished glomerular filtration; decreased hepatic metabolism of medications, resulting from reduced liver size and hepatic blood flow; decreased cardiac output; and altered activity and density of target receptors. Addi-

tionally, elderly persons are more likely to have multiple medical conditions and to be taking multiple medications (Mulsant and Pollock 2004).

5. What are the goals of treatment? The goal of treatment of affective disorders is to assist an elderly person in "staying well" (Charney et al. 2003), which implies a two-part standard: maintaining remission and attaining a clinical state that is better than simply no longer meeting the criteria for a full-fledged illness episode. In the Stanley Foundation Bipolar Network cohort (Post et al. 2003), the majority of the sample experienced mild or worse symptoms most of the time despite state-of-the-art care, meaning that true remission may be the exception. Treatment should therefore strive for the reduction of subsyndromal or breakthrough symptoms, as well as the prevention of suicide and suicidal ideation. Lithium, for example, may have a greater antisuicidal effect than divalproex (Goodwin et al. 2003). Moreover, *wellness* implies return to a previous level of functioning. Little is known about functional recovery in elderly patients. Most do experience remission of symptoms after their first episode, but far fewer have functional recovery (Tohen et al. 2003). Therefore, health-related quality of life should be a targeted outcome measure of pharmacotherapy for bipolar disorder.

MOOD STABILIZERS

Despite the common usage of the term *mood stabilizer* in the treatment of bipolar disorder, there is no single definition of what constitutes a "mood stabilizer" and no official recognition of the term by the U.S. Food and Drug Administration. Lithium was the first medication approved for the treatment of bipolar disorder, followed by carbamazepine, valproate, and, most recently, lamotrigine. While lithium continues to be recognized as a first-line treatment for acute mania in most treatment guidelines, K. Shulman and colleagues (2003) noted a rapid shift between 1993 and 2001 in the use of valproate among patients older than 65 years, using data from the Ontario Drug Benefit Program. The authors also noted a concurrent trend toward reduced use of lithium, even when patients with dementia were excluded from the analyses. This shift toward valproate occurred in the absence of empirical data on the effectiveness of this medication for elderly persons with mania.

Lithium

Lithium has been studied as a treatment for psychiatric disorders for more than 50 years. However, only three studies have reported the effectiveness of lithium for older patients with bipolar disorder, all using retrospective review of patient records

(Chen et al. 1999; Himmelhoch et al. 1980; Schaffer and Garvey 1984). All three reported on the treatment of acute mania in hospitalized patients. Of the 152 patients in all, the weighted average positive response was 72% (range 66–88), which is comparable to that (78%) reported for younger adults (Goodwin and Jamison 1990). In a sample of 30 inpatients aged 55 or older, Chen and colleagues (1999) found that lithium was more effective (a Clinical Global Impression score of much or very much improved) for those with typical manic symptoms than for those with mixed features. Himmelhoch and colleagues (1980) examined the effectiveness of lithium for 81 patients over age 55 with bipolar disorder and found that those with neurological comorbidity or substance abuse had a worse response. In that study and a more recent study (Wylie et al. 1999), age of onset did not seem to influence the effectiveness of lithium.

The relation between serum lithium levels and antimanic effectiveness in elderly patients remains unclear. Given the pharmacokinetic changes associated with aging, geriatric patients with mania may respond to lower lithium levels (e.g., 0.5–0.8 mEq/L) than those considered therapeutic for younger adults (e.g., 0.8–1.2 mEq/L). Although a few case series have supported the use of a lower lithium dose (G. P. Roose et al. 1979; Schaffer and Garvey 1984; Young et al. 2004), other studies have recommended achieving similar serum lithium concentrations regardless of age (Young et al. 2004). The length of time considered to be an adequate trial of lithium for treating mania in older adults is unclear, but it should be at least the same as for younger adults.

The use of lithium for older adults presents several clinical challenges related to pharmacokinetic alterations in aging. Renal clearance of lithium decreases with age, and lithium's elimination half-life increases to approximately double that in younger adults (Hardy et al. 1987; Young et al. 2004). These changes can lead to elevated lithium concentrations in geriatric patients and may place these older adults at increased risk for lithium toxicity. Other factors related to aging may also lead to higher lithium concentrations in older adults: increased fat-to-lean body mass, renal disease, cardiac insufficiency, and drug-drug interactions. Older adults are commonly prescribed several classes of somatic medications that can interact with lithium to cause increased serum lithium levels. These medications include thiazide diuretics, angiotensin-converting enzyme inhibitors, and nonsteroidal anti-inflammatory agents (Semla et al. 2003; Young et al. 2004).

In all patients, but especially geriatric patients, lithium is associated with some potentially adverse side effects. For older adults, the potential of lithium to cause cardiovascular effects and cognitive and neurological impairment can be significant. Mild tremor is the most common neurological side effect, although a range of neurological effects has been reported, including delirium. A recent review by Young and colleagues (2004) indicated that 16%–58% of patients in studies examining lithium toxicity reported neurological side effects (Chacko et al. 1987; Himmelhoch et al. 1980; Schaffer and Garvey 1984; Smith and Helms 1982; Stone 1989). A range of potential cardiovascular effects of lithium have also been reported (S. P. Roose et al. 1979; Young et al. 2004). Other common side effects in elderly patients (up to 30% of patients) include polyuria, polydipsia, edema, and altered thyroid function (hypothyroid > hyperthyroid) (Head and Dening 1998; Hewick et al. 1977; Young et al. 2004). In general, there seems to be a positive relation between lithium concentration and side effects, although such a relationship is primarily derived from data on younger adults. Supratherapeutic lithium concentrations clearly should be monitored to avoid or minimize side effects, but there are also reports of serious lithium toxicity in geriatric patients even at moderate lithium concentrations (0.5–0.8 mEq/L) (Arana and Rosenbaum 2000; Prien et al. 1972; Strayhorn and Nash 1977; Young et al. 2004).

Valproate

Valproate (i.e., valproic acid or divalproex sodium) seems to be beneficial in monotherapy for mania in elderly patients with bipolar disorder, in combination with lithium for individuals only partially responsive to lithium, and in treatment of rapid cycling (Goldberg et al. 2000; A. L. Schneider and Wilcox 1998; Sharma et al. 1993; Young et al. 2004). We found six open-label studies that examined the effectiveness of valproate in a series of more than six older patients (Chen et al. 1999; Kando et al. 1996; McFarland et al. 1990; Mordecai et al. 1999; Niedermier and Nasrallah 1998; Noaghiul et al. 1998). The weighted average of positive response to valproate (n = 103) was 67% (range 38–91), similar to that found for younger people (Bowden 2003). Chen and colleagues (1999) found a 38% rate of response, although when restricted to those with blood valproate levels above 65 μg/ml, the response rate was considerably higher (75%). Furthermore, these authors found that valproate was more effective in treating mania with mixed features (67%) than in typical mania (30%). One small case series reported the use of intravenous valproate for treating acute mania in two elderly patients with early-onset bipolar disorder (Regenold and Prasad 2001).

Again, no data exist to elucidate the relation between serum valproate levels and antimanic effectiveness. Nonetheless, several researchers have proposed target valproate concentration ranges, based on studies using varied methodology (including various ages of participants). Bowden (1998) recommended valproate concentrations of 50–120 µg/ml, and Chen and colleagues (1999) recommended 65–90 µg/ml. These recommendations do not differ substantially from those for younger adults, but given that the proportion of unbound valproate (i.e., active drug) increases with age, valproate concentrations at the lower end of these ranges might make good initial targets (L. A. Bauer et al. 1985; Young et al. 2004).

The pharmacological profile of valproate provides some advantages over lithium for elderly persons. Valproate therapy does not seem to be as affected by age-related pharmacokinetic/pharmacodynamic changes, although the elimination half-life of valproate may be increased in older persons (Bryson et al. 1983; Young et al. 2004). Furthermore, valproate has fewer drug-drug interactions than lithium, but valproate levels can be affected by aspirin, phenytoin, and carbamazepine, and valproate can inhibit the metabolism of lamotrigine (Arana and Rosenbaum 2000).

Valproate seems to be well tolerated by elderly adults with bipolar disorder, but side effects are a definite possibility. Although rates of neurological and/or cognitive side effects are less than for lithium, adverse effects such as tremor, sedation, and gait disturbance are frequently experienced. Other side effects reported in trials of valproate for older adults include nausea, diarrhea, weight gain, and dry mouth. The relation between valproate concentration and side effects remains unclear (Semla et al. 2003).

Carbamazepine/Oxcarbazepine

Carbamazepine has proved beneficial in the treatment of young and middle-aged adults with mania. This agent has generally been relegated to a second-line option because of its side-effect profile and its involvement in drug-drug interactions. Carbamazepine remains a second-line therapy for late-life bipolar disorder, given the lack of studies involving elderly patients and the drawbacks mentioned above (Kellner and Neher 1991; Young et al. 2004). Carbamazepine is a strong inducer of the hepatic enzymes that can reduce serum concentrations of various anticonvulsants and mood stabilizers, and it can also auto-induce its own metabolism (Arana and Rosenbaum 2000). Carbamazepine is associated with a variety of problematic side effects. It has some antiarrhythmic properties and has been associated with various bradycardias (Kasarkis et al. 1991; Young et al. 2004). Other side effects reported in trials of carbamazepine involving elderly adults include gastrointestinal side effects, hepatic toxicity, rash, and leukopenia (Tohen et al. 1995; Young et al. 2004). Oxcarbazepine has a better pharmacological profile than carbamazepine, including a lower-intensity induction of hepatic enzymes and a somewhat more benign side-effect profile. In an investigation of elderly patients with epilepsy treated with oxcarbazepine, the most common side effects were vomiting, dizziness, nausea, and somnolence. Hyponatremia was noted in a few patients (Kutluay et al. 2003).

Topiramate/Lamotrigine

Despite the popularity of second-generation anticonvulsants such as lamotrigine and, to a lesser extent, gabapentin and topiramate in the treatment of bipolar disorder, few data have been published on studies with older adults. Successful use of lamotrigine was described in a case series of five women (four with rapid cycling) with a mean age of 71 who were admitted for bipolar disorder with depression (Robillard and Conn 2002). This case series is unique in its focus on the treatment of bipolar depression. Three of the five patients experienced remission of symptoms (<50% on the Hamilton Depression Rating Scale) and were not rehospitalized within three months. One patient withdrew from lamotrigine treatment because of coarse hand tremor.

Topiramate is a less common mood stabilizer for younger adults. In a case study of a 65-year-old man with early-onset bipolar disorder who received topiramate to augment valproate, lorazepam, and olanzapine, the patient showed a substantial reduction in psychosis and mania symptom scores as well as an 8 pound weight loss (Madhusoodanan et al. 2002). Gabapentin has not proved effective for younger adults with bipolar disorder (M. S. Bauer and Mitchner 2004), despite its initial promise in open trials as a safer mood stabilizer. Again, only one case series could be found on the use of gabapentin for the inpatient treatment of mania in older adults (Sethi et al. 2003). No data are presently available for the treatment of older adults with so-called third-generation mood stabilizers, such as zonisamide and felbamate.

The utility of lamotrigine in bipolar depression must be balanced against its association with the serious cutaneous eruption Stevens-Johnson syndrome. This necessitates gradual dose titration and careful patient monitoring when prescribing lamotrigine. The effect of age on the occurrence of Stevens-Johnson syndrome as a side effect of lamotrigine is unclear. Information on the tolerability of lamotrigine in older adults must currently be drawn from controlled trials involving older adults with epilepsy. In these studies, investigators reported that lamotrigine was relatively well tolerated (Brodie et al. 1999; Giorgi et al. 2001; Mulsant and Pollock 2004). Somnolence, rashes, and headaches were observed in a significant number of patients in these investigations, but lamotrigine was noted to be better tolerated than the comparator medications, carbamazepine or phenytoin. The pharmacological profile of lamotrigine provides several advantages over many other mood stabilizers or antidepressants. For example, lamotrigine does not seem to be associated with weight gain (Morrell et al. 2003; Mulsant and Pollock 2004). Unlike some psychotropics associated with numerous drug-drug interactions resulting from hepatic metabolism via the cytochrome P450 (CYP) system, lamotrigine is metabolized primarily by hepatic glucuronide conjugation and is associated with fewer drug-drug interactions (Willmore 2000). Topiramate is also not without potentially bothersome side effects, especially in older adults. Topiramate has been associated with reports of fatigue, somnolence, dizziness, ataxia, and paresthesias (Arana and Rosenbaum 2000).

ANTIPSYCHOTICS

Only a few case reports are available on the use of atypical (or second-generation) antipsychotics in the treatment of acute mania in older adults; these drugs include quetiapine (Madhusoodanan et al. 2000), clozapine (R. Shulman et al. 1997), aripiprazole (Gupta et al. 2004), olanzapine (Beyer et al. 2001), and risperidone (Madhusoodanan et al. 1995). No data are available on ziprasidone. Nonetheless, these agents will probably become a viable and increasingly popular treatment option, as studies involving younger adults with bipolar disorder have shown the agents have consistent antimanic and antipsychotic effects. Currently, risperidone, olanzapine, quetiapine, ziprasidone, and aripiprazole are all indicated for the short-term treatment (as monotherapy or in combination with a mood stabilizer) of acute mania in adults. Olanzapine and aripiprazole are also indicated for maintenance treatment for bipolar disorder and quetiapine is indicated for bipolar depression. In general, the manufacturers recommend low antipsychotic doses when treating older adults. Recommendations for initial therapy with risperidone and olanzapine are 0.5 mg twice daily and 2.5–5 mg once daily, respectively. The FDA-approved dosage regimen for quetiapine in treating bipolar mania (initiate at 100 mg/day, titrate up to 400 mg/day by day 4, and a maximum dose of 800 mg/day) should be modified (i.e., titrate more slowly and lower the target dose) for elderly patients with mania. Serum concentrations of antipsychotics, unlike anticonvulsants, are not routinely measured.

Expert consensus guidelines have been published on the use of antipsychotic medications by older adults, including the use of these agents for bipolar disorder (Alexopoulos et al. 2004). Antipsychotics are not recommended for mild mania but are considered the treatment of choice for psychotic mania (in combination with a mood stabilizer). Clinicians also recommend the use of antipsychotics as adjunctive treatment in severe nonpsychotic mania. For patients requiring an antipsychotic, risperidone (1.25–3 mg/day) or olanzapine (5–15 mg/day) are recommended. Also recommended is waiting at least a week before changing the antipsychotic dose and observing a treatment response for at least 2–3 months before discontinuing the antipsychotic. In addition to recommending risperidone or olanzapine for elderly patients, the guidelines note situations in which to avoid certain antipsychotics. For instance, low- and mid-potency conventional antipsychotics, clozapine, and ziprasidone should be avoided for elderly patients who have corrected QT interval prolongation or heart failure. Additionally, avoidance of low- and mid-potency conventional antipsychotics, clozapine, and olanzapine are recommended for patients with diabetes, dyslipidemias, and/or obesity. These agent-specific recommendations are based primarily on the positive efficacy data for risperidone and olanzapine, along with the side effects associated with certain antipsychotic medications.

The selection of an antipsychotic must take into account the potential for side effects, the differences in side effects among antipsychotics (e.g., conventional vs. atypical), and the sensitivity of older adults to several common antipsychotic side effects. In general, atypical antipsychotics are preferred over conventional agents because of the reduced side-effect burden of the atypical agents. Conventional antipsychotics have been shown to produce sedation and impaired cognition, side effects that can be especially troubling in older adults. Sedation is less likely with atypical antipsychotics, but somnolence is a fairly common side effect with medications such as clozapine, olanzapine, and quetiapine. Low-potency conventional antipsychotics (e.g., chlorpromazine) and olanzapine have significant anticholinergic effects that may be problematic in older adults (Arana and Rosenbaum 2000; Semla et al. 2003; Young et al. 2004). These anticholinergic effects include constipation, urinary hesitancy, tachycardia, and cognitive impairment (Young et al. 2004). Conventional antipsychotics, especially high-potency agents such as haloperidol and fluphenazine, are associated with extrapyramidal side effects (parkinsonism, acute dystonia, akathisia) and tardive dyskinesia. Older adults treated with antipsychotic agents are at a substantially increased risk for developing these medication-induced side effects, especially tardive dyskinesia and parkinsonism. Fortunately, the atypical antipsychotics have been shown to place patients at a lower risk for developing these motor side effects compared with conventional antipsychotics (Caligiuri et al. 2000; Jeste 2004; Yassa et al. 1992; Young et al. 2004). Some antipsychotics (e.g., thioridazine, ziprasidone) also have the ability to prolong the QT interval, which can lead to life-threatening arrhythmias in susceptible individuals (Arana and Rosenbaum 2000; Glassman and Bigger 2001; Reilly et al. 2000; Young et al. 2004).

Although the use of atypical antipsychotics is generally preferred over conventional antipsychotics, the atypical agents are not without side effects. Clozapine and olanzapine, especially, have been associated with metabolic effects such as weight gain and diabetes. Although the likelihood of these side effects may be decreased with age, the potential for such effects during long-term treatment requires a base-line evaluation and follow-up monitoring for these patients (American Diabetes Association 2004; Meyer 2002). Recently, additional concerns have arisen about the safe and appropriate use of atypical antipsychotics by elderly persons, following the FDA's warning of an increased risk of death (related to cardiovascular and infectious disorders) in older patients with dementia-related behavioral disturbances who are treated with atypical antipsychotics (U.S. Food and Drug Administration 2005). The mortality risk associated with these agents has created therapeutic and ethical challenges: this use of atypical antipsychotics represents off-label prescribing, but there are limited pharmacological options with proven efficacy for treating behavioral disturbances in dementia. Clinicians must practice careful patient selection to decrease the risk of adverse events when treating older adults with behavioral disturbances in dementia. Although the use of most atypical antipsychotics by older adults with bipolar disorder does not represent off-label prescribing, caution and careful patient selection are still required because of the limited availability of data on treatment of bipolar disorder in such patients.

ANTIDEPRESSANTS

Reports of antidepressant use for bipolar depression in older adults are scarce. Antidepressants are an important component of the pharmacological treatment of bipolar disorder, especially bipolar depression. When selecting an antidepressant for treatment of bipolar disorder in late life, choosing the most appropriate patient-specific agent is important, because of the differences in side effects among classes of antidepressant and the sensitivity of older adults to some of the common side effects. The rational use of antidepressants for patients with bipolar disorder is important; as in younger patients, the use of antidepressants in later life is associated with the potential to induce mania (Young et al. 2003).

Tricyclic Antidepressants

Tricyclic antidepressants (TCAs) represent some of the oldest antidepressant agents approved for the treatment of depressive disorders. In general, the use of most TCAs for elderly patients is limited by the anticholinergic effects (blurred vision, constipation, urinary hesitancy, memory impairment, tachycardia, dry mouth), antihistaminic action (sedation), and alpha-adrenergic blocking properties (orthostasis) of these medications (Flint 1998). Orthostatic hypotension is of particular concern in older persons, as this side effect can lead to falls and hip fractures (Flint 1998;

Halper and Mann 1988). The TCAs differ in side effects and tolerability. Secondary amine TCAs (e.g., nortriptyline, desipramine) are less likely to cause the above-mentioned side effects than are tertiary amine TCAs (e.g., amitriptyline, imipramine). Thus, nortriptyline and desipramine are generally preferred for elderly patients requiring a TCA. Many of the side effects associated with TCAs are concentration dependent (Flint 1998; Preskorn 1993). This relation between side effects and plasma concentration creates the opportunity to monitor plasma TCA concentrations in order to minimize adverse effects. Unfortunately, all TCAs slow cardiac conduction and can have serious adverse effects for patients with existing cardiac conditions such as bundle branch block and ischemic heart disease (Flint 1998; S. P. Roose and Glassman 1994). In contrast to several mood-stabilizing agents and selective serotonin reuptake inhibitors (SSRIs), TCAs, although generally metabolized via the CYP system (isoenzyme 2D6), do not seem to have significant inhibitor or inducer effects on this enzyme (Crewe et al. 1992; Flint 1998; Pollock et al. 1994).

Selective Serotonin Reuptake Inhibitors

Generally, SSRIs have replaced TCAs and monoamine oxidase inhibitors as the first-line treatments for late-life depression (Alexopoulos et al. 2001), because of the efficacy of SSRIs combined with their ease of use, safety, and tolerability. In contrast to the tricyclic antidepressants, SSRIs have little effect on adrenergic, cholinergic, or histaminic receptors. The only exception to this is the modest anticholinergic properties of paroxetine (Flint 1998; Geretsegger et al. 1994; Thomas et al. 1987). The side effects of SSRIs reflect their ability to block serotonin reuptake centrally and peripherally, leading to side effects including nausea, anorexia, diarrhea, insomnia, sedation, nervousness, restlessness, dizziness, headaches, tremor, and sexual dysfunction (Arana and Rosenbaum 2000). Many of the side effects tend to be dose related and transient (Arana and Rosenbaum 2000; Rickels and Schweizer 1990). SSRIs have been reported to produce postural instability in older adults, as well as syndrome of inappropriate antidiuretic hormone secretion (SIADH) and hyponatremia (Flint 1998; Laghrissi-Thode et al. 1995; Liu et al. 1996). It is important to remember that despite the relatively low prevalence of side effects associated with SSRIs, a substantial percentage of older adults experience nausea, vomiting, dizziness, and drowsiness that can lead to drug intolerance. In a recent meta-analysis of SSRI and TCA side effects and discontinuation rates in older people, the authors concluded that SSRIs are less likely than TCAs to be withdrawn in general or withdrawn specifically because of side effects. Nevertheless, 17% of patients taking SSRIs withdrew because of side effects (Wilson and Mottram 2004).

As a group, SSRIs inhibit a variety of CYP isoenzymes (e.g., 1A2, 2C9, 2D6, and 3A4), although individual SSRIs differ in the inhibition (and extent of inhibition) of specific isoenzymes (Flint 1998; Harvey and Preskorn 1996; Kellner and Neher 1991; Nemeroff et al. 1996). The ability of SSRIs to inhibit CYP isoenzymes leads to many potential drug-drug interactions, although the clinical significance of many interactions is unclear. Nonetheless, the potential for drug interactions necessitates potential dosage adjustments and careful monitoring of patients — especially older adults, who are more likely to be prescribed multiple medications. Particular care should be taken when prescribing SSRIs along with medications that have narrow therapeutic indices, such as TCAs, antipsychotics, carbamazepine, theophylline, phenytoin, warfarin, and type 1C antiarrhythmics (Nemeroff et al. 1996).

Starting and maximum doses of SSRIs for older patients should generally be lower than those for younger individuals because of age-related pharmacokinetic changes. The starting dosages for older adults are generally half those for younger adults; the dosage is usually doubled after 1 week. In addition, SSRIs have a flat dose-response curve, meaning that increases in dose above the minimum effective dose often do not substantially increase efficacy but do increase the potential for medication side effects (Flint 1998). For the SSRIs available in the United States (citalopram, escitalopram, fluoxetine, fluvoxamine, paroxetine, and sertraline), trial data have demonstrated that all have similar efficacy and tolerability in the treatment of both younger and older adults with depression (Kroenke et al. 2001; Mulsant and Pollock 2004; L. S. Schneider and Olin 1995; Solai et al. 2001). Expert consensus guidelines for the use of antidepressants in older adults reported a preference for citalopram, escitalopram, or sertraline, largely because these agents have a lower potential for clinically relevant drug interactions (Alexopoulos et al. 2001; Mulsant et al. 2001).

Other Antidepressants

Despite the limited availability of controlled data, the newer antidepressants bupropion, mirtazapine, and venlafaxine are considered the preferred alternatives to SSRIs for older adults (Alexopoulos et al. 2001). Venlafaxine has serotonergic and noradrenergic reuptake inhibitory properties similar to those of TCAs, but it does not have appreciable anticholinergic, antihistaminic, and alpha-adrenergic blockade activity. In addition, venlafaxine does not significantly affect cardiac conduction. The most common side effects reported with venlafaxine include nausea, somnolence, dry mouth, dizziness, nervousness, constipation, and sexual dysfunction. Some patients may experience modest elevations in blood pressure. The side-effect profile of venlafaxine can be affected by the dose of the medication. At low doses, venlafaxine mostly inhibits serotonergic reuptake; at higher doses it inhibits reuptake of both serotonin and norepinephrine. Additionally, venlafaxine is only a weak inhibitor of CYP2D6 and is not associated with many significant drug-drug interactions (Feighner 1994; Flint 1998; Nemeroff et al. 1996).

Bupropion is an antidepressant with an unclear mechanism of action. It has minimal anticholinergic, antihistaminic, or cardiovascular effects, although at high doses it does increase a patient's risk of seizure. Bupropion should not be prescribed for persons with preexisting or at risk for seizure disorders. Case reports have also noted the onset of psychosis in patients treated with bupropion (Howard and Warnock 1999; Mulsant and Pollock 2004). The most common side effects associated with bupropion include agitation, headaches, dizziness, insomnia, anorexia, and nausea. This agent is generally not associated with sexual dysfunction (Arana and Rosenbaum 2000).

Mirtazapine is thought to produce its antidepressant effects by increased norepinephrine and serotonin neurotransmission via blockade of alpha-2 autoreceptors. Mirtazapine also inhibits 5-HT2 and 5-HT3 receptors. This action, opposite to that of SSRIs, could make mirtazapine useful for patients who cannot tolerate the sexual dysfunction, tremor, or nausea associated with SSRIs (Gelenberg et al. 2000; Montejo et al. 2001; Mulsant and Pollock 2004; Pedersen and Klysner 1997). Unlike SSRIs, mirtazapine has substantial histaminergic activity, which leads to its most common side effect, sedation. Mirtazapine is also associated with constipation, dry mouth, increased appetite, weight gain, and increased cholesterol levels (Arana and Rosenbaum 2000; Thompson 2000).

OTHER TREATMENTS

Older adults with bipolar disorder may also receive other treatments, in particular electroconvulsive therapy and sedative medications. ECT is an indicated treatment for bipolar disorder, for both mania and depression, and may be particularly useful for individuals who are refractory to medications. Unfortunately, there are no studies comparing ECT to pharmacotherapy among older adults with bipolar disorder and relatively few studies of ECT in older adults with bipolar disorder. A comprehensive review of ECT in late-life depression concluded that ECT is an effective and generally safe treatment option, but the authors could identify only four randomized trials of ECT in late-life depression (van der Wurff et al. 2003). With little information available on the use of ECT in late-life depression, and even less on its use in late-life bipolar depression, data from other populations must guide treatment choices.

A considerable body of literature supports the efficacy of ECT for treatment of major depression in younger adults. These trials have also suggested that ECT is the most rapid and effective treatment for major depression, with effects that extend to both unipolar and bipolar depression. In several trials involving primarily younger adults, ECT has also proved to be an effective treatment for bipolar mania, with response rates similar to those produced by lithium. Among older adults with unipolar depression, ECT is generally regarded as effective, perhaps even more so than in younger adults (Greenberg and Kellner 2005; Weiner and Krystal 2004). In a small retrospective chart review, investigators examined the efficacy and safety of bifrontal ECT in 14 older adults (mean age 74 years) with a depressive disorder. Five of the patients had bipolar depression. Overall, 12 of the 14 patients were considered responders after a mean of nine treatments. Five of the 14 patients experienced cognitive side effects, and during a mean follow-up period of 19 months, 1 patient had a relapse (Little et al. 2004).

In all patients, but especially older adults, the most common and concerning side effect of ECT is cognitive impairment, which may include disorientation, anterograde amnesia, and retrograde amnesia (Greenberg and Kellner 2005). Generally, confusion and anterograde amnesia dissipate within the first few weeks after ECT, but retrograde amnesia (memory for previous events) may be a persistent and troubling problem, particularly for those with preexisting cognitive deficits. Patients with preexisting cerebral disease (e.g., space-occupying cerebral lesions, recent stroke, history of aneurysms, dementia) seem to be at greater risk for ECT-related cognitive side effects. Careful patient selection and the tailoring of ECT therapy to minimize such side effects are essential. It is important to note that age itself does not seem to increase the medical and neurological risks of ECT. Instead, older adults are more likely to have comorbid medical conditions that can increase the risks associated with ECT (Weiner and Krystal 2004).

Sedatives are frequently used in inpatient settings for acute mania, as well as in the treatment of comorbid anxiety or agitation. A considerable body of evidence warrants the cautious and time-limited use of these medications for elderly persons, given the associated increased risk of hypotension and falls.

In the treatment of bipolar disorder in older adults, other therapeutic considerations include concomitant disease states such as dementia, psychosis and agitation associated with dementia, and insomnia. Although nonpharmacological treatment should be initiated, many patients will also require medication therapy. For such patients, clinicians should consider the use of complementary medications or the use of a single medication that targets multiple psychiatric symptoms, in an attempt to maximize efficacy while minimizing medication burden. For instance, low-dose atypical antipsychotics would be a rational choice for a patient with both psychotic mania and psychosis or agitation associated with dementia. An SSRI could be used to target aggression and bipolar depression in a patient with dementia. And valproate might be appropriate as a mood stabilizer for a patient with bipolar disorder and be-havioral disturbances associated with dementia. Other agents may be initiated in such cases, but medications with low central anticholinergic properties, without ad-verse effects on cognition, and with low risk of orthostasis are preferable (Mulsant and Pollock 2004).

Insomnia is common in older adults and has negative consequences for health. When treating older adults with insomnia, clinicians must identify whether the con-dition is a primary or secondary sleep disorder. Sleep apnea and restless leg syndrome are prevalent in older adults and can lead to sleep complaints. It is important to iden-tify and treat the underlying condition rather than merely prescribing a sleeping aid. If pharmacological therapy is prescribed, one should, if possible, avoid medications with problematic side effects for elderly persons (e.g., long-acting benzodiazepines, highly anticholinergic medications). Agents such as zolpidem, zaleplon, eszopi-clone, and trazodone may be initiated; however, nonpharmacological interventions should be tried first, such as changes in diet, exercise, light exposure, and sleep hy-giene. Sleep disorders in patients with Alzheimer disease are also common. Sun-downing — evening or nocturnal arousal accompanied by agitation and confusion — may also lead to sleep abnormalities. In addition to nonpharmacological treatments, low-dose atypical antipsychotics and nonbenzodiazepines (zolpidem, zaleplon) may be effective (Krystal et al. 2004).

CONCLUSIONS

Young and colleagues' review (2004) of the pharmacological treatment of older adults with bipolar disorder and the American Psychiatric Association's bipolar dis-order treatment guidelines (2002) together provide recommendations for the treat-ment of bipolar disorder in late life. A baseline clinical and laboratory evaluation is critical before initiating therapy. Assessments such as standing and lying blood pres-sure, pulse rate, an electrocardiogram, neurological examination, and a cognitive as-sessment should be part of routine care for older adults with bipolar disorder.

Despite the proliferation and growing popularity of novel treatments for bipolar mania, the available data support lithium as a first-line treatment for mania in older adults. To reduce potential side effects and toxicities, clinicians should target moderate plasma concentration ranges (0.4–0.8 mEq/L); however, higher concentrations may be necessary. Dose adjustments to lithium therapy should be made gradually. Valproate should also be considered a first-line therapy for elderly patients with mania. Clinicians should target drug concentrations comparable to those used for younger patients (50–100 μg/ml). Carbamazepine should be considered a second-line treatment for mania. Given the potential for hematological and hepatic side effects associated with carbamazepine, baseline and follow-up liver-function tests and complete blood counts are essential. The role of other anticonvulsants in the treatment of mania in elderly patients is unclear at this time.

Monotherapy with a mood stabilizer is a reasonable initial therapy in the management of late-life bipolar mania. Barring the initial development of any serious or extremely bothersome side effects, three to four weeks (including any necessary dosage adjustments) is the minimum duration needed to assess the effectiveness of treatment. If a partial response is noted to the initial therapy, the addition of an atypical antipsychotic or another mood stabilizer should be considered. A lack of response warrants discontinuation of the initial medication and addition of another mood stabilizer with or without an atypical antipsychotic.

The potential benefits of monotherapy in the treatment of older adults with bipolar depression, especially the minimization of side effects, make initial treatment with a mood stabilizer attractive. Lithium or lamotrigine should be considered for the initial treatment of bipolar depression. These agents may also be used later in combination with antidepressants such as selective serotonin reuptake inhibitors.

In general, pharmacotherapy that has proved effective for mania or bipolar depression should be continued for 6–12 months. Gradual discontinuation of adjunct antidepressant, antipsychotic, or antianxiety agents may then be attempted if remission is maintained. Maintenance mood-stabilizer treatment should be continued.

Finally, although pharmacotherapy should be considered the "backbone" of treatment for bipolar disorder, and for many older adults is sufficient to restore high-level functioning in the community, medication should be seen as part of a comprehensive rehabilitation strategy. Collaboration with case managers, community support, and augmentation with psychoeducational/psychotherapeutic interventions (Zaretsky 2003) together provide the highest probability of the older patient's ultimate goals: getting well and staying well.

REFERENCES

Alexopoulos, G. S., Katz, I. R., Reynolds, C. F., et al. 2001. Pharmacotherapy of depression in older patients: a summary of the expert consensus guidelines. *J Psychiatr Pract* 7:361–376.

Alexopoulos, G. S., Streim, J. E., and Carpenter, D. 2004. Expert consensus guidelines for using antipsychotic agents in older patients. *J Clin Psychiatry* 65(suppl. 2):24–41.

American Diabetes Association and American Psychiatric Association. 2004. Consensus development conference on antipsychotic drugs and obesity and diabetes. *Diabetes Care* 27:596–561.

American Psychiatric Association. 2002. Practice guideline for the treatment of patients with bipolar disorder. www.psych.org/psych_pract/treatg/pg/bipolar_revisebook_index.cfm

Arana, G. W., and Rosenbaum, J. F. 2000. *Handbook of psychiatric drug therapy* (4th ed.). Philadelphia: Lippincott Williams and Wilkins.

Bauer, L. A., Davis, R., Wilensky, A., et al. 1985. Valproic acid clearance: unbound fraction and diurnal variations in young and elderly adults. *Clin Pharmacol Ther* 37:697–700.

Bauer, M. S., and Mitchner, L. 2004. What is a "mood stabilizer"? An evidence-based response. *Am J Psychiatry* 161:3–18.

Beyer, J. L., Siegal, A., Kennedy, J. S., et al. 2001. Olanzapine, divalproex, and placebo treatment, non-head-to-head comparisons of older adults with acute mania (abstract). Institute of Psychiatric Services Annual Meeting, Florida, USA, October 2001.

Bowden, C. 1998. Anticonvulsants in bipolar elderly. In Nelson, J. C. (ed.), *Geriatric psychopharmacology* (pp. 285–299). New York: Marcel Dekker.

Bowden, C. L. 2003. Valproate. *Bipolar Disord* 5:189–202.

Brodie, M. J., Overstall, P. W., and Giorgi, L. 1999. Multicentre, double-blind, randomized comparison between lamotrigine and carbamazepine in elderly patients with newly diagnosed epilepsy. *Epilepsy Res* 37:81–87.

Bryson, S. M., Verma, N., Scott, P. J. W., et al. 1983. Pharmacokinetics of valproic acid in young and elderly subjects. *Br J Clin Psychiatry* 16:104–105.

Caligiuri, M. R., Jeste, D. V., and Lacro, J. P. 2000. Antipsychotic-induced movement disorders in the elderly: epidemiology and treatment recommendations. *Drugs Aging* 17:363–384.

Chacko, R. C., Marsh, B., Marmion, J., et al. 1987. Lithium side effects in elderly bipolar outpatients. *J Clin Psychiatry* 9:79–88.

Charney, D. S., Reynolds, C. F. 3rd, Lewis, L., et al. 2003. Depression and Bipolar Support Alliance consensus statement on the unmet needs in diagnosis and treatment of mood disorders in late life. *Arch Gen Psychiatry* 60:664–672.

Chen, D., Altshuler, L., Melnyk, K., et al. 1999. Efficacy of lithium vs. valproate in the treatment of mania in the elderly: a retrospective study. *J Clin Psychiatry* 60:181–188.

Crewe, H. K., Lennard, M. S., Tucker, G. T., et al. 1992. The effect of selective serotonin reuptake inhibitors on cytochrome P450 2D6 (CYP2D6) activity in human liver microsomes. *Br J Clin Pharmacol* 34:262–265.

Depp, C., and Jeste, D. V. 2004. Bipolar disorder in older adults: a critical review. *Bipolar Disord* 6:343–367.

Feighner, J. P. 1994. The role of venlafaxine in rational antidepressant therapy. *J Clin Psychiatry* 55(suppl. A):62–68.

Flint, A. J. 1998. Choosing appropriate antidepressant therapy in the elderly: a risk-benefit assessment of available agents. *Drugs Aging* 13:269–280.

Gelenberg, A. J., Laukes, C., McGahuey, C., et al. 2000. Mirtazapine substitution in SSRI-induced sexual dysfunction. *J Clin Psychiatry* 61:356–360.

Geretsegger, C., Bohmer, F., and Ludwig, M. 1994. Paroxetine in the elderly depressed patient: randomised comparison with fluoxetine of efficacy, cognitive and behavioural effects. *Int Clin Psychopharmacol* 9:25–29.

Giorgi, L., Gomez, G., O'Neill, F., et al. 2001. The tolerability of lamotrigine in elderly patients with epilepsy. *Drugs Aging* 18:621–630.

Glassman, A. H., and Bigger, J. T. Jr. 2001. Antipsychotic drugs: prolonged QTc interval, torsades de pointes, and sudden death. *Am J Psychiatry* 158:1774–1782.

Goldberg, J. F., Sacks, M. H., and Kocsis, J. H. 2000. Low-dose lithium augmentation of divalproex in geriatric mania. *J Clin Psychiatry* 61:304.

Goodwin, F. K., Fireman, B., Simon, G., et al. 2003. Suicide risk in bipolar disorder during treatment with lithium and divalproex. *JAMA* 290:1467–1473.

Goodwin, F., and Jamison, K. 1990. *Manic-depressive illness*. Oxford: Oxford University Press.

Greenberg, R. M., and Kellner, C. H. 2005. Electroconvulsive therapy: a selected review. *Am J Geriatr Psychiatry* 13:268–281.

Gupta, S., Chohan, M., and Madhusoodanan, S. 2004. Treatment of acute mania with aripiprazole in an older adult with noted improvement in coexisting Parkinson's disease. *Prim Care Companion J Clin Psychiatry* 6:50–51.

Halper, J. P., and Mann, J. J. 1988. Cardiovascular effects of antidepressant medications. *Br J Psychiatry Suppl* 153:87–98.

Hardy, B. G., Shulman, K. I., Mackenzie, S. E., et al. 1987. Pharmacokinetics of lithium in the elderly. *J Clin Psychopharmacol* 7:153–158.

Harvey, A. T., and Preskorn, S. H. 1996. Cytochrome P450 enzymes: interpretation of their interactions with selective serotonin reuptake inhibitors: part II. *J Clin Psychopharmacol* 16:345–355.

Head, L., and Dening, T. 1998. Lithium in the over-65s: who is taking it and who is monitoring it? A survey of older adults on lithium in the Cambridge Mental Health Services catchment area. *Int J Geriatr Psychiatry* 13:164–171.

Hewick, D. S., Newburg, P., Hopwood, S., et al. 1977. Age as a factor affecting lithium therapy. *Br J Clin Pharmacol* 4:201–205.

Himmelhoch, J., Neil, J. R., May, S. J., et al. 1980. Age, dementia, dyskinesias, and lithium response. *Am J Psychiatry* 137:941–945.

Howard, W. T., and Warnock, J. K. 1999. Bupropion-induced psychosis. *Am J Psychiatry* 156:2017–2018.

Jeste, D. V. 2004. Tardive dyskinesia rates with atypical antipsychotics in older adults. *J Clin Psychiatry* 65(suppl. 9):21–24.

Johnson, R. E., and McFarland, B. 1996. Lithium use and discontinuation in a health maintenance organization. *Am J Psychiatry* 153:993–1000.

Kando, J., Tohen, M.., Castillo, J., et al. 1996. The use of valproate in an elderly population with affective symptoms. *J Clin Psychiatry* 57:238–240.

Kasarkis, E. J., Kuo, C. S., Berger, R., et al. 1991. Carbamazepine-induced cardiac dysfunction: characterization of two distinct clinical syndromes. *Arch Intern Med* 152:186–191.

Kellner, M. B., and Neher, F. 1991. A first episode of mania after age 80. *Can J Psychiatry* 36:607–608.

Kroenke, K., West, S. L., Swindle, R., et al. 2001. Similar effectiveness of paroxetine, fluoxetine, and sertraline in primary care: a randomized trial. *JAMA* 286:2947–2955.

Krystal, A. D., Edinger, J. K., Wohlgemuth, W. K., et al. 2004. Sleep and circadian rhythm disorders. In Blazer, D. G., Steffens, D. C., and Busse, E. W. (eds.), *The American psychiatric publishing textbook of geriatric psychiatry* (3rd ed., pp. 339–350). Washington, DC: American Psychiatric Press.

Kutluay, E., McCague, K., D'Souza, J., et al. 2003. Safety and tolerability of oxcarbazepine in elderly patients with epilepsy. *Epilepsy Behav* 2:175–180.

Laghrissi-Thode, F., Pollock, B. G., Miller, M. C., et al. 1995. Double-blind comparison of paroxetine and nortriptyline on the postural stability of late-life depressed patients. *Psychopharmacol Bull* 31:659–663.

Little, J. D., Atkins, M. R., Munday, J., et al. 2004. Bifrontal electroconvulsive therapy in the elderly: a 2-year retrospective. *J ECT* 20:139–141.

Liu, B. A., Mittman, N., Knowles, S. R., et al. 1996. Hyponatremia and the syndrome of inappropriate secretion of antidiuretic hormone associated with the use of selective serotonin reuptake inhibitors: a review of spontaneous reports. *CMAJ* 155:519–527.

Madhusoodanan, S., Brenner, R., Araujo, L., et al. 1995. Efficacy of risperidone treatment for psychoses associated with schizophrenia, schizoaffective disorder, bipolar disorder, or senile dementia in 11 geriatric patients: a case series. *J Clin Psychiatry* 56:514–518.

Madhusoodanan, S., Brenner, R., and Alcantra, A. 2000. Clinical experience with quetiapine in elderly patients with psychotic disorders. *J Geriatr Psychiatry Neurol* 13:28–32.

Madhusoodanan, S., Bogunovic, O., Brenner, R., et al. 2002. Use of topiramate as an adjunctive medication in an elderly patient with treatment-resistant bipolar disorder. *Am J Geriatr Psychiatry* 10:759.

McFarland, B., Miller, M., and Staurmfjord, A. 1990. Valproate use in the older manic patient. *J Clin Psychiatry* 51:479–481.

Meyer, J. M. 2002. A retrospective comparison of weight, lipid, and glucose changes between risperidone- and olanzapine-treated inpatients: metabolic outcomes after 1 year. *J Clin Psychiatry* 63:425–433.

Montejo, A. L., Llorca, G., Izquierdo, J. A., et al. 2001. Incidence of sexual dysfunction associated with antidepressant agents: a prospective multicenter study of 1022 outpatients. *J Clin Psychiatry* 62(suppl. 3):10–21.

Mordecai, D., Sheikh, J., and Glick, I. 1999. Divalproex for the treatment of geriatric bipolar disorder. *Int J Geriatr Psychiatry* 14:494–496.

Morrell, M. J., Isojarvi, J., Taylor, A. E., et al. 2003. Higher androgens and weight gain with valproate compared with lamotrigine for epilepsy. *Epilepsy Res* 54:189–199.

Mulsant, B. H., Alexopoulos, G. S., Reynolds, C. F. III, et al. 2001. Pharmacological treatment of depression in older primary care patients: the PROSPECT algorithm. *Int J Geriatr Psychiatry* 16:585–592.

Mulsant, B. H., and Pollock, B. G. 2004. Psychopharmacology. In Blazer, D. G., Steffens, D. C., and Busse, E. W. (eds.), *The American Psychiatric Publishing textbook of geriatric psychiatry* (3rd ed., pp. 387–411). Washington, DC: American Psychiatric Press.

Nemeroff, C. B., DeVane, C. L., and Pollock, B. G. 1996. Newer antidepressants and the cytochrome P450 system. *Am J Psychiatry* 153:311–320.

Niedermier, J., and Nasrallah, H. 1998. Clinical correlates of response to valproate in geriatric inpatients. *Ann Clin Psychiatry* 10:165–168.

Noaghiul, S., Narayan, M., and Nelson, J. 1998. Divalproex treatment of mania in elderly patients. *Am J Geriatr Psychiatry* 6:257–262.

Pedersen, L., and Klysner, R. 1997. Antagonism of selective serotonin reuptake inhibitor–induced nausea by mirtazapine. *Int Clin Psychopharmacol* 12:59–60.

Pollock, B. G., Perel, J. M., Paradis, C. F., et al. 1994. Metabolic and physiologic consequences of nortriptyline treatment in the elderly. *Psychopharmacol Bull* 30:145–150.

Post, R., Leverich, G. S., Altshuler, L. L., et al. 2003. An overview of recent findings of the Stanley Foundation Bipolar Network (part I). *Bipolar Disord* 5:310–319.

Preskorn, S. H. 1993. Recent pharmacologic advances in antidepressant therapy for the elderly. *Am J Med* 94(suppl. 5A):2S–12S.

Prien, R. F., Caffey, E. M. Jr., and Klett, C. J. 1972. Relationship between serum lithium level and clinical response in acute mania treated with lithium. *Br J Psychiatry* 120:409–414.

Regenold, W., and Prasad, M. 2001. Uses of intravenous valproate in geriatric psychiatry. *Am J Geriatr Psychiatry* 9:306–308.

Reilly, J. G., Ayis, S. A., Ferrier, I. N., et al. 2000. QT-interval abnormalities and psychotropic drug therapy in psychiatric patients. *Lancet* 355:1048–1052.

Rickels, K., and Schweizer, E. 1990. Clinical overview of serotonin reuptake inhibitors. *J Clin Psychiatry* 51(suppl. B):9–12.

Robillard, M., and Conn, D. 2002. Lamotrigine use in geriatric patients with bipolar depression. *Can J Psychiatry* 47:767–770.

Roose, G. P., Bone, S., Haidorfer, C., et al. 1979. Lithium treatment in older patients. *Am J Psychiatry* 136:843–844.

Roose, S. P., and Glassman, A. H. 1994. Antidepressant choice in the patient with cardiac disease: lessons from the Cardiac Arrhythmia Suppression Trial (CAST) studies. *J Clin Psychiatry* 55(suppl. A):83–87.

Roose, S. P., Nurnberger, J. I., Dunner, D. L., et al. 1979. Cardiac sinus node dysfunction during lithium treatment. *Am J Psychiatry* 136:804–806.

Schaffer, C. B., and Garvey, M. J. 1984. Use of lithium in acutely manic elderly patients. *Clin Gerontol* 3:58–60.

Schneider, A. L., and Wilcox, C. S. 1998. Divalproate augmentation in lithium-resistant rapid cycling mania in four geriatric patients. *J Affect Disord* 47:201–205.

Schneider, L. S., and Olin, J. T. 1995. Efficacy of acute treatment for geriatric depression. *Int Psychogeriatr* 7(suppl.):7–25.

Scott, J., and Pope, M. 2002. Non-adherence with mood-stabilizers: prevalence and predictors. *J Clin Psychiatry* 63:384–389.

Semla, T. P., Beizer, J. L., and Higbee, M. D. 2003. *Geriatric dosage handbook* (8th ed.). Hudson, OH: Lexi-Comp.

Sethi, M., Mehta, R., and Denanand, D. 2003. Gabapentin in geriatric mania. *J Geriatr Psychiatry Neurol* 16:117–120.

Sharma, V., Prasad, E., Mazmanian, D., et al. 1993. Treatment of rapid cycling bipolar disorder with combination therapy of valproate and lithium. *Can J Psychiatry* 38:137–139.

Shulman, K., Rochon, P., Sykora, K., et al. 2003. Changing prescription patterns for lithium and valproic acid in old age: shifting practice without evidence. *BMJ* 326:960–961.

Shulman, R., Singh, A., and Shulman, K. 1997. Treatment of elderly institutionalized bipolar patients with clozapine. *Psychopharmacol Bull* 33:113–118.

Smith, R. E., and Helms, P. M. 1982. Adverse effects of lithium therapy in the acutely ill elderly patient. *J Clin Psychiatry* 43:94–99.

Snowdon, J. 2000. The relevance of guidelines for treatment of mania in old age. *Int J Geriatr Psychiatry* 15:779–783.

Solai, L. K., Mulsant, B. H., and Pollock, B. G. 2001. Selective serotonin reuptake inhibitors for late-life depression: a comparative review. *Drugs Aging* 18:355–368.

Stone, K. 1989. Mania in the elderly. *Br J Psychiatry* 155:220–224.

Strayhorn, J. M. Jr., and Nash, J. L. 1977. Severe neurotoxicity despite "therapeutic" serum lithium levels. *Dis Nerv Syst* 38:107–111.

Thomas, D. R., Nelson, D. R., and Johnson, A. M. 1987. Biochemical effects of the antidepressant paroxetine, a specific 5-hydroxytryptamine uptake inhibitor. *Psychopharmacology* 93:193–200.

Thompson, D. S. 2000. Mirtazapine for the treatment of depression and nausea in breast and gynecological oncology. *Psychosomatics* 41:356–359.

Tohen, M., Castillo, J., Baldessarini, R. J., et al. 1995. Blood dyscrasias with carbamazepine and valproate: a pharmacoepidemiological study of 2,228 patients at risk. *Am J Psychiatry* 152:413–418.

Tohen, M., Zarate, C., Hennen, J., et al. 2003. The McLean-Harvard first-episode mania study: prediction of recovery and first recurrence. *Am J Psychiatry* 160:2099–2107.

U.S. Food and Drug Administration. 2005. Public health advisory: deaths with antipsychotics in elderly patients with behavioral disturbances. April 11. www.fda.gov/cder/drug/advisory/antipsychotics.htm

van der Wurff, F. B., Stek, M. L., Hoogendijk, W. L., et al. 2003. The efficacy and safety of ECT in depressed older adults: a literature review. *Int J Geriatr Psychiatr* 18:894–904.

Weiner, R. D., and Krystal, A. D. 2004. Electroconvulsive therapy. In Blazer, D. G., Steffens, D. C., and Busse, E. W. (eds.), *The American Psychiatric Publishing textbook of geriatric psychiatry* (3rd ed., pp. 413–426). Washington, DC: American Psychiatric Press.

Willmore, L. J. 2000. Choice and use of newer anticonvulsant drugs in older patients. *Drugs Aging* 17:441–452.

Wilson, K., and Mottram, P. 2004. A comparison of side effects of selective serotonin reuptake inhibitors and tricyclic antidepressants in older depressed patients: a meta-analysis. *Int J Geriatr Psychiatry* 19:754–762.

Wylie, M., Mulsant, B., Pollock, B., et al. 1999. Age at onset in geriatric bipolar disorder. *Am J Geriatr Psychiatry* 7:77–83.

Yassa, R., Nastase, C., and Dupont, D. 1992. Tardive dyskinesia in elderly psychiatric patients: a 5-year study. *Am J Psychiatry* 149:1206–1211.

Young, R. C., Jain, H., Kiosses, D. N., et al. 2003. Antidepressant-associated mania in late life. *Int J Geriatr Psychiatry* 18:421–424.

Young, R. C., Gyulai, L., Mulsant, B., et al. 2004. Pharmacotherapy of bipolar disorder in old age. *Am J Geriatr Psychiatry* 12:342–357.

Zaretsky, A. 2003. Targeted psychosocial interventions for bipolar disorder. *Bipolar Disord* 5(suppl. 2):80–87.

CHAPTER SIX

Psychosocial Interventions for Older Adults with Bipolar Disorder

Navigating Terra Incognita

LINDA McBRIDE, M.S.N., AND MARK S. BAUER, M.D.

What is it like to grow old with bipolar disorder? What new challenges present themselves to individuals growing old with this illness? What new coping skills are required? What types of psychosocial intervention are effective in improving outcomes for older individuals with bipolar disorder?

We have few systematic answers to these questions. A comprehensive vision of a research agenda for bipolar disorder in elderly persons has yet to be formulated, despite the fact that the population of the developed world is rapidly aging. Historically, most research on bipolar disorder in late life has been neurobiologically driven, focusing on late-onset mania and its relation to cerebrovascular factors (Almeida and Fenner 2002; Hays et al. 1998; Stone 1989; Tohen et al. 1994; Wylie et al. 1999) (see also chapter 4).

Taking a broader and more catholic view of this issue, the recent excellent review by Depp and Jeste (2004) provides a comprehensive survey of topics of relevance to bipolar disorder in older adults. Among the major conclusions drawn from their scholarly review are the following:

— Contrary to some perceptions, bipolar disorder does not "burn out" with age.
— Rather, recurring symptoms are the rule. And few older persons show full functional recovery, as is true for younger ages.
— There seems to be an association of cerebrovascular disease with late-onset mania.
— However, medical comorbidity of all types is substantial in older age groups with bipolar disorder, as it is for the older population in general.

— Substance use disorders as a comorbidity are less common in older than in younger individuals.

— Little is known about other psychiatric comorbidities in older individuals with bipolar disorder.

Simultaneously, several database and clinical studies have begun to explore the interrelated issues of bipolar disorder, aging, and medical comorbidity. Many reports derive from studies of veterans who receive care in the medical centers of the U.S. Department of Veterans Affairs (VA), a system on the forefront of clinical care for older individuals with serious mental illness (Fenn et al. 2005; Kilbourne et al. 2004; Sajatovic et al. 1996, 2004, 2005). Such studies, and this book, represent the needed broadening of perspective on research involving this important and growing population.

What is known specifically about psychosocial interventions for aging individuals with bipolar disorder? In short, very little. To our knowledge, there are no published studies of psychosocial treatment targeted toward older individuals with this illness. Numerous clinical trials of psychosocial interventions for adults with bipolar disorder have been published (reviewed in Otto et al. 2003; Bauer 2001), but none of these interventions has been applied specifically to older individuals. Similarly, none of the studies published to date has reported post hoc analyses of subsets of older persons with bipolar disorder; this is undoubtedly because the sample sizes, modest to begin with, become vanishingly small in the older decades.

When older individuals with bipolar disorder come to us for treatment, where are we to look for guidance? When quantitative data fail us, qualitative data may help.

Accordingly, in this chapter we first review some recently published quantitative data from our clinical study of U.S. veterans hospitalized for bipolar disorder as part of VA Cooperative Study #430 (Bauer et al. 2006a, 2006b; Fenn et al. 2005). These are cross-sectional data, obtained at intake of participants into this three-year randomized controlled trial. As such, the data can only provide hints, though we think valuable ones, to characterize this population. We then describe the Life Goals Program (Bauer and McBride 1996, 2003), a psychoeducational intervention widely used for veterans, including older veterans, with bipolar disorder (Yatham and Kennedy 2005), and provide some case vignettes of individuals participating in this program. Some key themes emerge from our observations on these, and similar, older individuals with bipolar disorder whom we have treated.

NEW QUANTITATIVE DATA ON AGING AND MEDICAL / PSYCHIATRIC COMORBIDITY IN BIPOLAR DISORDER

As part of VA Cooperative Study #430, we obtained clinical research assessments and structured medical chart reviews for 290 veterans hospitalized for treatment of bipolar disorder on acute psychiatric wards across 11 participating VA medical centers (Fenn et al. 2005). Consistent with Depp and Jeste's review (2004), bipolar disorder does not seem to "burn out" with age. There was no difference across age decades in the number of manic or depressive episodes in the year before entry into the study. Not surprisingly, medical comorbidity was highly prevalent in the sample and is certainly not limited to neurovascular disorders (table 6.1). The median number of active comorbidities was 2 (quartiles [25th and 75th percentiles] 1–3), with a median of 4 for lifetime comorbidities (quartiles 2–6). It was equally striking, and expected, that both current and lifetime prevalence of medical illness increased with increasing age (fig. 6.1). In contrast, interestingly, the prevalence rates of substance use disorders and anxiety comorbidities decreased with increasing age (table 6.2) — though, in the overall sample, the prevalence rates of these comorbidities were, respectively, 34% and 38%.

Physical health-related quality of life (HRQOL) declined with age (fig. 6.2), as it does in individuals with schizophrenia (Friedman et al. 2002; Sciolla et al. 2003).

TABLE 6.1
*Medical comorbidities in bipolar disorder in 290 veterans
hospitalized at Veterans Affairs medical centers*

Medical disorder	Current	Lifetime
Autoimmune	4 (1.4%)	7 (2.4%)
Cardiovascular/cerebrovascular	101 (34.8%)	141 (48.6%)
Dermatological	20 (6.9%)	59 (20.3%)
Endocrine	66 (22.8%)	83 (28.6%)
Eyes, ears, nose, throat (EENT)	26 (9.0%)	67 (23.1%)
Gastrointestinal	52 (17.9%)	114 (39.3%)
Genitourinary	26 (9.0%)	62 (21.4%)
Hematological	11 (3.8%)	25 (8.6%)
Hepatic	49 (16.9%)	61 (21.0%)
HIV/AIDS	4 (1.4%)	4 (1.4%)
Dyslipidemias	65 (23.4%)	81 (28.9%)
Musculoskeletal	68 (23.4%)	144 (37.9%)
Neurological	50 (17.2%)	110 (49.7%)
Pulmonary	38 (13.1%)	70 (24.1%)
Renal	7 (2.4%)	19 (6.6%)
Any medical comorbidity	235 (81%)	272 (94.1%)

Source: Fenn et al. 2005.

TABLE 6.2
Rates of psychiatric comorbidity in bipolar disorder across the lifespan

	Number (rate) by age decade							
	≤30 (n = 13)	31–40 (n = 69)	41–50 (n = 128)	51–60 (n = 51)	61–70 (n = 23)	>70 (n = 6)	χ_2 (df)	Univariate p-value
Substance use disorders								
Current	8 (61.5%)	28 (40.6%)	44 (34.4%)	16 (31.4%)	3 (13.0%)	0 (0.0%)	13.7 (5)	.018
Lifetime	9 (69.2%)	47 (68.1%)	105 (82.0%)	34 (66.7%)	14 (60.9%)	1 (16.7%)	18.2 (5)	.003
Anxiety disorders								
Current	4 (30.8%)	30 (43.5%)	58 (45.3%)	17 (33.3%)	2 (8.7%)	0 (0.0%)	16.7 (5)	.005
Lifetime	6 (46.2%)	32 (46.4%)	63 (49.2%)	22 (43.1%)	2 (8.7%)	0 (0.0%)	18.5 (5)	.002

Source: Fenn et al. 2005.

This decrement in Physical Component Score (PCS) is associated with medical comorbidity but not with age per se. Thus, decrements in physical HRQOL in this population are not an inevitable aspect of aging. Rather, adequate attention to medical comorbidity at any age may have a tangible effect on HRQOL.

Surprisingly, mental HRQOL *increased* rather than declined with age (fig. 6.2), associated with a lower likelihood of presentation in a depressed/mixed episode, a lower number of depressive episodes in the prior year, and a lower prevalence of current anxiety disorder. Our research group continues to debate the meaning of the apparently better mental HRQOL among older individuals with bipolar disorder, with several working hypotheses: underreporting of symptoms with age (Zingmond et al. 2003), accommodation to symptoms and disability with age (Vaillant and Mukamal 2001), higher mortality rate among the most ill, secular trends associated with increasingly complex and disabling bipolar disorder, and more substance abuse and anxiety comorbidities among the younger individuals. Longitudinal studies will be required to differentiate among these possibilities.

Thus, the older population with bipolar disorder emerges as distinct from the younger population, based on distinctive patterns of medical and psychiatric comorbidities and HRQOL. Consequently, the clinical needs of these populations are likely to differ. How, then, do these quantitative data help us in structuring psychosocial treatments for older individuals with bipolar disorder?

First and most obviously, continued attention to bipolar disorder throughout older ages is critical, as the disease clearly does not remit with age. Second, attention to medical comorbidities must play a substantial role if quality of life is to be maximized for these individuals. The good news is that the age-related decline in physical HRQOL may be due to physical illnesses, and therefore a more effective treatment of these illnesses will reduce that decline. Third, although the prevalence

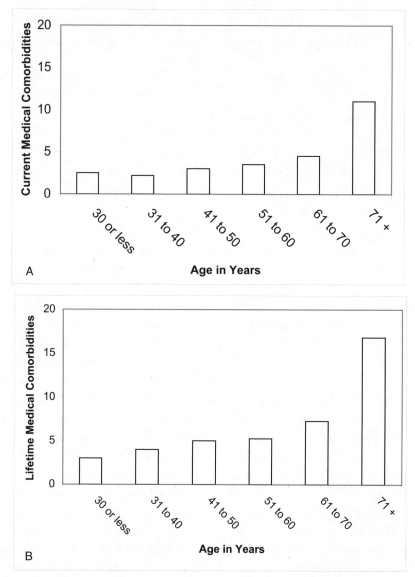

Fig. 6.1. Medical comorbidities across the adult age span, showing the number of (A) current and (B) lifetime comorbid medical diagnoses by age decade ($p < .001$ for both). *Source:* Fenn et al. 2005.

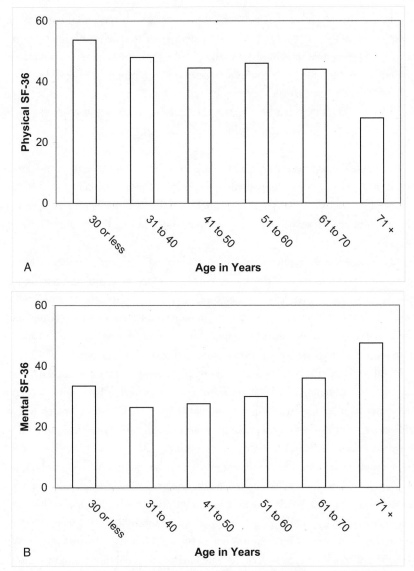

Fig. 6.2. Physical and mental health-related quality of life (HRQOL) across the adult age span were measured using the SF-36 (Ware et al. 1994). (A) Physical HRQOL was measured as the Physical Component Score of the SF-36 (PCS; $p = .003$), and (B) mental HRQOL as the Mental Component Score of the SF-36 (MCS; $p < .001$). PCS decreased significantly with increasing age ($p = .003$), whereas MCS increased with increasing age ($p < .001$). See text for interpretation and clinical significance of these differences. *Source*: Fenn et al. 2005.

of substance abuse and anxiety comorbidities declines with age—whether through selective mortality, adaptation, or lower incidence due to cohort effects—a not insignificant prevalence remains even in the older age group. Attention to both these comorbidities, therefore, will continue to be important throughout the lifespan.

QUALITATIVE DATA FROM THE LIFE GOALS PROGRAM
Overview of the Life Goals Program

In the early 1990s we recognized the need for more comprehensive and structured psychoeducation for individuals with bipolar disorder. At that time, few psychosocial modalities of any type were available for this disorder, yet it was clear that pharmacotherapy alone was failing to optimize outcomes for these patients (Bauer et al. 2001; Keller et al. 1986).

Accordingly, we developed a structured, manual-based group intervention to improve illness-management skills, using a psychoeducational, problem-solving approach in a group format. The manual, *Structured Group Psychotherapy for Bipolar Disorder: The Life Goals Program,* was initially published in 1996 (Bauer and McBride 1996), translated into French (Aubry 2001) and Spanish (Xochitl Alvarez, unpublished), and reissued in a second edition (Bauer and McBride 2003).

The Life Goals Program took a primarily psychoeducational approach because our clinical experience and feedback from patients, as well as from clinicians and researchers experienced with bipolar disorder, suggested that this approach would address the critical need for optimizing medical-model care. We added more traditional cognitive-behavioral methods where appropriate (Bauer and McBride 1996), and we recognized many commonalities with motivational interviewing techniques (Miller and Rollnick 2002) as we updated the program (Bauer and McBride 2003). Additionally, the Life Goals Program integrates principles of the biopsychosocial model developed by George Engel (1977), who recognized that all aspects of the individual have an impact on health—not just mental but also physical health. We view the collaborative approach of the Life Goals Program as an attempt to implement treatment based on the full spectrum of Engel's approach to biopsychosocial assessment.

The group format was adopted for two reasons. First, we reasoned that individuals with bipolar disorder could be effective teachers and role models for others, as well as providing support and destigmatization and combating the isolation endemic in this population. Second, we wished to minimize cost and maximize the dissemination potential of the intervention.

The Life Goals Program consists of two phases, typically conducted in weekly 60-

to 75-minute sessions. The therapist is usually a psychiatric clinical nurse specialist (CNS), though we have successfully trained therapists who are trainees in social work and psychiatry (Bauer et al. 1998). To enter a group, individuals need not be experiencing a complete remission of their bipolar or comorbid symptoms or substance use; however, manic symptoms should be under reasonable control, as detailed in the therapist directions in the manual, and intoxicated patients are turned away at the door to return when sober.

The purpose of Phase 1 is to improve individuals' illness-management skills so that they may be more effective collaborators with medical and other practitioners in the management of their own illness. The purpose of Phase 2 is to improve social and occupational functions in ways that individuals themselves identify as meaningful.

In Phase 1, the therapist works from a structured agenda and is provided with specific probes to facilitate educational work in each session. The therapeutic approach in each of these sessions is to work from a discussion of topics in "nonpersonalized" terms toward an application of knowledge and insights to one's own illness. Group-generated lists and discussions are supplemented by individual work in the group member's own workbook. Phase 1 consists of six sessions:

— Session 1: An overview of the definition of bipolar disorder, its possible causes, and the effects of psychiatric stigma on illness-management skills
— Session 2: A general overview of symptoms, triggers, and personalization of the information from session 2 through the construction of a *personal illness profile* of (hypo)mania for the specific individual
— Session 3: Development of an *action plan* for dealing with the onset of a (hypo)manic episode. This approach relies heavily on constructing a *personal cost-benefit analysis* for a variety of coping responses to symptoms, similar in orientation to that of the motivational interviewing techniques of Miller and Rollnick (2002).
— Session 4: An introduction to depression, using an approach similar to session 2
— Session 5: Development of an action plan for dealing with depression, similar to session 3
— Session 6: Added in the second edition of the manual (Bauer and McBride 2003) to review medical and psychosocial treatments for bipolar disorder and construct an integrated treatment plan

It is intriguing that this core agenda — development of a basic understanding of the illness, followed by identification of individual-specific symptom patterns and triggers and formulation of a plan to address them — seems to be common to most of the psychotherapies developed for bipolar disorder, although the core agenda may be embedded in very different interventions and overall agendas (Bauer 2001).

Phase 2 focuses on achieving *social role function goals* that the individual, because of bipolar symptoms, may have been unable to achieve thus far. It is open-ended and agenda-driven, and continues the weekly format. Phase 2 takes a strongly behavioral approach, with group members working jointly with the therapist to identify functional goals that are concrete, specific, and achievable. Such goals may range from those as apparently straightforward as getting a driver's license reinstated to improving one's social life according to specified parameters. A key therapist task is to assist group members in operationalizing their goals in behavioral terms and constructing a series of feasible subgoals and steps to achieving them. The general approach guiding this behavioral plan for group members is to "set them up for success" with each step, attempting to facilitate a sense of mastery and self-efficacy (see Bandura 2001 on social cognitive theory), which is so often missing in people with chronic mental illnesses. Accordingly, a variety of cognitive, behavioral, and group process tools are used to encourage progress. The group member continues to work on his or her agenda until a goal is reached, and then either chooses another goal or terminates participation. The therapist uses a combination of individual work with members and group sharing and feedback about individual plans.

George was a 72-year-old divorced man, a former police officer, with bipolar disorder type 1 and a medical history of osteoarthritis and benign prostatic hypertrophy. He was diagnosed with bipolar disorder at age 35, and at that time lost his job and marriage. George's baseline mood was typically hyperthymic. He was in a relationship with Mary, with whom he had lived for eight years. He had frequent contact with his four adult children, who lived nearby. Mary also had a depressive illness and frequent hospitalizations. George had a difficult time accepting his own bipolar disorder diagnosis and Mary's diagnosis of major depressive disorder.

George did not understand the medical basis of bipolar disorder or other mental illness. He had difficulty accepting that he had a serious mental illness, though he did adhere to his medication regimen of lithium carbonate 900 mg at bedtime and kept scheduled appointments. He never took illicit drugs and had stopped drinking alcohol 25 years ago at the suggestion of his physician.

Nevertheless, George had a succession of severe depressive episodes that increased in severity as he aged. He believed depression was something that could be overcome with endurance and motivation to "do better." He took pride in his self-reliance. Typically his depressions began slowly and increased in severity over several weeks.

During a major depressive episode in 2001, George became critically ill. He was found lethargic and confused at home, and on admission to the intensive care unit was found to have weight loss, delirium, severe dehydration, lithium toxicity, and a cardiac arrhythmia. Once medically stabilized, he was transferred to the inpatient psychiatric unit. He was severely depressed, with neurovegetative symptoms and poor appetite, interest, and insight. His lithium was restarted at 300 mg three times a day; his serum lithium level reached 0.8 mEq/L, and after several days he began taking the antidepressant bupropion. Electroconvulsive therapy was suggested when George did not respond to medications after three weeks of treatment, but he refused. He made slow continuous progress over the following four weeks, and eventually his depression remitted.

When George was evaluated in the Bipolar Clinic following his hospital discharge, he was able to recognize that he had been seriously ill and nearly died, but he could not associate his recent illness with "depression." Underlying his denial was his thinking that depression represented weakness, and this conflicted significantly with his pride in his self-reliance and independence. He also said that he never felt "depressed," but did identify that he lost his energy, interest, and appetite and slept more than his routine six hours a night. The stigma of having a depressive illness was embedded in his cultural beliefs.

However, George was motivated to avoid becoming seriously ill again. He demonstrated a need to be in control and responded well to the collaborative treatment approach practiced in the Bipolar Clinic. He agreed to participate in individual appointments for medication management and in psychoeducation in the Life Goals Program.

During Phase 1 of the program, George learned about the medical basis of bipolar disorder, heard other members openly discuss their feelings and experiences with psychiatric stigma, developed personal profiles of his hypomanic and depressive episodes, and learned his early warning signs. He identified stress-related triggers and their relation to episode recurrence, and developed action plans to respond to symptoms by seeking treatment early. He also learned about the purpose, dose, and side effects of medications to treat bipolar disorder.

In Phase 2, George settled into the low-intensity interpersonal style of the group, with members sharing and (with permission — a Life Goals Program procedure) providing feedback about topics discussed in Phase 1 and setting goals on topics related to managing their lives. These topics included, in particular, substance abuse and other psychiatric comorbidities, interpersonal relationships, structuring a daily routine, employment, finances, and coping with losses associated with having bipolar disorder. George began using the group as a central point for his medication-management needs. After observing how other group members made their treatment choices, by weighing the potential costs and benefits, he now translated his self-reliance into self-management and collaborative care for his bipolar disorder.

About two years after his previous hospitalization for depression, George called to cancel his group appointment, reporting that he had a loss of energy and appetite and had been sleeping on and off throughout the day for the past week. He was seen later that day for an assessment of his medical and psychiatric symptoms. He was diagnosed with a urinary tract infection (UTI) and mild dehydration, and immediately received fluid replacement and antibiotics. He continued to take the prescribed antibiotic and his UTI cleared; however, his depressive symptoms continued.

George came to several group sessions, where his goal was to "be myself again." We operationalized this goal as "resolving the depression." The steps to reach his goal were as follows:

1. To have brief visits, following the group session, to manage his medications
2. To attend the group weekly
3. To report any additional medical problems immediately
4. To continue a minimum of three small, nourishing meals a day and maintain fluid intake, and to keep a record of his intake

At a subsequent Bipolar Clinic visit, his laboratory studies revealed a lithium level of 0.8 mEq/L at a dose of 600 mg/day (formerly, he had a lithium level of 0.8 mEq/L at a dose of 900 mg/day); blood urea nitrogen (an index of kidney function) mildly elevated at 28 mg/dl; and creatinine in the normal range, at 1.2 mg/dl. A decision was made to increase his dose of bupropion and to continue weekly group appointments. Despite his adherence to treatment, George's depression gradually worsened, and he agreed to admission to the inpatient psychiatric unit for stabilization. During the ensuing two weeks he eventually responded to the milieu and his medications. His interest, appetite, and energy improved; he began gaining weight and was discharged home.

He resumed his weekly group appointments, and his goal was "to maintain

my mood" at his hyperthymic baseline and to work on "getting Mary to stop going into the hospital." George described how Mary would leave for "a drive to
the store and not come back." He would later learn she was in the hospital.
That goal was redefined as "inviting Mary to participate in two or three couple's
appointments" with George and his clinician (which she agreed to attend).

During those couple's appointments Mary was able to disclose to George
that she avoided telling him about her depression and desire for inpatient treatment because she thought he'd insist she stay home and give her other advice,
when she felt sure she needed hospital-based care. Mary and George partici-
pated in learning more about each other's illnesses, reviewed symptom lists,
and planned how and when to seek treatment.

Several months later, George was admitted to the hospital medical unit with
a diagnosis of congestive heart failure. While in the hospital, he was maintained on his lithium and bupropion. During this hospitalization the medical
staff prescribed lisinopril, and he went home with a plan to return within one
week for a serum lithium level check because of the potential for lisinopril to
increase lithium levels. The Bipolar Clinic staff was not notified of the admission.

George missed his weekly group meeting, and the Bipolar Clinic staff then
discovered that he had been hospitalized over the weekend, had started taking
lisinopril, and had not come in for his serum lithium check. He did not respond to outreach telephone calls and several messages left by the CNS. His
son was notified, and he found his father confused and brought him to the
emergency room, where George was diagnosed as having lithium toxicity with
a serum level of 2.5 mEq/L.

George was admitted to the medical ward, and the staff contacted the Bipolar Clinic CNS for consultation and information about his baseline cognitive
functioning. George was observed to be picking at his clothes, incontinent, and
disoriented about place and time. The CNS's diagnosis was delirium due to
lithium toxicity and possible interaction with lisinopril. The lisinopril and
lithium were discontinued, George was given an alternative antihypertensive
agent and fluid replacement, and, once his lithium level decreased, his lithium
dose was restarted at 300 mg/day with a target level of 0.4–0.6 mEq/L.
Lithium was continued as a mood stabilizer for George because he tolerated it
well and it was effective before the recent drug interaction with lisinopril. During the following week George's lithium level stabilized at 0.45 mEq/L, his
mental status cleared, and he became independent in his self-care. He was discharged home, with continued follow-up in the Bipolar Clinic.

Comment. George's story illustrates several common themes we have encountered in working with individuals with bipolar disorder in late life. These themes run the biopsychosocial gamut from the management of comorbid medical illnesses and medications to the important psychosocial issues of stigma and overreliance on stoicism as a coping style. Learning from peers in a group setting assisted George in addressing these issues, which for this patient would have been much more difficult with therapist-based, one-on-one counseling. Another common theme is the need to recognize and help deal with a significant other's disability from a chronic illness — in George's case, Mary's psychiatric disorder.

Paul, a 69-year-old married man with an eighth grade education, was referred to the Bipolar Clinic by the mental health clinic's new patient assessment team. He had been diagnosed with bipolar disorder at a private hospital where he was admitted with a manic episode 25 years earlier. He had bipolar type I with rapid cycling that was fairly well stabilized with 900 mg of lithium and 30 mg of temazepam at bedtime. Paul had mild memory deficits and hearing loss. He had had an injury to his left arm, surgery, and an infection that later developed into chronic osteomyelitis with chronic pain. His other medical problems included a left inguinal hernia and a history of myocardial infarction with a coronary artery bypass graft. He also had multiple stresses that seemed to increase the intensity and frequency of his mood episodes, most notably the stress caused by a daughter with bipolar disorder who had become addicted to heroin. His daughter was divorced, with one child, and had undergone multiple hospitalizations and treatments for both psychotic mixed episodes and substance dependence. Paul and his wife were very involved in trying to help their daughter overcome her illnesses. He spent a great amount of time coaching her to adhere to her medication regimens and attend treatments for her substance abuse, and he helped her to function in her home and to parent her child. The daughter gradually lost control of her addiction and sold household items to purchase drugs; she left her child unattended and eventually lost custody of the child to her spouse. Paul was very focused on her problems, at times to the detriment of his own care.

Paul agreed to participate in the Life Goals Program to better manage the stresses in his life. During the Phase 1 sessions he listened attentively, attempted to complete the workbook entries, and often offered support to younger group members. The group leader recognized his limited education and hearing impairment and would often gently ask if "anyone had any questions or needed more time" with the written segments of the program.

Once in Phase 2, Paul identified a goal to "decrease my lithium hand tremor." He felt "embarrassed in the coffee shop" where he met his friends in the morning, because he could barely lift the cup to his mouth without spilling coffee. He told the group he had tried to lower his lithium "on my own," but when he did, he felt more depressed and his mood cycles were more of a problem. Initially, Paul said he did not want to burden the group or his health care provider with his problems: "A lot of other people need care and I am better off than they are." With the group coaching him and pointing out his own worth and his value to them, he took the time to arrange treatment for himself. His lithium level was 0.7 mEq/L while taking 300 mg three times a day. He began to work more closely with the Bipolar Clinic staff to adjust his medications, and because a prior trial of a lower dose of lithium had resulted in recurrence of his bipolar symptoms, he began taking 12.5 mg of atenolol twice daily to treat his lithium-induced hand tremor. When he later discussed his progress, he told the group that although the tremor was better, he felt dizzy and lightheaded at times. He recognized that continued dialogue with his prescriber was another step toward his goal, and he and his prescriber discussed the issue and agreed to try a lower dose of atenolol, 6.25 mg twice daily. His tremor remained improved and he had no further medication side effects.

During subsequent sessions Paul encouraged and supported other group members as they described personal goals and life challenges. He did not share personal information regularly, except for medical matters. During one group session he complained he had a severe pain in his "left side." Knowing about his reticence to complain, the Bipolar Clinic staff took Paul to the emergency room, where his left inguinal hernia was reduced and a surgical consultation was planned for the following week. Paul had his hernia repaired without complications.

After some months in the group, Paul shared his problem coping with his daughter's addiction and described his feelings about this. He hadn't talked about this problem with anyone outside his family and treatment team, and he expressed feeling ashamed that he'd failed to restore his daughter's functioning. Group members greeted his disclosure with much support and empathy. Several members shared their personal experiences with addictions, and another member spoke of his own adult child with alcoholism. He told Paul that he'd learned not to blame himself for his child's problem, and he described his own struggles to love her and yet accept that she was responsible for her choices. Another member suggested Paul attend Al-Anon and shared his personal experiences in that group. Paul remarked that he felt better knowing he was not alone, because others in the group shared a similar problem.

Given this positive initial experience, clearly outside his "comfort zone," in subsequent sessions Paul continued to share his feelings and problems coping with his daughter. However, during her times of crisis he found it difficult to think about anything else, and he told the group he was feeling angry and was more often depressed. He was not "ready" to go to Al-Anon because he "didn't want to tell more people" about his daughter. The group suggested he could; he could consider going to Al-Anon meetings and simply listen to how other people coped, without speaking about his personal issues. Paul also became interested in a suggestion of setting up scheduled time to spend with his wife and in other pleasant activities, and to partition and limit the time spent thinking about his daughter's problems. He thought this might help him feel less angry and resentful.

During subsequent group sessions Paul described his progress in reaching his goal to structure his time in this way. He talked more about his disappointment that his daughter was so impaired, and group members listened and spoke more about addictions and the feeling of powerlessness about the addictions of the people one loves. Paul continues to attend the group program, speaking more easily on sensitive topics in a nonjudgmental environment and using the group as a support system.

Comment. Paul's story illustrates the importance of facilitating individuals' dialogue with their clinicians to manage side effects and emerging medical problems. Psychosocially, note also the importance of understanding older individuals' roles with regard to adult offspring. In Paul's case the issue was not the more common fear of being a burden, but rather having to continue to act as parent to an adult child and having to come to terms with regrets and feelings of failure about her upbringing.

Hal was a 60-year-old married man who came to the Bipolar Clinic in 1995 for an initial assessment. He was diagnosed with bipolar type I (vs. schizoaffective disorder, post-traumatic stress disorder, obsessive compulsive disorder, and panic disorder with agoraphobia). He described psychotic bizarre delusions, and he wore a helmet "to stop the radio waves from penetrating my brain" during major depressive episodes. Hal had been housebound because of the panic disorder. He had cycles of mania with rushing thoughts, sleeplessness, intense anxiety, and flashbacks of a jungle war where he had witnessed mass casualties and "the stench of death." He checked his home for safety repeatedly day and night, locking and relocking doors and windows for up to three hours a day.

Hal's condition partially stabilized on a combination of divalproex, risperidone, lithium, and clonazepam, and he began the Life Goals Program. He attended all Phase 1 sessions, and he read information about bipolar disorder on
the Internet, including information on his medications and the advantages and
disadvantages of taking them. He became very committed to participating in
managing his illness and adhered to his medication regimens and appointments.

During Phase 2 of the group program Hal's initial goals were "to stabilize
my symptoms" and to "leave the house for bike rides." "To stabilize my symptoms" was further operationalized into steps, including adherence to medication and appointments, getting care early when experiencing warning signs of
impending depression and/or mania, and following a structured daily activity
and sleep schedule. His mood was extremely sensitive to stress. Even mild viral
symptoms could lead to significant mood cycling and depressive episodes. A
subgoal for his goal "to stabilize my symptoms" was to continue the list, begun
in Phase 1, of his potential triggers of mania and depression and to learn more
about the stressors that led to mood instability.

Hal began riding his bike, and one day he had a panic attack on a bridge
along the bike route. During a group session he discussed his treatment options, which included challenging the anxiety repeatedly with multiple bridge
crossings, having his medication adjusted to reduce his panic symptoms, or
changing his bike route. He chose to select an alternative route.

He later identified a goal to volunteer in a nearby hospital two days a week,
and he did this for approximately one month. He was well liked and enthusias-
tic, but he did not tolerate the pressures of a fixed volunteer schedule; his mood
cycled to a mild mania followed by a major depression. Hal became unable to
function outside his home once again.

Hal gained weight and was often depressed during the following two years.
During that time he attended the weekly groups, and his goal became to focus
more directly on symptom management. He focused on learning more about
his mood symptoms, patterns, and stressors, and he made changes in his lifestyle. He created a highly structured routine of daily activity and sleep, a diet of
strictly nutritional foods, and weight management that included walking his
dog four to six times a day and joining and "working out" at a gym.

Hal experienced difficulty going to the gym. Each week he would come to
the group upset with himself for not following through. The group jointly recognized that there was an underlying barrier to reaching this step, or the step
was too advanced and needed modification. A group member suggested Hal

might benefit from adding a step to reaching his goal, to "take a walk through the gym." It worked. After completing that step, he was able to work out at the gym regularly. Whenever a medical illness or other issue interrupted his routine of working out at the gym, Hal would again face the challenge of reapproaching the gym and overcoming his anxiety. It sometimes took several weeks to get back on track.

Over the following two years, as Hal's condition stabilized and he learned to avoid stress that triggered mood instability, he and his provider coordinated a gradual taper of his medications, which he tolerated well. He is currently doing well, taking 1,500 mg of divalproex, 0.5 mg of risperidone, and 600 mg of lithium at bedtime, and 0.25 mg of clonazepam twice daily. His most recent major depressive episode was two years ago.

Comment. Hal's story illustrates the common situation of multiple psychiatric comorbidities complicating the course of bipolar disorder. In fact, Hal's panic and agoraphobic symptoms were arguably at least as disabling as his mania, depression, and psychosis. A thorough psychiatric review of systems is warranted in all assessments. Several guides exist that can assist the clinician in this type of screening process, even in such complicated cases (Bauer 2003).

Ted was a 62-year-old divorced man with bipolar disorder type II, obsessive-compulsive disorder, and alcohol dependence. He also had multiple medical problems: he'd had a heart attack and a coronary artery bypass graft with stent placement, and had hypertension, abdominal aortic aneurysm, hyperlipidemia, osteoarthritis with right knee replacement, and spinal stenosis. He walked slowly, with a cane.

Ted had two adult children who lived in Washington State, and aged parents who lived in a nearby town. He had a driver's license but did not drive. He was estranged from his children. He had restricted his communication with them to e-mail only. He discouraged visits from them because of his severe obsessions about their safety on aircraft. He had a system in place that blocked calls to his answering machine unless the caller knew a complex code to access the machine, which he set up because he chose to avoid calls from his mother. When Ted was a child, his mother's behavior had been unpredictable and verbally abusive, and he was hit by her car and suffered multiple fractures. They had never discussed the accident and he was never sure it was an accident.

Following his divorce, Ted did not have another close relationship. He had no friends, did not participate in Alcoholics Anonymous or other community-based groups, and lived a solitary life. He had been admitted multiple times to inpatient psychiatry for depression, alcohol dependence, and suicide attempts by impulsive overdose.

Ted was referred to the Bipolar Clinic and agreed to attend the Life Goals Program. This was a difficult decision, but he decided to give the group a try once he learned it was "low intensity" and he was not expected to share personal information unless he felt ready. He could also decide whether to continue attending or not. During Phase 1, Ted learned that he had rapid cycling and that his alcohol relapses were associated with mild mania. During the manic episodes he felt an initial euphoria that soon became more anxious, depressed, and paranoid, and he drank to relieve his symptoms. When Ted drank alcohol he became more impulsive and would take an overdose of his medication.

He projected a "harsh parent" image to his health care providers and avoided self-disclosure. During the group sessions Ted received consistent positive reinforcement from the therapist (a practice intrinsic to the Life Goals Program). He was assigned an individual therapist for time-limited therapy to enhance his ability to build relationships and decrease his interpersonal parent-child transactional paradigm. He slowly began sharing personal information with the group, as he observed other members build stability, participate in the management of their psychiatric symptoms, and set goals.

Ted began to realize that his estrangement from his adult children was self-imposed, and partially due to his behavior while intoxicated. He gradually spoke more openly about his alcoholism and received feedback from other group members with a history of alcoholism, with the suggestion to consider alcoholism treatment as a goal. He contemplated the potential benefits and disadvantages, and he elected to attend an six-week outpatient daily substance abuse program. He successfully completed the program and moved on to follow-up in substance abuse aftercare.

After periodic alcohol relapses and medication overdoses early in his treatment, Ted gradually learned more effective coping strategies for his symptoms and responded to the addition of low-dose antipsychotic and antidepressant medication. His relationships with his adult children grew closer. He talked during groups about his parents and his difficulty with his mother's inconsistent behavior toward him: at times she was happy to see him, and at other times verbally abusive and rejecting. Group members gave feedback that he was not responsible for her actions. During the subsequent year of participating in this comprehensive treatment plan, Ted achieved abstinence from alcohol. He changed his phone system and allowed direct calls to his message machine.

He set a goal to attend his daughter's wedding, but he was extremely anxious about navigating air travel, anxious that his plane would crash or he would not be able to walk through the air terminals. Multiple steps were organized for his travel goal. It was arranged that he would have low-dose benzodiazepines to manage his anxiety during the journey, and he arranged to have wheelchair service to escort him to the gates during his flight transfers. When he returned to the group, he talked about how good he had felt reuniting with his children and how he'd walked his daughter down the aisle to give her to the groom.

Ted terminated the sessions with his individual therapist and now maintains strict medication adherence, keeps scheduled group appointments, and is playing cribbage with a new friend. He recently purchased a car and, with a new sense of mastery over his alcohol dependence, when a friend recently called him in crisis at 2 a.m., he drove the friend to the emergency room for an admission for detoxification.

Comment. Ted's story illustrates the often neglected fact that psychodynamic issues can affect one's life — and one's participation in treatment — throughout the life cycle. This vignette also reflects the Life Goals Program approach of not delving psychodynamically but rather maintaining a nonjudgmental, behaviorally based approach. This nonprovocative, supportive stance has the benefit of providing a modicum of corrective emotional experience with a stable "object," the Life Goals Program therapist, which is usually enough to at least allow an individual to participate effectively in treatment of his or her other mental health issues.

SUMMARY: COMMON THEMES ON PSYCHOSOCIAL INTERVENTIONS FOR OLDER INDIVIDUALS WITH BIPOLAR DISORDER

These vignettes demonstrate several aspects of the biopsychosocial assessment and treatment of aging individuals with bipolar disorder. For example, the older population, perhaps even more than younger generations, was taught to think about mental illness and addictions as signs of weakness and that such symptoms are shaming and disgraceful. Assisting elderly persons to overcome the culture of psychiatric stigma and overreliance on a stoic coping style is a critical step toward educating them about bipolar disorder and engaging them in their treatment. For example,

George had a self-image tarnished by his psychiatric hospitalizations, divorce, and job loss. He became an active participant in psychoeducation, psychotherapy, and illness management, knowing his responsibilities and contributions to the treatment plan were confidential, valued, and respected and that the roles of the clinic staff in his treatment were well defined. Paul and Ted learned they were not alone and that addictions were a problem faced by many people.

For some (e.g., George), low-intensity approaches, including a focus on "psychoeducation" and "illness management" rather than "psychotherapy," may be essential to engage individuals whose cultural background makes them less accepting of explicitly mental health interventions. This approach may lead to an individual (e.g., Ted) eventually accepting needed psychotherapy, which would not have been acceptable initially.

Older individuals may have nontypical symptoms and often, at the very least, do not "speak the same language" as their providers, who are clinically trained and usually younger by a generation (or two). George could not identify with the term "depressed" during a major depressive episode. He did learn — and accept — that for him, what we refer to as depression he experienced as changes in appetite, sleep, energy, interest, and daily functioning. Treating bipolar disorder in elderly persons may require flexibility and some modifications in the terms used to describe their personal experience.

Moreover, psychiatric comorbidity, though less prevalent, does not disappear with age. Attention not only to substance abuse comorbidity but also to anxiety comorbidity (e.g., Hal and Ted) is essential to the successful treatment of older individuals with bipolar disorder.

As in younger persons, suicidality must be kept in mind when treating the elderly individual with bipolar disorder. Overall, the suicide attempt rate for individuals with bipolar disorder approaches 2% per year (Baldessarini et al. 2001). Put another way, of 50 individuals with bipolar disorder, 1 will attempt suicide within the next 12 months. Aging is also associated with additional, independent risk factors for suicide, including chronic illness and psychosocial loss. Chronic pain, a frequent co-traveler with age, can be systematically managed even within the psychiatric setting (Bauer 2003).

Aging individuals with bipolar disorder are often disconnected, lonely, and socially isolated. Many do not have family members living nearby, or they may be socially disconnected as a result of prior manic and depressive episodes. They may fear burdening the family and friends who are available, and may themselves be burdened by sick spouses or adult children who remain dependent on them. Notably, the aging population fears a loss of independence, institutionalization, and separation from familiar routines, people, and environments. Many underreport medical and psychiatric symptoms, for all of the reasons noted above. Addressing relationships with significant others, and where possible involving significant others directly in treatment, is of great importance for the elderly patient. There are often three generations of active (or silent) partners in care, increasing the complexity. For example, compare the cases of Paul, with his need to address his daughter's substance use disorder, and George, with his evolving relationship with his similarly aging companion Mary as they struggle to become co-caregivers for each other.

One of Freud's more enduring contributions was his response to the question, "What makes life worth living?" His response: "*Leiben und arbeiten,*" love and work. What, then, is "work" for elderly persons? Paid activities are often a thing of the past for people aged 65 or older. However, decades of sedentary, isolated activity are not likely to maximize quality of life. Creative approaches to alternative, life-enhancing work are essential. The case of Hal illustrates the persistence necessary on the part of both patients and clinicians in maximizing "work" function — for Hal, initially volunteer work and then regular gym "work."

Comorbid medical illnesses make assessment and treatment of bipolar disorder in elderly individuals more complex. As the population ages, skills in assessing and treating individuals with multiple illnesses are increasingly important. George had symptoms of depression, but his primary illness at one point was a urinary tract infection. Less astute clinicians might be ready to ascribe George's change in mental status to "dementia," whereas in reality he had a delirium, probably brought on in part by the interaction of medical and psychiatric medications. Moreover, for frail older persons, depression as a stand-alone illness may be fatal, as these individuals are likely to succumb more easily to fluid and electrolyte imbalance and other metabolic instability due to decreased fluid intake. For a person living in isolation, such dysregulation is likely to be more advanced before they get clinical attention. Given the complexities of psychotropic regimens for elderly patients and the increased potential for medical and psychiatric medication interactions, deft management is essential (see chapter 5 for more information on this topic). Assessment and treatment of elderly persons must include comprehensive collaboration among psychiatric and other medical care providers.

Why include such "medical" issues in a chapter on psychosocial interventions for bipolar disorder? As is well documented in numerous randomized controlled trials, psychosocial interventions — particularly collaborative chronic care models (CCMs) — are efficacious in improving outcomes for chronic medical illnesses such as diabetes and in managing multiple illnesses in frail elderly persons (Coleman et al. 1999; Diabetes Complications and Control 1993; Leveille et al. 1998; Rich et al.

1995; Stuck et al. 1995; Wagner et al. 2001). Such models have also proved useful in treating depression in primary care settings (Badamgarav et al. 2003; Sherbourne et al. 2001; Simon et al. 2001; Unützer et al. 2001).

The crux of CCMs, simply stated, is (1) to prepare patients to collaborate better in their own treatment by helping them improve their illness self-management skills, (2) to facilitate the flow of information to support evidence-based decision-making by providers, and (3) to redesign systems to enhance patients' access to and continuity of care (Von Korff et al. 1997; Wagner et al. 1996; on bipolar disorder specifically, see Bauer et al. 2006a; Simon et al. 2002). Evidence is beginning to accumulate that these models are also useful in treating bipolar disorder (Bauer et al. 1997, 2006b; Simon et al. 2006). CCMs for bipolar disorder serve as a central point for accessing specialized psychiatric care, treatment for substance abuse, and other medical care.

In general, navigating the complexities of the health care system can be overwhelming for elderly persons, and those who have chronic mental illnesses are particularly at risk for fragmented care and undertreatment, according to the President's New Freedom Commission (Hogan 2003). Continuity of care allows the health care professional to observe and intervene on behalf of patients with complex psychiatric and medical illness, and this may improve psychiatric stability and social, family, and medical outcomes, as well as decrease health care costs. Clearly, enhancing continuity of care was important in Paul's case, in which his decline in mental status was recognized to be acute and not chronic; that is, his clinician's longitudinal perspective led to the assessment that Paul was not at a new, more impaired baseline but rather experiencing a reversible delirium.

Yet, optimal responsivity and continuity of care can have little impact on outcome for any illness if the patient is not a willing and skilled collaborator in his or her own care. Psychoeducational interventions such as the Life Goals Program and others (Colom et al. 2003; Perry et al. 1999) give individuals an opportunity to learn about and become active in self-management of their bipolar disorder, as well as any comorbid psychiatric or medical disorders. As a person ages, these illness-management skills become more rather than less essential, and a comprehensive biopsychosocial approach by caregivers also becomes more important.

REFERENCES

Almeida, O., and Fenner, S. 2002. Bipolar disorder: similarities and differences between patients with illness onset before and after 65 years of age. *Int Psychogeriatr* 14:311–322.

Aubrey, J. M. 2001. *Thérapie de groupe pour le trouble bipolaire: un approche structurée.* Geneva: Editions Médecine et Hygiene.

Badamgarav, E., Weingarten, S. R., Henning, J. M., et al. 2003. Effectiveness of disease management programs in depression. *Am J Psychiatry* 160:2080–2090.

Baldessarini, R. J., Tondo, L., and Hennen, J. 2001. Treating the suicidal patient with bipolar disorder: reducing suicide risk with lithium. *Ann N Y Acad Sci* 932:24–43.

Bandura, A. 2001. Social cognitive theory: an agentic perspective. *Ann Rev Psychol* 52:1–26.

Bauer, M. S. 2001. The collaborative practice model for bipolar disorder: design and implementation in a multi-site randomized controlled trial. *Bipolar Disord* 3:233–244.

Bauer, M. S. 2003. Suicidality and assaultiveness. In *The field guide to psychiatric assessment and treatment* (pp. 55–66). Philadelphia: Lippincott Williams and Wilkins.

Bauer, M. S., and McBride, L. 1996. *Structured group psychotherapy for bipolar disorder: the Life Goals Program.* New York: Springer.

Bauer, M. S., and McBride, L. 2003. *Structured group psychotherapy for bipolar disorder: the Life Goals Program* (2nd ed.). New York: Springer.

Bauer, M. S., McBride, L., Shea, N., et al. 1997. Impact of an easy-access clinic-based program for bipolar disorder. *Psychiatr Serv* 48:491–496.

Bauer, M. S., McBride, L., Chase, C., et al. 1998. Manual-based group psychotherapy for bipolar disease: a feasibility study. *J Clin Psychiatry* 59:449–455.

Bauer, M. S., Williford, W. O., Dawson, E. E., et al. 2001. Principles of effectiveness trials and their implementation in VA Cooperative Study #430: "Reducing the Efficacy-Effectiveness Gap in Bipolar Disorder." *J Affect Disord* 67:61–78.

Bauer, M. S., McBride, L., Williford, W. O., et al. 2006a. Collaborative care for bipolar disorder: part I. Intervention and implementation in a randomized effectiveness trial. The CSP #430 Study Team. *Psychiatr Serv* 57:927–936.

Bauer, M. S., McBride, L., Williford, W. O., et al. 2006b. Collaborative care for bipolar disorder: part II. Impact on clinical outcome, function, and costs. The CSP #430 Study Team. *Psychiatr Serv* 57:937–945.

Coleman, E. A., Grothaus, L. C., Sandhu, N., et al. 1999. Chronic care clinics: a randomized controlled trial of a new model of primary care for frail older adults. *J Am Geriatr Soc* 47:908–909.

Colom, F., Vieta, E., Martinez-Aran, A., et al. 2003. A randomized trial on the efficacy of group psychoeducation in the prophylaxis of recurrences in bipolar patients whose disease is in remission. *Arch Gen Psychiatry* 60:402–407.

Depp, C. A., and Jeste, D. V. 2004. Bipolar disorder in older adults: a critical review. *Bipolar Disord* 6:343–367.

Diabetes Complications and Control Trial Research Group (DCCT). 1993. The effect of intensive treatment of diabetes on the development and progression of long-term complication in insulin-dependent diabetes mellitus. *N Engl J Med* 329:977–986.

Engel, G. L. 1977. The need for a new medical model: a challenge for biomedicine. *Science* 196:129–136.

Fenn, H. H., Bauer, M. S., Altshuler, L., et al. 2005. Medical comorbidity and health-related quality of life in bipolar disorder across the adult age span. *J Affect Disord* 86:47–60.

Friedman, J. I., Harvey, P. D., McGurk, S. R., et al. 2002. Correlates of change in functional status of institutionalized geriatric schizophrenic patients: focus on medical morbidity. *Am J Psychiatry* 159:1388–1394.

Hays, J., Krishnan, K., George, L. et al., 1998. Age at first onset of bipolar disorder: demographic, family history, and psychosocial correlates. *Depress Anxiety* 7:76–82.

Hogan, M. F. 2003. The President's New Freedom Commission: recommendations to transform mental health care in America. *Psychiatr Serv* 54:1467–1474.

Keller, M., Lavori, P., Klerman, G., et al. 1986. Low levels and lack of predictors of somatotherapy and psychotherapy received by depressed patients. *Arch Gen Psychiatry* 43:458–466.

Kilbourne, A. M., Cornelius, J. R., Han, X., et al. 2004. Burden of general medical conditions among individuals with bipolar disorder. *Bipolar Disord* 6:386–373.

Leveille, S. G., Wagner, E. H., Davis, C., et al. 1998. Preventing disability and managing chronic illness in frail older adults: a randomized trial of a community-based partnership with primary care. *Am Geriatr Soc* 46:1191–1198.

Miller, W. R., and Rollnick, S. 2002. *Motivational interviewing: preparing people for change* (2nd ed.). New York: Guilford Press.

Otto, M. W., Reilly-Harrington, N., and Sachs, G. S. 2003. Psychoeducational and cognitive-behavioral strategies in the management of bipolar disorder. *J Affect Disord* 73:171–181.

Perry, A., Tarrier, N., Morriss, R., et al. 1999. Randomised controlled trial of efficacy of teaching patients with bipolar disorder to identify early symptoms of relapse and obtain treatment. *BMJ* 318:149–153.

Rich, M. W., Beckham, V., Wittenberg, C., et al. 1995. A multidisciplinary intervention to prevent the readmission of elderly patients with congestive heart failure. *N Engl J Med* 333:1130–1195.

Sajatovic, M., Popli, A., and Semple, W. 1996. Ten year use of hospital based services by geriatric veterans with schizophrenia and bipolar disorder. *Psychiatr Serv* 47:961–965.

Sajatovic, M., Blow, F. C., Ignacio, R. V., et al. 2004. Age-related modifiers of clinical presentation and health service use among veterans with bipolar disorder. *Psychiatr Serv* 55:1014–1021.

Sajatovic, M., Blow, F. C., Ignacio, R. V., et al. 2005. New-onset bipolar disorder in later life. *Am J Geriatr Psychiatr* 13:282–289.

Sciolla, A., Patterson, T. L., Wetherell, J. L., et al. 2003. Functioning and well-being of middle-aged and older patients with schizophrenia. *Am J Geriatr Psychiatry* 11:629–637.

Sherbourne, C. D., Wells, K. B., Duan, N., et al. 2001. Long-term effectiveness of disseminating quality improvement for depression in primary care. *Arch Gen Psychiatry* 58:696–703.

Simon, G. E., Katon, W. J., Von Korff, M., et al. 2001. Cost-effectiveness of a collaborative care program for primary care patients with persistent depression. *Am J Psychiatry* 158:1638–1644.

Simon, G. E., Ludman, E. J., Unützer, J., et al. 2002. Design and implementation of a randomized trial evaluating systematic care for bipolar disorder. *Bipolar Disord* 4:226–236.

Simon, G. E., Ludman, E. J., Bauer, M. S., et al. 2006. Long-term effectiveness and cost of a systematic care management program for bipolar disorder. *Arch Gen Psychiatry* 63:500–508.

Stone, K. Mania in the elderly. 1989. *Br J Psychiatry* 55:220–224.

Stuck, A. E., Aronow, H. U., Steiner, A., et al. 1995. A trial of annual in-home comprehensive geriatric assessments for elderly people living in the community. *N Engl J Med* 333:1184–1190.

Tohen, M., Shulman, K., and Satlin, A. 1994. First-episode mania in late-life. *Am J Psychiatry* 150:130–132.

Unützer, J., Rubenstein, L., Katon, W. J., et al. 2001. Two-year effects of quality improvement programs on medication management for depression. *Arch Gen Psychiatry* 58:935–942.

Vaillant, G. E., and Mukamal, K. 2001. Successful aging. *Am J Psychiatry* 158:839–847.

Von Korff, M., Gruman, J., Schaefer, J., et al. 1997. Collaborative management of chronic illness. *Ann Intern Med* 127:1097–1102.

Wagner, E. H., Austin, B. T., and Von Korff, M. 1996. Organizing care for patients with chronic illness. *Milbank Q* 74:511–544.

Wagner, E. H., Grothaus, L. C., Sandhu, N., et al. 2001. Chronic care clinics for diabetes in primary care. *Diabetes Care* 25:695–700.

Ware, J., Kosinksi, J., and Keller, S. D. 1994. *SF-36 physical and mental health summary scales: a user's manual.* Boston: Health Institute, New England Medical Center.

Wylie, M., Mulsant, B., Pollock, B., et al. 1999. Age at onset in geriatric bipolar disorder. *Am J Geriatr Psychiatry* 7:77–83.

Yatham, L. N., and Kennedy, S. H. 2005. Canadian Mood and Anxiety Network (CANMAT) guidelines for the management of patients with bipolar disorder: consensus, controversies, and international commentaries. *Bipolar Disord* 7(suppl. 3):1–88.

Zingmond, D. S., Kilbourne, A. M., Justice, A. C., et al. 2003. Differences in symptom expression in older HIV-positive patients: the veterans aging cohort 3 site study and HIV cost and service utilization study experience. *J Acquir Immune Defic Syndr* 33:84–92.

CHAPTER SEVEN

Adherence to Treatment

A *Life-Course Perspective*

MARCIA VALENSTEIN, M.D.,

AND MARTHA SAJATOVIC, M.D.

A cornerstone of medical treatment for bipolar disorder is mood-stabilizing medication. Mood stabilizers have been defined as medications that decrease the duration, frequency, or severity of at least one phase of bipolar disorder without adversely affecting other phases (Calabrese et al. 2002). Regular use of mood-stabilizing medications, in conjunction with psychosocial interventions, allows many individuals with bipolar disorder to have fewer and less-severe acute mood episodes, fewer subthreshold symptoms, and fewer relapses into new episodes of depression or mania. Current practice guidelines recommend the long-term use of mood stabilizers for persons with bipolar I disorder (American Psychiatric Association 2002).

Lithium has long been a cornerstone of pharmacological treatment for bipolar disorder (Burgess et al. 2001; Geddes et al. 2004). However, in the last few decades, medications used to control seizure disorders, such as valproate/divalproex, carbamazepine, and lamotrigine, have also become widely used to control symptoms of bipolar disorder (American Psychiatric Association 2002; Keck 2004). For many patient populations, valproate now is prescribed more commonly than lithium (Blow et al. 2006; Goodwin et al. 2003).

Many second-generation antipsychotic compounds have also received approval for the treatment of specific phases of bipolar disorder. The U.S. Food and Drug Administration (2005) has approved all second-generation antipsychotic agents for the treatment of mania and has also approved aripiprazole and olanzapine for maintenance treatment of bipolar disorder. Other atypical antipsychotics will probably soon gain FDA approval for additional phases of bipolar disorder.

Many individuals with bipolar disorder receive several mood-stabilizing medications concurrently to control their symptoms, with polytherapy now considered an important treatment approach for individuals who still have symptoms when receiving monotherapy (Keck 2004; Keck and McElroy 2002).

However, while the expansion of treatment options for persons with bipolar disorder offers the potential for improving outcomes, a growing body of literature suggests that nonadherence to prescribed treatments is widespread (Colom et al. 2000; Greenhouse et al. 2000; Johnson and McFarland 1996; Keck et al. 1997; Lingam and Scott 2002; Perlick et al. 2004; Scott and Pope 2002a; Svarstad et al. 2001). As a result, many patients with bipolar disorder treated in the community do not enjoy the full benefits of their prescribed mood-stabilizing medications.

BIPOLAR DISORDER AND ADHERENCE TO TREATMENT: REVIEW OF STUDIES

Numerous studies have examined adherence to lithium medication regimens among persons with bipolar disorder (Connelly et al. 1982; Johnson and McFarland 1996; Licht et al. 2001; Maarbjerg et al. 1988; Schumann et al. 1999). Several groups of investigators have also examined adherence among individuals taking anticonvulsant medications and those taking a variety of mood-stabilizing medications (Colom et al. 2000; Keck et al. 1997; Li et al. 2002). According to these studies, approximately 20%–70% of patients adhere poorly to medication regimens (Colom et al. 2000; Connelly 1984; Keck et al. 1997; Licht et al. 2001; Lingam and Scott 2002; Perlick et al. 2004). Johnson and McFarland (1996) reported that for 1,594 patients receiving lithium in a large health maintenance organization, pharmacy data indicated that, on average, they had medication coverage for only 32% of observed days. The median duration of continuous lithium use was 72 days.

In an analysis of California Medicaid claims, Li and colleagues (2002) also found very low rates of continuous use of mood stabilizers by persons with bipolar disorder. In two reviews of adherence among individuals taking a variety of medications for bipolar disorder, Lingham and Scott (2002) and Perlick and colleagues (2004) found median rates of nonadherence of 41% and 42%, respectively. These figures are similar to the median rates of poor adherence noted by Cramer and Rosenheck (1998) in their review of studies examining adherence to antipsychotic medications (42%) but somewhat higher than the median rates of poor adherence among individuals taking antidepressants (35%) or medications for chronic medical (nonpsychiatric) disorders (24%). Estimates of poor adherence among persons with bipolar disorder are also substantially higher than the median rate of poor adherence (25%) reported for individuals with chronic medical disorders in a large-scale review by DiMatteo (2004). The authors noted that adherence to prescribed medications among persons with nonpsychiatric chronic illnesses seemed to be improving over time; however, to date, few studies have indicated that adherence is improving among persons with mood disorders. Blow and colleagues (2006) have reported modest increases in rates of adherence among persons with schizophrenia between 2000 and 2005, during a time when many were switched from first- to second-generation antipsychotics.

Poor adherence to mood-stabilizing medication treatments has been associated with adverse clinical outcomes for patients with bipolar disorder. Colom and colleagues (2000) found that in a two-year follow-up of 200 patients with bipolar disorder, those who adhered to medication regimens had fewer psychiatric hospitalizations. Scott and Pope (2000b) reported that among 98 patients with mood disorders, rates of hospitalization were significantly lower for those who were fully adherent and whose mood stabilizers were at therapeutic blood levels than for partially adherent patients with subtherapeutic levels. A study by Johnson and McFarland (1996) found that discontinuation of lithium use among patients in a large health maintenance organization was associated with increased rates of psychiatric hospitalization and use of psychiatric emergency services.

Determinants of Adherence to Medication Regimens

Adherence to prescribed medication use is a multidetermined, complex phenomenon and is influenced by a number of illness, patient, provider, and system-level factors (Aagaard and Vestergaard 1990; Aagaard et al. 1988; Coldham et al. 2002; Colom et al. 2000; Maarbjerg et al. 1988; Miklowitz 1992). Demographic factors that seem to be associated with adherence in bipolar disorder include patient's age, marital status, gender, and educational level (Aagaard et al. 1988; Berk et al. 2004; Lingam and Scott 2002). Most studies indicate that individuals who are younger, unmarried, male, and with fewer years of education are more likely to adhere poorly to mood-stabilizing medication treatments (Connelly 1984; Keck et al. 1997; Maarbjerg et al. 1988). Levels and types of psychiatric symptoms are also associated with treatment adherence (Keck et al. 1996; Nose et al. 2003). Persons with earlier onset of the disorder are noted to have more difficulties with adherence (Aagaard et al. 1988).

Concurrent substance abuse and comorbid psychiatric disorders seem to strongly influence adherence to treatment (Aagaard and Vestergaard 1990; Keck et al. 1997; Perlick et al. 2004). Several groups of investigators have noted that concurrent substance use disorders are associated with poorer adherence (Keck et al. 1997; Maarb-jerg et al. 1988; Perlick et al. 2004; K. A. Weiss et al. 2002; R. D. Weiss et al. 1998). Unfortunately, substance abuse is common among individuals with bipolar disorder, with prevalence rates much higher than those observed in the general population. Approximately 40% of people with bipolar disorder meet the criteria for alcohol de-pendence (American Psychiatric Association 2002). R. D. Weiss and colleagues (1998) reported that more than 14% of individuals with bipolar disorder gave "want-ing to take drugs or alcohol" as an explanation for treatment nonadherence. Other studies have reported that comorbid personality disorders are associated with poorer adherence among persons with bipolar disorder (Colom et al. 2000; Maarbjerg et al. 1988; Perlick et al. 2004).

Treatment factors such as medication side effects or tolerability may affect ad-herence. Some studies have noted that poorer adherence is associated with a higher reported side-effect burden from medications (Maarbjerg et al. 1988), although other studies find no relation between poor adherence and reported medication side ef-fects (Connelly et al. 1982; Lingam and Scott 2002). A few investigators suggest that individuals may be less likely to adhere to lithium than valproate treatment (R. D. Weiss et al. 1998). However, other investigators have found no differences in adher-ence among individuals with bipolar disorder treated with a variety of mood-stabilizing agents (Colom et al. 2000).

Other treatment and environmental factors, such as psychosocial support, access to care, and the complexity of the medication regimen, are reported to be associated with adherence to medication regimens (Colom et al. 2000; Frank et al. 1985; Maarb-jerg et al. 1988; Miklowitz 1992; Schumann et al. 1999). Some investigators suggest that use of multiple agents to stabilize mood is associated with poorer adherence (Keck et al. 1996; R. D. Weiss et al. 1998). Other researchers have not found increased rates of poor adherence to polytherapy (Danion et al. 1987). A recent report noted that higher treatment intensity (more classes of medication in the treatment regi-men) is associated with *better* treatment adherence (Sajatovic et al. 2006).

Models of health behaviors that focus on proximal determinants of treatment ad-herence — such as the Health Belief Model, Health Decision Model, Theory of Planned Behavior, and Protection Motivation Theory — note the influence of the above factors on patients' perceptions of their susceptibility to the illness, the sever-ity of their illness, the benefits of treatment, and the costs of treatment (side effects, time, monetary outlay). These beliefs, in turn, influence adherence behaviors (Flay and Petraitis 1994; Leventhal and Cameron 1987). The importance of family support and of "cues to action" is also recognized in these models (Becker 1990; Madden and

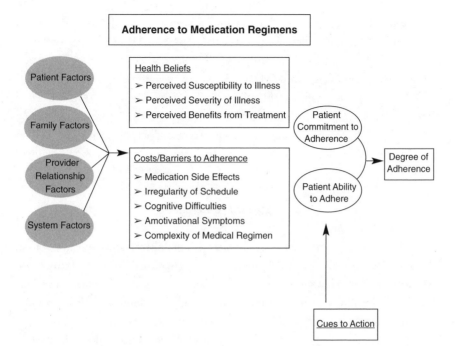

Fig. 7.1. Factors affecting adherence to medication regimens.

Ellen 1992). Figure 7.1 summarizes the interaction of factors involved in adherence to medication regimens.

Although there are likely to be special considerations in schizophrenia and bipolar disorder, medication adherence among persons with these illnesses seems to be affected by many of the same factors that affect adherence by individuals with other types of illness (Adams and Scott 2000; Budd et al. 1996). Several studies have demonstrated that the constructs included in the Health Belief Model predict medication adherence among patients with a variety of serious mental disorders, including schizophrenia and bipolar disorder (Adams and Scott 2000; Budd et al. 1996; Coldham et al. 2002; Corrigan et al. 1990; Cuffel et al. 1996; Owen et al. 1996; Scott 2002). Adams and Scott (2000) reported that for 39 patients with a variety of serious mental illnesses, including affective disorders and schizophrenia, constructs of the Health Belief Model predicted 43% of the variance in adherence to medication treatment. Patients who were highly adherent perceived their illnesses to be more severe and perceived the benefits of treatment to be greater than did those with poorer adherence. In a study by Coldham and colleagues (2002) of patients experiencing a first episode of psychosis, those with little insight into their illness were more likely to be poorly adherent to treatment. Connelly (1984) found that among patients treated with lithium, adherence was negatively associated with the perceived costs of treatment. In a series of 32 patients with bipolar disorder, Greenhouse and colleagues (2000) found that those who minimized the severity of their illness were least likely to adhere to treatment. Finally, Kleindienst and Greil (2004) reported that among 171 patients with bipolar disorder receiving maintenance treatment over 2.5 years, those who received lithium were more likely to adhere to treatment if they had "greater trust" in the medication and fewer negative expectations about the treatment.

Age and Adherence

Most studies indicate that older persons are more likely than younger persons to adhere to mood-stabilizing medication regimens (Berk et al. 2004). The reasons for this are unclear. A lower prevalence of substance abuse may play a role. There may also be a "healthy survivor" effect, with treatment-adherent individuals being more likely to survive to old age. Few studies have explicitly examined whether demographic or clinical factors have differential effects on adherence among older versus younger individuals.

ADHERENCE STUDIES AT THE SERIOUS MENTAL ILLNESS TREATMENT RESEARCH AND EVALUATION CENTER

Our investigative team has evaluated adherence to several mood-stabilizing medications among U.S. Department of Veterans Affairs (VA) patients with bipolar disorder, including those treated with the second-generation antipsychotic medications, lithium, and anticonvulsant medications.

Data for these studies are from the VA National Psychosis Registry (NPR), which is maintained by the Serious Mental Illness Treatment Research and Evaluation Center (SMITREC) in Ann Arbor, Michigan. The NPR is compiled from annual extracts from several VA administrative databases, including the National Patient Care Database and the VA Pharmacy Benefits Management Strategic Healthcare Group database. The NPR includes records for all patients who have received a diagnosis indicating a psychotic disorder, including bipolar disorder, at any time during inpatient stays from fiscal year (FY) 1988 onward or during outpatient visits from FY 1997 onward. (A full description of the NPR is available at www.va.gov/annarbor-hsrd.)

For our studies on medication adherence among patients with bipolar disorder, we identified patients in the NPR who received VA treatment during FY 2003 and had International Classification of Diseases–Ninth Revision (ICD-9) diagnoses of 296.0 (bipolar manic, single episode), 296.1 (manic disorder, recurrent episode), 296.4 (bipolar manic/hypomanic), 296.5 (bipolar I depressed), 296.6 (bipolar I mixed), or 296.7 (bipolar I unspecified) during the majority of clinical encounters resulting in diagnoses indicating psychotic disorders. The total sample size for these studies was 73,964 patients.

We measured adherence to treatment by using the medication possession ratio (MPR), the ratio of "number of days' supply of the medication that a patient has received" to "number of days' supply of the medication that would be needed for continuous outpatient use." We and other investigative teams have used the MPR successfully in previous studies of adherence to antipsychotic medication regimens by persons with schizophrenia (Gilmer et al. 2004; Valenstein et al. 2002; Weiden et al. 2004). An MPR of 1, or 100%, indicates that the patient has received all medications needed to take the medication as prescribed; an MPR of 0.5, or 50%, indicates that the patient has received medications sufficient to take only half of the prescribed dose.

In the first of two studies of medication adherence among patients with bipolar disorder, we calculated the MPR for those receiving antipsychotic medications. In the second study, we calculated MPRs for patients receiving lithium or anticonvulsant medications. The MPR was calculated for FY 2003 (October 1, 2002, through September 30, 2003), using the days following patients' first prescription for the specified medication during the year. MPR calculations included only those patients with 90 or more days of observation during the fiscal year. Days spent in institutional settings following the first prescription fill were subtracted from the "number of days' supply of the medication that would be needed for continuous outpatient use." In cases where an individual was taking more than one anticonvulsant medication, or both lithium and an anticonvulsant medication, the average MPR was calculated for the two drugs. Patients who received three or more mood-stabilizing medications during the year were excluded from the MPR calculations.

The patients were categorized into three clinical groups based on their MPRs: patients with MPRs ≥ 0.80 were considered fully adherent to the specified medication; those with MPRs of 0.50–0.80, partially adherent; and those with MPRs < 0.50, nonadherent (i.e., nonadherence means using less than half the medication needed for continuous use). Several previous investigative groups have categorized adherence to treatment by individuals with serious mental illness in a similar manner (Gilmer et al. 2004; Svarstad et al. 2001).

Statistical analysis. In both studies, descriptive statistics were used to characterize patients' demographic and clinical characteristics and the overall prevalence of poor adherence to the specified mood-stabilizing agents. Bivariate and multivariate analyses were used to compare patients prescribed and not prescribed lithium, anticonvulsant medications, and antipsychotic medications. Bivariate and multivariate analyses were also used to evaluate patients' characteristics associated with poor adherence. In these multivariate analyses, patients' gender, age, race/ethnicity, marital status, type of bipolar disorder, and presence/absence of substance abuse, comorbid post-traumatic stress disorder (PTSD), and homelessness were included as covariates in the models. Finally, we used multivariate regression analyses to examine the relation between psychiatric hospitalization and good adherence to treatment, adjusting for other patient factors.

FINDINGS FROM THE ADHERENCE STUDIES AT SMITREC

In our large, naturalistic studies examining pharmacy data for more than 70,000 patients, we found that poor adherence to prescribed mood-stabilizing medications was a major issue for nearly half of the individuals with bipolar disorder. While the slight majority (54.1%) of individuals fully adhered to lithium or anticonvulsant use, a substantial proportion were only partially adherent (24.5%) or nonadherent (21.4%). Likewise, for individuals prescribed antipsychotic medications, 52% were fully adherent, 21% were partially adherent, and 27% were nonadherent.

Our results reinforce previous smaller studies indicating that poor adherence is a major problem in translating the demonstrated efficacy of mood-stabilizing medications into effective treatments for persons with bipolar disorder in the community. As in most, but not all, previous studies, our results also reveal few differences in rates of adherence across the various mood stabilizers. The mean MPRs for lithium, carbamazepine, valproate, lamotrigine, and the second-generation antipsychotic medications ranged between 0.75 and 0.84. Thus, the general side-effect profiles of these specific medications seem to make little difference in clinical settings, where clinicians and patients work to find a medication that is most tolerable for the individual.

Congruent with previous studies, we also found that demographic factors such as age, marital status, and race/ethnicity were associated with adherence to medication regimens. Younger, unmarried, nonwhite individuals had poorer adherence to prescribed mood-stabilizing medications. Among patients with bipolar disorder who were receiving antipsychotic medications, African Americans had an odds ratio (OR) of 0.58 for adherence compared with whites; younger individuals had an OR of 0.77 compared with older individuals. Clinical factors, such as comorbid substance abuse, were also associated with poorer adherence. Those with a diagnosis of co-morbid substance abuse had an OR of 0.76 for adherence to antipsychotic compared with those without this diagnosis.

Like previous studies, our study also found that in bivariate analyses, full adherence to use of antipsychotic medications and anticonvulsants was associated with reduced rates of hospitalization. However, in multivariate analyses that included other important factors in the model, such as substance abuse, homelessness, and previous psychiatric hospitalization, better adherence was *not* substantially associated with the likelihood of psychiatric admission. Compared with nonadherent patients, those who fully adhered to antipsychotic medication regimens had an OR of 1.0 for psychiatric admission, and those who fully adhered to anticonvulsants had an OR of 1.1. In contrast, substance abuse, homelessness, and preexisting psychiatric severity were strongly associated with psychiatric admission, with ORs of approximately 4.0, 2.2, and 3.5, respectively, in these models. These findings suggest that among individuals with bipolar disorder, the relation between poor adherence and increased rates of hospitalization may be mediated through greater long-term illness severity and/or higher levels of substance abuse.

Treatment Adherence across the Lifespan

In the study sample, there were differences both in the types of medication prescribed to older individuals and in levels of adherence to the prescribed medications. Older individuals were more likely than younger individuals to be prescribed lithium and less likely to be prescribed an antipsychotic or anticonvulsant medication. These differences in use of alternative mood stabilizers may be due to secular prescribing patterns. In recent years, for patients with newly diagnosed bipolar disorder or with new affective episodes, physicians have prescribed mood-stabilizing medications other than lithium. Because older patients have often been in treatment for longer periods than younger patients, they are more likely to have received a lithium trial at some point in their treatment, and responders to lithium may have continued with this medication.

Older patients in our study sample were also more likely than younger patients to be fully and partially adherent to treatment across all mood-stabilizing medications. Approximately 62% of older patients fully adhered to prescribed antipsychotic medication, 19% were partially adherent, and 19% were nonadherent. Similarly, 64% fully adhered to lithium and anticonvulsant treatment, 23% were partially adherent, and 13% were nonadherent.

Interestingly, the smallest difference in adherence between older patients and younger patients was among those taking lithium. Adjusting for race/ethnicity, marital status, type of bipolar disorder, previous psychiatric hospitalization, and concurrent substance abuse or PTSD, patients aged 65 years or older had an OR of 1.3 for adherence to prescribed antipsychotic medications compared with younger patients, an OR of 1.4 for adherence to anticonvulsant medications, and an OR of 1.1 for adherence to lithium.

We examined several interactions to determine whether adherence among older versus younger patients was differentially affected by race/ethnicity, marital status, previous psychiatric hospitalization, or concurrent substance abuse. For the most part, these interactions were nonsignificant, suggesting that demographic and clinical factors have similar associations with adherence across age groups. Thus, for example, concurrent substance abuse was associated with similar decreases in observed adherence among older and younger patients. However, among patients taking antipsychotic medications, the race/ethnicity and age group interaction was significant ($p = .003$). This indicates that being in the older age group (=65 years) was associated with greater increases in adherence to antipsychotic treatment among African American than among white patients.

Health Beliefs and Medication Attitudes among Older and Younger Persons with Bipolar Disorder

In a third study, we examined potential differences in health beliefs and attitudes toward medications among older and younger individuals with serious mental illness and poor adherence to antipsychotic medications (n = 125; 88 with schizophrenia, 37 with bipolar disorder) (M. Valenstein et al., unpublished data). Patients were included in this study if their pharmacy data indicated an MPR < 0.80 for prescribed antipsychotic medication in the previous 12 months and their physician indicated the individual was receiving long-term antipsychotic treatment.

At enrollment, all participants completed the Health Belief Questionnaire (HBQ), the Ratings of Medication Influence (ROMI), the Awareness of Illness (AOI) questionnaire, and the Weschler Memory Scale III (WMS-III), Logical Memory and Family Pictures subscales.

The HBQ is designed to measure patients' beliefs about their illness and treatment, and includes four subscales that measure perceptions about susceptibility to the illness, severity of illness, benefits of treatment, and costs of treatment. The ROMI is a multidimensional instrument with subscales that measure factors possibly influencing patients' adherence or nonadherence to medication regimens. These subscales measure concerns and beliefs about preventing the illness, the influence of significant others on promoting adherence to treatment, positive attitudes toward the medications, denial or dysphoria about the medication or illness, logistical problems in taking the medication, rejection of the illness label, family influences that impede adherence, and a negative therapeutic alliance. The AOI measures patients' insight about psychiatric illness, using a summary score derived from an eight-item interviewer-administered questionnaire. The interviewer asks questions related to several dimensions of insight, including patients' beliefs about the nature of their illness and the helpfulness of their medications. The interviewer-rater then uses the instrument's anchors to rate the responses on a reverse five-point scale, from most to least insight. Finally, the WMS-III Logical Memory and Family Pictures subscales measure the retention and recall of auditory and visual material.

In multivariate analyses adjusting for age, race/ethnicity, and substance abuse, we found no significant differences between individuals with bipolar disorder and those with schizophrenia in their health beliefs as measured by the HBQ or insight into their illness as measured by the AOI scale. There were also no significant differences on the subscales of the ROMI. Finally, we found no significant differences on the WMS-III subscales, measuring new learning and ability to recall complex, meaningful conceptual material presented in the auditory and visual modalities. These findings suggest that among patients with serious mental illness and poor medication adherence, there are few differences in health beliefs or attitudes toward medications by diagnostic group (schizophrenia or bipolar disorder).

In multivariate analyses examining differences between older (≥ 60 years) and younger patients on these scales, we found that older individuals perceived themselves as less susceptible to becoming ill ($p = .02$) on the HBQ than did younger individuals. On the ROMI, older patients scored significantly lower on the denial subscale ($p < .03$), which assesses denial of illness or helpfulness of medications, and they showed a trend ($p = .09$) toward more positive attitudes about medication. Older patients also showed a nonsignificant trend ($p = .08$) toward less insight about their illness on the AOI scale. The WMS-III results showed a nonsignificant difference in cognitive abilities between patients in the older and younger age groups.

These findings suggest that older patients with poor adherence to medication regimens may be less likely than younger patients to believe they are more susceptible to an illness episode but more likely to have less insight about their illness. Clinicians attempting to improve adherence to treatment may need to pay particular attention to these issues when working with older individuals.

MONITORING AND IMPROVING ADHERENCE TO TREATMENT

The data from our study and from previous studies indicate that clinicians must remain alert for and vigorously address poor adherence to medication regimens by patients with bipolar disorder. To successfully accomplish this, strategies and systems for monitoring adherence must be in place, in addition to intervention strategies to improve adherence.

Monitoring Adherence

Although clinicians have been repeatedly advised about the high prevalence of poor adherence to medication regimens and have become increasingly concerned about this problem, detecting poor adherence and intervening to improve it remain challenging. Patients may fail to report poor adherence, and clinicians may fail to recognize when patients take their medications intermittently or not at all. To improve detection, clinicians may wish to make frequent nonjudgmental inquires about medication use, see patients at risk for poor adherence more frequently, and work with family members to detect cessation of medications as soon as possible. If measures of serum levels are available (e.g., for lithium, valproate, carbamazepine), regular serum level monitoring may be appropriate clinically and also helpful in evaluating adherence. While there is no established "gold standard" for measuring adherence to treatment for bipolar disorder, a mixed methodology that combines selected measures (self-report, family report, serum levels, selective use of rating scales) is most likely to provide the most accurate assessment of adherence among this group of patients (Colom and Vieta 2002; Colom et al. 2003; Lam et al. 2003).

Given the limits to individual clinicians' time and ability to detect poor adherence, however, organizational approaches to monitoring adherence may also be needed. One approach is to use organizational pharmacy data to monitor adherence. Many patients with serious mental illness are enrolling in managed Medicaid or Medicare programs (Essock and Goldman 1995). These organizations — and the other public sector organizations that have traditionally cared for patients with serious mental illness, such as the Veterans Health Administration (VHA) and community mental health organizations — now have access to comprehensive pharmacy data and sophisticated information systems. In previous work, we have shown that these data and information systems could be used to assist clinicians in identifying patients with poor adherence to medication regimens (Valenstein et al. 2002).

Systematically reviewing pharmacy data may be one of the few practical approaches for monitoring adherence to treatment for large patient populations. This procedure is less costly and intrusive than other methods, such as pill counts, medication blood levels, or electronic monitoring devices (e.g., MEMS-4; Aprex, division of Aardex, Union City, CA) (Farmer 1999; Steiner and Prochazka 1997). Poor adherence as determined through review of pharmacy data has been associated with important intermediate outcomes for patients with hypertension and epilepsy (Steiner and Prochazka 1997; Steiner et al. 1988). Pharmacy data indicating poor adherence are also strongly associated with psychiatric hospitalization among both VA and Medicaid patients with schizophrenia (Gilmer et al. 2004; Svarstad et al. 2001; Valenstein et al. 2002; Weiden et al. 2004). In our VA studies, individuals with schizophrenia who adhered poorly to medication regimens were 2.4 times more likely to be hospitalized during the year than those with better adherence, and they also had longer hospital stays once admitted (Valenstein et al. 2002). Similar levels of risk have been noted for Medicaid patients with schizophrenia in subsequent studies (Gilmer et al. 2004; Weiden et al. 2004).

Unlike other studies (Johnson and McFarland 1996; Svarstad et al. 2001), we did not find that pharmacy data indicating poorer adherence to prescribed medication were associated with increased rates of hospitalization for patients with bipolar disorder, when other important factors, such as substance abuse, homelessness, and previous psychiatric hospitalization, were included in the model. This suggests that the effects of poor adherence on hospitalization for individuals with bipolar disorder may be mediated through longer-term illness severity and higher levels of substance abuse.

Currently, few health systems are using their extensive pharmacy data to systematically identify poor adherence among patients with schizophrenia or bipolar disorder. Further efforts must be made to use such data to identify these at-risk patients and begin efforts to intervene to improve adherence.

Interventions to Improve Adherence

Once patients have been identified as having poor adherence to medication regimens, targeted interventions are needed to improve adherence and reduce the risks of adverse outcomes. These interventions may include specific psychosocial interventions, increased levels of observation, and alternative methods for drug delivery. For a variety of medical disorders, simple didactic approaches are not as successful as more individualized, multicomponent, behavioral, and family interventions in improving patients' adherence to treatment (Fenton et al. 1997; Haynes et al. 1996). This may also be true for persons with bipolar disorder.

Researchers have studied the effectiveness of several individual and family interventions for improving adherence to treatment for bipolar disorder. Evidence is emerging that cognitive-behavioral therapies (CBTs), social rhythm therapy, and interpersonal therapy may improve both adherence and symptom management among these patients (Craighead and Miklowitz 2000). Kelly and Scott (1990) reported that among psychiatric outpatients, an intervention that engaged significant others as active participants in patients' aftercare and an intervention that trained patients to become more active participants in their health care increased adherence to medication. Kemp and colleagues (1998) found in a small controlled trial (N = 74) that inpatients with psychosis who underwent compliance therapy (a group-based CBT) had increased adherence to medication regimens in the 18 months following inpatient admission. According to Scott (2001), difficulties with adherence to prescribed medication among patients with bipolar disorder may be tackled via an exploration of barriers to adherence and by using cognitive and behavioral techniques to enhance adherence (e.g., challenging automatic thoughts about medications). More recent studies in the literature on bipolar disorder use standardized or manual-driven psychoeducational interventions, with specific formats and goals that may potentially be replicated in other treatment settings (Craighead and Miklowitz 2000).

Several of these psychosocial interventions require specialized training of therapists (in CBT and motivational techniques) and may require frequent visits by patients and/or their family members, making dissemination potentially challenging in many mental health systems. These systems will need to make concerted efforts to train their clinicians and find efficient ways to deliver the key components of these interventions.

Other approaches to improving adherence to treatment among patients with bipolar disorder include alternative methods of drug delivery, such as depot medication injections or implantable devices. With the recent FDA approvals of second-generation agents for the treatment of bipolar disorder, depot antipsychotic medications may become an important treatment option for individuals with bipolar disorder, as they have long been for those with schizophrenia. Currently, only one second-generation agent is available as a depot preparation, but additional depot preparations are in development. Depot antipsychotic medications are usually injected every few weeks, eliminating the need for daily oral doses and preventing *covert* noncompliance. Patients who fail to appear for their scheduled injections are readily identified, and early outreach efforts can then be initiated. The preponderance of research evidence suggests that depot medications increase compliance and reduce relapse among patients with schizophrenia (Lehman and Steinwachs 1998);

studies on the effectiveness of depot antipsychotics for patients with bipolar disorder have yet to be completed. Alternative drug delivery methods, such as surgically implanted long-term delivery systems, may soon become available and could also increase adherence (Irani et al. 2004).

However, clinicians and patients in the United States have been relatively reluctant to use depot antipsychotics to treat schizophrenia. This may also be true for bipolar disorder. Only 5%–20% of U.S. patients with schizophrenia receive depot agents, compared with 40%–60% in the United Kingdom and Europe (Glazer and Kane 1992; Lindstrom et al. 1996). In a large sample of VA patients with schizophrenia, 49% were judged to be poorly compliant by their clinicians, but only 18% were receiving depot medications (Valenstein et al. 2001). This reluctance to use depot medications may have several causes. Injections may be perceived as coercive, painful, or stigmatizing. Clinicians may be even more reluctant to prescribe depot antipsychotic medications for patients with bipolar disorder than for those with schizophrenia. There are few data on the acceptability of surgically implanted medication devices, although a recent study reported that approximately half of patients with psychiatric disorders had potentially favorable attitudes toward these devices (Irani et al. 2004).

Another common approach to addressing poor adherence to medication regimens by patients with serious mental illness is to increase the level of direct supervision. One possibility is to place patients in adult foster care or other supervised settings. Individuals also may be offered frequent clinical contacts in the community, usually in the form of intensive case-management services or assertive community treatment. However, providing these services to individuals with bipolar disorder may present challenges and require flexibility. In bipolar disorder, functional levels may vary over time, with periods of low functioning alternating with periods of higher functioning. Individuals may not need or want high levels of supervision or intensive services during periods of higher functioning. In addition, both supervised settings and intensive case-management services are expensive and in limited supply.

Potentially, lower-cost pharmacy-based services involving reminders for patients and physicians and "cues to action" may increase patients' adherence to medication regimens. Reminders to patients have been shown to increase attendance at appointments and use of preventive measures such as immunizations (Macharia et al. 1992; Szilagyi et al. 2000). Reminders may also improve refilling of medication prescriptions. Prompt notification of clinicians when their patients fail to refill their medications may also increase adherence. One of the hypotheses about improvement in adherence to antipsychotic treatment with the use of depot preparations is that clinicians know immediately when their patients stop their antipsychotic use and can make early efforts to reengage them in treatment. Prompt clinician notification of missed refills of oral medications may not be as timely as noting a "missed" injection, but it would allow clinicians to act more quickly when patients stop their oral medications than is possible with current clinical procedures.

Interventions that include reminders about medication refills in conjunction with other "cues to action," such as unit-of-use medication packaging, have successfully increased adherence to oral hypoglycemic and antihypertensive medication regimens among patients with diabetes and hypertension. Skaer and colleagues (1993b) assigned 258 Medicaid beneficiaries with diabetes who were taking oral hypoglycemic medications to one of four treatment groups: (1) usual care (control group), (2) medication-refill reminders, (3) unit-of-use packaging, and (4) a combination of mailed reminders and unit-of-use packaging. Patients who received mailed reminders, unit-of-use packaging, or a combination of both achieved a significant increase in mean MPR for oral hypoglycemics compared with controls. In addition, the combination of refill reminders and unit-of-use packaging resulted in a significant increase in mean MPR compared with all other groups. The mean MPR was 0.58 for patients in the control group and 0.87 for patients receiving both unit-of-use packaging and refill reminders. A second randomized controlled trial examining adherence among 304 Medicaid beneficiaries treated for hypertension with an oral antihypertensive medication reported similar results (Skaer et al. 1993a). Again, patients receiving mailed prescription-refill reminders, unit-of-use packaging, or a combination of both interventions achieved a significant increase in their MPRs relative to controls.

Cramer and Rosenheck (1999) conducted a small randomized controlled trial that demonstrated the effectiveness of other "cues to action" in increasing adherence to medication among patients with schizophrenia and other psychiatric illnesses. The researchers worked with patients to develop cues for remembering antipsychotic doses and gave patients MEMS pill bottles (Aprex), which had caps that digitally displayed the number of bottle openings. The researchers also gave patients feedback about the regularity of their bottle openings (and presumably medication dosing). Adherence, as measured by the proportion of days in which the number of bottle openings matched the number of prescribed doses, was 57% among controls and 76% among individuals receiving cues to action and feedback.

Our investigative team is currently conducting a randomized controlled trial of a low-cost pharmacy-based intervention designed to improve adherence to antipsychotic medication by persons with schizophrenia and bipolar illness. Like the interventions described above, this intervention includes unit-of-use packaging of all the medications taken by a patient, an education session about the medications, re-fill reminders mailed to patients, and notification of clinicians when patients fail to refill their medication in a timely fashion. Preliminary results indicate that this in-tervention is highly acceptable to enrolled patients.

Because individuals have a unique constellation of factors affecting their adher-ence to medication regimens, we expect this pharmacy-based approach to be most helpful for older patients or those with cognitive difficulties, and less helpful for in-dividuals with intact cognitive functioning but little insight into their illness or with negative attitudes toward medications. Individuals in the latter group will require other interventions to improve their adherence.

CONCLUSIONS

There are many efficacious treatments for persons with bipolar disorder. How-ever, poor adherence to treatment with mood stabilizers limits the benefits available from these medications for patients in the community. In our studies, we found poor adherence to be common among individuals with bipolar disorder, with 48% demonstrating less than full adherence.

As in previous studies, we also found that poor adherence is associated with de-mographic and clinical factors. Older age is associated with better adherence, al-though poor adherence remains an important issue for older patients, with 38% of older individuals with bipolar disorder being less than fully adherent. Demographic factors and clinical factors seem to have similar effects on adherence among young and old patients. For example, although substance abuse is less prevalent in older persons, when substance abuse does occur in this group it is associated with de-creases in adherence that are similar to those observed for younger adults. Health beliefs among older and younger individuals with poor adherence are also quite sim-ilar, although older adults may be less likely to perceive themselves as being sus-ceptible to an episode of illness.

Systematic monitoring of adherence to treatment and timely interventions to im-prove adherence are likely to be key in improving outcomes for patients with bipo-lar disorder.

REFERENCES

Aagaard, J., and Vestergaard, P. 1990. Predictors of outcome in prophylactic lithium treatment: a 2-year prospective study. *J Affect Disord* 18:259–266.

Aagaard, J., Vestergaard, P., and Maarbjerg, K. 1988. Adherence to lithium prophylaxis: II. Multivariate analysis of clinical, social, and psychosocial predictors of nonadherence. *Pharmacopsychiatry* 21:166–170.

Adams, J., and Scott, J. 2000. Predicting medication adherence in severe mental disorders. *Acta Psychiatr Scand* 101:119–124.

American Psychiatric Association. 2002. Practice guideline for the treatment of patients with bipolar disorder (revision). *Am J Psychiatry* 159(4 suppl.):1–50.

Becker, M. H. 1990. Theoretical models of adherence and strategies for improving adherence. In Shumaker, S. A., Schron, E. B., and Ockene, J. K. (eds.), *The handbook of health behavior change*. New York: Springer.

Berk, M., Berk, L., and Castle, D. 2004. A collaborative approach to the treatment alliance in bipolar disorder. *Bipolar Disord* 6:504–518.

Blow, F. C., McCarthy, J. F., Valenstein, M., et al. 2006. *Care in the VHA for veterans with psychosis: FY05. Sixth annual report on veterans with psychoses*. Ann Arbor, MI: Serious Mental Illness Treatment Research and Evaluation Center.

Budd, R. J., Hughes, I. C. T., and Smith, J. A. 1996. Health beliefs and compliance with antipsychotic medication. *Br J Clin Psychol* 35(pt. 3):393–397.

Burgess, S., Geddes, J., Hawton, K., et al. 2001. Lithium for maintenance treatment of mood disorders. *Cochrane Database Syst Rev* 3:CD003013.

Calabrese, J. R., Shelton, M. D., Rapport, D. J., et al. 2002. Bipolar disorders and the effectiveness of novel anticonvulsants. *J Clin Psychiatry* 63(suppl. 3):5–9.

Coldham, E. L., Addington, J., and Addington, D. 2002. Medication adherence of individuals with a first episode of psychosis. *Acta Psychiatr Scand* 106:286–290.

Colom, F., and Vieta, E. 2002. Treatment adherence in bipolar patients. *Clin Approach Bipolar Disord* 1:49–56.

Colom, F., Vieta, E., Martinez-Aran, A., et al. 2000. Clinical factors associated with treatment noncompliance in euthymic bipolar patients. *J Clin Psychiatry* 61:549–555.

Colom, F., Vieta, E., Martinez-Aran, A., et al. 2003. A randomized trial on the efficacy of group psychoeducation in the prophylaxis of recurrences in bipolar patients whose disease is in remission. *Arch Gen Psychiatry* 60:402–407.

Connelly, C. E. 1984. Compliance with outpatient lithium therapy. *Perspect Psychiatr Care* 22:44–50.

Connelly, C. E., Davenport, Y. B., and Nurnberger, J. I. Jr. 1982. Adherence to treatment regimen in a lithium carbonate clinic. *Arch Gen Psychiatry* 39:585–588.

Corrigan, P. W., Liberman, R. P., and Engel, J. D. 1990. From noncompliance to collaboration in the treatment of schizophrenia. *Hosp Community Psychiatry* 41:1203–1211.

Craighead, W. E., and Miklowitz, D. J. 2000. Psychosocial interventions for bipolar disorder. *J Clin Psychiatry* 61(supp. 13):58–64.

Cramer, J. A., and Rosenheck, R. 1998. Compliance with medication regimens for mental and physical disorders. *Psychiatr Serv* 49:196–201.

Cramer, J. A., and Rosenheck, R. 1999. Enhancing medication compliance for people with serious mental illness. *J Nerv Ment Dis* 187:53–55.

Cuffel, B. J., Alford, J., Fischer, E. P., et al. 1996. Awareness of illness in schizophrenia and outpatient treatment adherence. *J Nerv Ment Dis* 184:653–659.

Danion, J. M., Neunreuther, C., Krieger-Finance, F., et al. 1987. Compliance with long-term lithium treatment in major affective disorders. *Pharmacopsychiatry* 20:230–231.

DiMatteo, M. R. 2004. Variations in patients' adherence to medical recommendations: a quantitative review of 50 years of research. *Med Care* 42:200–209.

Essock, S. M., and Goldman, H. H. 1995. States' embrace of managed mental health care. *Health Aff (Millwood)* 14(3):34–44.

Farmer, K. C. 1999. Methods for measuring and monitoring medication regimen adherence in clinical trials and clinical practice. *Clin Ther* 21:1074–1090; discussion 1073.

Fenton, W. S., Blyler, C. R., and Heinssen, R. K. 1997. Determinants of medication compliance in schizophrenia: empirical and clinical findings. *Schizophr Bull* 23:637–651.

Flay, B. R., and Petraitis, J. 1994. The theory of triadic influence: a new theory of health behavior with implications for preventive interventions. *Adv Med Sociol* 4:19–44.

Frank, E., Prien, R. F., Kupfer, D. J., et al. 1985. Implications of noncompliance on research in affective disorders. *Psychopharmacol Bull* 21:37–42.

Geddes, J. R., Burgess, S., Hawton, K., et al. 2004. Long-term lithium therapy for bipolar disorder: systematic review and meta-analysis of randomized controlled trials. *Am J Psychiatry* 161:217–222.

Gilmer, T. P., Dolder, C. R., Lacro, J. P., et al. 2004. Adherence to treatment with antipsychotic medication and health care costs among Medicaid beneficiaries with schizophrenia. *Am J Psychiatry* 161:692–699.

Glazer, W. M., and Kane, J. M. 1992. Depot neuroleptic therapy: an underutilized treatment option. *J Clin Psychiatry* 53:426–433.

Goodwin, F. K., Fireman, B., Simon, G. E., et al. 2003. Suicide risk in bipolar disorder during treatment with lithium and divalproex. *JAMA* 290:1467–1473.

Greenhouse, W. J., Meyer, B., and Johnson, S. L. 2000. Coping and medication adherence in bipolar disorder. *J Affect Disord* 59:237–241.

Haynes, R. B., McKibbon, K. A., and Kanani, R. 1996. Systematic review of randomised trials of interventions to assist patients to follow prescriptions for medications. *Lancet* 348:383–386.

Irani, F., Dankert, M., Brensinger, C., et al. 2004. Patient attitudes towards surgically implantable, long-term delivery of psychiatric medicine. *Neuropsychopharmacology* 29:960–968.

Johnson, R. E., and McFarland, B. H. 1996. Lithium use and discontinuation in a health maintenance organization. *Am J Psychiatry* 153:993–1000.

Keck, P. E. Jr. 2004. Defining and improving response to treatment in patients with bipolar disorder. *J Clin Psychiatry* 65(suppl. 15):25–29.

Keck, P. E. Jr., and McElroy, S. L. 2002. Carbamazepine and valproate in the maintenance treatment of bipolar disorder. *J Clin Psychiatry* 63(suppl. 10):13–17.

Keck, P. E. Jr., McElroy, S. L., Strakowski, S. M., et al. 1996. Factors associated with pharmacologic noncompliance in patients with mania. *J Clin Psychiatry* 57:292–297.

Keck, P. E. Jr., McElroy, S. L., Strakowski, S. M., et al. 1997. Compliance with maintenance treatment in bipolar disorder. *Psychopharmacol Bull* 33:87–91.

Kelly, G. R., and Scott, J. E. 1990. Medication compliance and health education among outpatients with chronic mental disorders. *Med Care* 28:1181–1197.

Kemp, R., Kirov, G., Everitt, B., et al. 1998. Randomised controlled trial of compliance therapy: 18-month follow-up. *Br J Psychiatry* 172:413–419.

Kleindienst, N., and Greil, W. 2004 Are illness concepts a powerful predictor of adherence to prophylactic treatment in bipolar disorder? *J Clin Psychiatry* 65:966–974.

Lam, D. H., Watkins, E. R., Hayward, P., et al. 2003. A randomized controlled study of cognitive therapy for relapse prevention of bipolar affective disorder. *Arch Gen Psychiatry* 60:145–162.

Lehman, A. F., and Steinwachs, D. M. 1998. At issue: translating research into practice. The Schizophrenia Patient Outcomes Research Team (PORT) treatment recommendations. *Schizophr Bull* 24:1–10.

Leventhal, H., and Cameron, L. 1987. Behavioral theories and the problem of compliance. *Patient Educ Counseling* 10:117–138.

Li, J., McCombs, J. S. and Stimmel, G. L. 2002. Cost of treating bipolar disorder in the California Medicaid (Medi-Cal) program. *J Affect Disord* 71(1–3):131–139.

Licht, R. W., Vestergaard, P., Rasmussen, N. A., et al. 2001. A lithium clinic for bipolar patients: 2-year outcome of the first 148 patients. *Acta Psychiatr Scand* 104:387–390.

Lindstrom, E., Widerlov, B., and von Knorring, L. 1996. Antipsychotic drug—a study of the prescription pattern in a total sample of patients with a schizophrenic syndrome in one catchment area in the county of Uppland, Sweden, in 1991. *Int Clin Psychopharmacol* 11:241–246.

Lingam, R., and Scott, J. 2002. Treatment non-adherence in affective disorders. *Acta Psychiatr Scand* 105:164–172.

Maarbjerg, K., Aagaard, J., and Vestergaard, P. 1988. Adherence to lithium prophylaxis: I. Clinical predictors and patient's reasons for nonadherence. *Pharmacopsychiatry* 21:121–125.

Macharia, W. M., Leon, G., Rowe, B. H., et al. 1992. An overview of interventions to improve compliance with appointment keeping for medical services. *JAMA* 267:1813–1817.

Madden, T. J., and Ellen, P. S. A. I. 1992. A comparison of the theory of planned behavior and the theory of reasoned action. *Pers Soc Psychol Bull* 18:3–9.

Miklowitz, D. J. 1992. Longitudinal outcome and medication noncompliance among manic patients with and without mood-incongruent psychotic features. *J Nerv Ment Dis* 180:703–711.

Nose, M., Barbui, C., and Tansella, M. 2003. How often do patients with psychosis fail to adhere to treatment programmes? A systematic review. *Psychol Med* 33:1149–1160.

Owen, R. R., Fischer, E. P., Booth, B. M., et al. 1996. Medication noncompliance and substance abuse among patients with schizophrenia. *Psychiatr Serv* 47:853–858.

Perlick, D. A., Rosenheck, R. A., Kaczynski, R., et al. 2004. Medication non-adherence in bipolar disorder: a patient-centered review of research findings. *Clin Approach Bipolar Disord* 3:56–64.

Sajatovic, M., Bauer, M., Kilbourne, A., et al. 2006. Self-reported medication adherence among veterans with bipolar disorder. *Psychiatr Serv*. In press.

Schumann, C., Lenz, G., Berghofer, A., et al. 1999. Non-adherence with long-term prophylaxis: a 6-year naturalistic follow-up study of affectively ill patients. *Psychiatry Res* 89:247–257.

Scott, J. 2001. Cognitive therapy as an adjunct to medication in bipolar disorder. *Br J Psychiatry* 178:s164–s168.

Scott, J. 2002. Using Health Belief Models to understand the efficacy-effectiveness gap for mood stabilizer treatments. *Neuropsychobiology* 46(suppl. 1):13–15.

Scott, J., and Pope, M. 2002a. Nonadherence with mood stabilizers: prevalence and predictors. *J Clin Psychiatry* 63:384–390.

Scott, J., and Pope, M. 2002b. Self-reported adherence to treatment with mood stabilizers, plasma levels, and psychiatric hospitalization. *Am J Psychiatry* 159:1927–1929.

Skaer, T. L., Sclar, D. A., Markowski, D. J., et al. 1993a. Effect of value-added utilities on prescription refill compliance and health care expenditures for hypertension. *J Hum Hypertens* 7:515–518.

Skaer, T. L., Sclar, D. A., Markowski, D. J., et al. 1993b. Effect of value-added utilities on prescription refill compliance and Medicaid health care expenditures—a study of patients with non-insulin-dependent diabetes mellitus. *J Clin Pharm Ther* 18:295–299.

Steiner, J. F., and Prochazka, A. V. 1997. The assessment of refill compliance using pharmacy records: methods, validity, and applications. *J Clin Epidemiol* 50:105–116.

Steiner, J. F., Koepsell, T. D., Fihn, S. D., et al. 1988. A general method of compliance assessment using centralized pharmacy records. *Med Care* 26:814–823.

Svarstad, B. L., Shireman, T. I., and Sweeney, J. K. 2001. Using drug claims data to assess the relationship of medication adherence with hospitalization and costs. *Psychiatr Serv* 52:805–811.

Szilagyi, P. G., Bordley, C., Vann, J. C., et al. 2000. Effect of patient reminder/recall interventions on immunization rates: a review. *JAMA* 284:1820–1827.

U.S. Food and Drug Administration. 2005. Searchable database. www.fda.gov/

Valenstein, M., Copeland, L. A., Owen, R., et al. 2001. Adherence assessments and the use of depot antipsychotic medications in patients with schizophrenia. *J Clin Psychiatry* 62:545–554.

Valenstein, M., Copeland, L. A., Blow, F. C., et al. 2002. Pharmacy data identifies poorly adherent patients at increased risk for admission. *Med Care* 40:630–639.

Weiden, P. J., Kozma, C., Grogg, A., et al. 2004. Partial compliance and risk of rehospitalization among California Medicaid patients with schizophrenia. *Psychiatr Serv* 55:886–891.

Weiss, K. A., Smith, T. E., Hull, J. W., et al. 2002. Predictors of risk of nonadherence in outpatients with schizophrenia and other psychotic disorders. *Schizophr Bull* 28:341–349.

Weiss, R. D., Greenfield, S. F., Najavits, L. M., et al. 1998. Medication compliance among patients with bipolar disorder and substance use disorder. *J Clin Psychiatry* 59:172–174.

PART THREE

Complexity and Comorbidity

CHAPTER EIGHT

Substance Abuse among Older Adults with Bipolar Disorder

STEPHEN T. CHERMACK, PH.D.,

JOHN M. WRYOBECK, PH.D.,

AND FREDERIC C. BLOW, PH.D.

Only recently have efforts been made to increase our understanding of the impact of aging on bipolar disorder (Chen et al. 1998; Depp and Jeste 2004; Young 1997). This development comes at an appropriate time, as the aging of the "baby boom" cohort is likely to increase the need and demand for mental health care for older adults generally (Day 1996) and for those with bipolar disorder specifically. Given this expected growth in the older population with bipolar disorder and expansion of services to help care for them, it is important to develop a better understanding of the disorder and its relation to aging. This will allow treatment outcomes to be optimized within a health care system that will probably be under significant financial constraints.

One factor shown to contribute to poor mental health outcomes across age groups is a co-occurring Axis I disorder. McElroy and colleagues (2001) reported that 65% of individuals with bipolar disorder meet *Diagnostic and Statistical Manual of Mental Disorders*, Fourth Edition (DSM-IV) criteria for at least one comorbid lifetime Axis I disorder. Compared with individuals with other Axis I diagnoses, those with bipolar disorder have the highest lifetime rates of alcohol use disorders (Regier et al. 1990) and are at increased risk for other substance use disorders (SUDs). The presence of a co-occurring SUD with bipolar disorder raises concerns because of its adverse effects on the course, treatment, and prognoses of both disorders. Comorbid substance use is particularly problematic and common among individuals with bipolar disorder (Bauer et al. 2005; McElroy et al. 2001). These problems are likely to be magnified in older adults.

Relatively little is known about the effects of co-occurring SUDs for older adults with bipolar disorder. In this chapter we review what is known about the prevalence and correlates of bipolar disorder and SUDs in older adults, their co-occurrence (bipolar disorder–substance use disorder [BPD-SUD]) in mixed-age samples, and likely problems when these psychiatric illnesses co-occur in a geriatric population. We address how aging likely complicates the clinical features and outcomes for individuals with BPD-SUD and how problems specific to older adulthood are likely to complicate engagement with treatment and thus outcomes for this population.

PREVALENCE AND CORRELATES OF BIPOLAR DISORDER IN ELDERLY PERSONS

Bipolar disorder is thought to be present in 1%–2% of the general U.S. population (Bebbington and Ramana 1995; Kessler et al. 1994; Regier et al. 1990). Among individuals over 65 years of age, prevalence estimates drop to between 0.01% and 0.5% (Hirschfeld et al. 2003; Weissman et al. 1991). Treatment prevalence, however, remains high (4%–18%) in the general older population (Cassano et al. 2000; Weissman et al. 1988; Yassa et al. 1988).

Although it is commonly believed that bipolar disorder first occurs primarily in young adulthood, recent work shows that many individuals first experience a manic episode as an older adult (≥60 years). Shulman (1994) identified two clinically distinct types of bipolar disorder: early-onset (first affective illness before midlife) and late-onset (first affective illness in late life). Studies examining the occurrence of bipolar disorder in recently hospitalized older adults have found that the average age of onset of the mood disorder is between 47 and 57 years, with the first manic episode occurring between ages 58 and 71 (Shulman and Post 1980; Snowden 1991; Yassa et al. 1988). Older adults with late-onset bipolar disease often present with milder manic symptoms and with mixed manic dysphoric or agitated states (Cassano et al. 2000). They are more likely to display irritable behavior (James 1977) and have cognitive symptoms that complicate both diagnosis and treatment (Shulman 1997).

Distinguishing between early- and late-onset bipolar disorder is important because the two may have different etiologies and potentially different clinical manifestations, which will affect outcomes. Early-onset bipolar disorder is considered to be more often associated with specific biological/genetic vulnerabilities (Baron et al. 1981; James 1977; Taylor and Abrams 1973) and stressful life events, whereas later onset is more likely associated with organic factors (Hays et al. 1998). Further, earlier age of onset seems to be associated with poorer functioning (Meeks 1999; Sajatovic et al. 2005). This association is mediated by length and frequency of depressive episodes — those who have experienced frequent, lengthy episodes of depression have worse global functioning. In terms of pharmacological treatment, lithium is considered a first-choice medication for early-onset mania (American Psychiatric Association 2002), whereas anticonvulsants may be a better first-choice medication for those with late-onset mania (McDonald 2000). When examining the association between bipolar and substance use disorders, few researchers have made a distinction between early- and late-onset bipolar disorder. Consequently, the findings we present here refer to the older adult with a diagnosis of bipolar disorder of early or late onset, unless "late onset" is specifically mentioned.

To date, then, research has not examined differences in rates of SUD among persons with early- versus late-onset bipolar disorder. Our understanding of the high rates of substance misuse by individuals with bipolar disorder might be enhanced if we knew whether there were differences in patterns or temporal sequencing of substance use and in depressive/manic symptoms between individuals with early- and late-onset bipolar disorder.

Late-life (as opposed to late-onset) bipolar disorder is associated with greater chronicity (Ameblas 1987; Angst 1980), greater resistance to treatment (Young and Falk 1989), and higher mortality rates (James 1977; Shulman and Tohen 1994). Mortality among older adults with bipolar disorder is high. Follow-up studies show a 34% mortality rate after 5 years and a 50% mortality rate over a 3–10 year period (Dhingra and Rabbins 1991; Shulman and Tohen 1994). Suicide and medical illness are two primary mechanisms for increased mortality among this older population. Dhingra and Rabins (1991) observed that the survival rate for their sample of older persons with bipolar disorder was significantly lower than the expected rate calculated from census data for older adults without bipolar illness.

Medication use by elderly persons can be complicated and problematic, particularly the use of antipsychotics (Neil et al. 2003). Older adults are at increased risk of experiencing drug interactions, side effects, and toxicity, even at low medication doses. Although lithium is being used successfully by older adults, it is important to consider and manage several issues, including lithium's interactions with other drugs and potential toxicity even at "normal" doses. A study examining older adults (ages 67–84) found that the use of lithium was associated with a 2.1-fold increased risk of injury in a vehicle accident (Etminan et al. 2004). Whether pharmacological interventions involve lithium, other prescribed medication, or over-the-counter drugs, older adults are at increased risk of experiencing adverse reactions to their medications. The use of alcohol and other drugs only compounds this problem.

PREVALENCE AND CORRELATES OF SUBSTANCE USE IN ELDERLY PERSONS

The lifetime prevalence of substance use disorders in the general population is high: 17% for alcohol dependence or abuse and 6% for other types of substance abuse (Regier et al. 1990). Six-month prevalence rates for persons aged 60 and older who meet *Diagnostic and Statistical Manual of Mental Disorders*, Third Edition Revised (DSM-III-R) criteria for alcohol abuse or dependence were shown to range from 1.4% to 3.7% (Adams et al. 1993). Rates of current substance use have been reported to range from 15% to 58% among older adults seeking treatment in hospitals, primary care clinics, and nursing homes (Blow 1998). According to one study examining a community-based population, approximately 15% of men and 12% of women aged 60 and older drank in excess of the limits recommended by the National Institute on Alcohol Abuse and Alcoholism (1995) for older adults (Adams et al. 1996; Saunders 1994).

The prevalence of problematic substance use among older adults will probably increase as the baby boom cohort ages (Blow 1998). Although many studies (typically cross-sectional) indicate that the use of alcohol and illicit drugs declines with age (National Institute on Alcohol Abuse and Alcoholism 2000; Substance Abuse and Mental Health Services Administration 2000), there is some evidence that lower levels of use among older adults today is due, at least in part, to cohort effects rather than an actual decline in use with aging (Glynn et al. 1985). For example, two age-related cohorts were compared on substance use in the late 1990s. Forty-nine percent of the baby boom cohort (ages 31–49) reported using illicit drugs in their lifetime, compared with 11% of older adults (age 50 or older) (Substance Abuse and Mental Health Services Administration 1996). Further, it has been reported that drinking patterns remain stable over the life course and that birth cohorts experiencing high substance use as young adults show high rates of use as they age, relative to other cohorts (National Institute on Alcohol Abuse and Alcoholism 1988; Substance Abuse and Mental Health Services Administration 2000). Taken together, such data suggest that future cohorts of older adults will probably have higher rates of alcohol and drug use than the present cohort. With the increases in life expectancy and the size of the baby boom cohort, there will also be a larger population of older adults in the coming decades. Thus, estimates indicate that the number of older adults with substance abuse problems will increase from 2.5 million in 1999 to 5.0 million by 2020 (Gfroerer et al. 2002). Given such trends, it is reasonable to expect increased rates as well as higher overall numbers of older adults with co-morbid bipolar disorder and problematic substance use.

Taking a broader view of "at-risk" drinking and drug use behavior among older adults is important for several reasons. Most older adults who experience problems related to their alcohol consumption do not meet DSM-IV criteria for alcohol abuse or dependence (Barry et al. 2001; Blow 1998). Specifically, older adults may have fewer vocational and social responsibilities that could be affected by substance use, and relatively low levels of use can present unique problems for older persons (Blow 1998). Problems stemming from substance misuse by elderly persons include injuries sustained at home and in motor vehicle accidents (DuFour et al. 1992), cognitive changes (Pfefferbaum et al. 1997), and exacerbation of several medical conditions (e.g., high blood pressure, liver disease, hemorrhagic stroke, chronic obstructive pulmonary disease [Criqui et al. 1981; Umbricht-Schneiter et al. 1991]). Further, older adults are at increased risk for adverse reactions to substance use that is combined with prescribed and over-the-counter medications (Korrapati and Vestal 1995), because of their greater number of medical conditions, greater use of medications, and aging-related changes in the metabolism of medications, illicit drugs, and alcohol. Thus, for some older adults, any alcohol or other drug use can increase adverse health consequences and influence treatment outcomes.

The effect of moderate or at-risk substance use on mental disorders, then, is important in terms of its implications for the course and treatment of such disorders. Substance use in the presence of psychiatric illness is associated with more severe symptoms, increased suicidality, poor compliance with medication regimens and treatment interventions, and generally negative mental health outcomes (Hasegawa et al. 1990; Schuckit et al. 1997; Tsuang et al. 1995). There is a paucity of research on the impact of relatively low-level substance use on the course of psychiatric symptoms/disorders in older adulthood. On the basis of evidence from younger population samples, however, it is highly likely that even relatively low levels of substance use can complicate the clinical course of bipolar disorder for older adults. Clearly, research is needed to obtain more detailed information on the effects of the type of drug (alcohol vs. other drugs) and patterns of use on bipolar symptoms among older adults.

PREVALENCE AND CORRELATES OF CO-OCCURRING
BIPOLAR DISORDER AND SUBSTANCE USE

According to the Epidemiological Catchment Area Study, the lifetime prevalence of substance use disorders across age groups is 61% for bipolar I disorder and 41% for bipolar II disorder (Reiger et al. 1990). The National Comorbidity Survey found that persons with mania have an increased risk for both alcohol dependence (odds ratio [OR] = 9.7) and drug dependence (OR = 8.4) (Kessler et al. 1996). The prevalence of bipolar disorder in individuals with SUD is also high: 6% in men and 7% in women (Regier et al. 1990). In a small sample of treatment-seeking cocaine-dependent individuals, an estimated 16%–30% had a lifetime bipolar spectrum disorder (Gawin and Kleber 1986). Further, Sbrana and colleagues (2005) found that 46% of individuals with bipolar disorder had a co-occurring SUD, with an additional 8% having "subthreshold" substance use. Other disorders (panic disorder, obsessive compulsive disorder) had lower rates of co-occurring SUD (<8%) and higher levels of subthreshold use (~26%). Finally, there is evidence of some common risk factors for developing bipolar and substance use disorders, as well as factors related to their co-occurrence, such as genetic influences (Schuckit et al. 2004) and a history of childhood physical/emotional abuse (Brown et al. 2005). These studies suggest that high rates of SUDs can be expected in individuals with bipolar illness, and that individuals with bipolar disorder who misuse substances are at an elevated risk of developing SUDs compared with those with other psychiatric disorders.

Most current knowledge about the impact of substance use on bipolar disorder comes from mixed-age studies. To our knowledge, no studies have specifically examined the correlates of this co-occurrence in an older adult population. Given this paucity of research involving older adults, we summarize what is known about the co-occurrence of these disorders in mixed-age and/or younger samples and discuss how aging might further affect this comorbidity.

Overall, individuals with BPD-SUD are more likely to be male and single/divorced/widowed, to have a low level of education, and to have additional Axis I disorders and medical problems (Sonne et al. 1994; Weiss et al. 2005). The presence of a co-occurring SUD has a significant adverse effect on the presentation and course of bipolar disorder. Studies report the co-occurrence of SUD to be associated with dysphoric mood, mixed mood states, and rapid cycling (Himmelhoch et al. 1976), along with a greater number of overall symptoms, impulsivity, and violence (Salloum et al. 2002b). A review examining the effect of substance use on bipolar disorder reported that use was associated with shorter latency between bipolar episodes, delayed recovery, more frequent relapse, and an increased number of episodes (Salloum and Thase, 2000). It also found increased disability and mortality. Figure 8.1 provides a summary of how the course of bipolar symptoms and substance use may be interrelated and how such interrelationships are affected by both individual and social/contextual risk factors.

An issue that deserves additional research attention is how the order of onset of bipolar and substance use disorders may affect the clinical course, particularly for older adults. For example, Strakowski and colleagues (2005) found among a younger patient sample (age range 12–45 years) that those with the onset of an alcohol use disorder preceding bipolar disorder tended to be older and recover more quickly than those with the onset of bipolar disorder preceding or concurrent with onset of alcohol use disorder, or those with bipolar disorder alone. It is unclear whether such a pattern would be found for older adults, given the increased sensitivity to alcohol and drug effects associated with aging (Cassano et al. 2000; James 1977; Shulman 1997). Finally, studies that have not focused primarily on a diagnosis of SUD have demonstrated that substance use levels (e.g., number of drinks per drinking day, marijuana use) are similarly related to clinical course (McKowen et al. 2005; Salloum et al. 2005). The presence of SUDs or lower-level substance use takes on added importance for elderly persons because, as previously noted, older adults with bipolar illness are already at increased risk of death and disability. The addition of substance use probably adds to this risk.

Results from a small number of studies suggest that older adults with bipolar disorder generally have lower rates of co-occurring SUD than younger adults with bipolar disorder (Cassidy et al. 2001; Sajatovic et al. 2004). In a large sample of hospitalized individuals with bipolar disorder (N = 392), using DSM-III-R criteria, Cassidy and colleagues (2001) found a lifetime SUD in 29% of patients over 60 years of age. Similarly, in a geropsychiatric unit, examination of 378 consecutive admissions showed that 19% of older adults with bipolar disorder had a current SUD (Ponce et al. 1999). In a small population of older veterans (N = 23), 25% of those with bipolar disorder also had a current SUD (Sajatovic et al. 1996). Thus, although these are lower rates than in younger samples, the presence of SUD seems to be common in samples of older adults treated for bipolar disorder. It should be noted, however, that these studies did not examine "at-risk" alcohol or illicit drug use behavior in this patient population, or measure consequences of use that are more specific to older adulthood. Therefore, among older adults with bipolar disorder who are in treatment, rates of problematic substance use could be higher than estimates from the studies described above. Further, because future cohorts of older adults may have higher rates of alcohol and other substance use, rates of co-occurring SUDs and

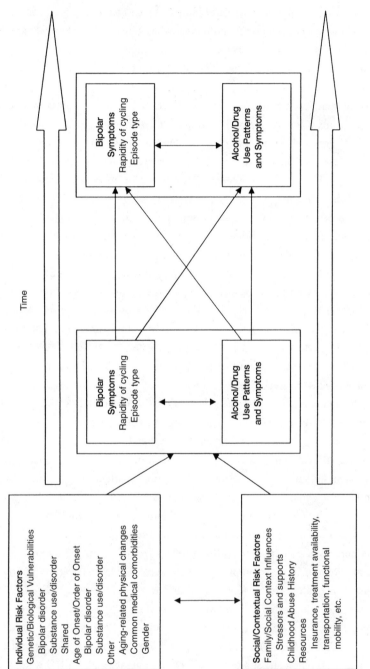

Individual Risk Factors
Genetic/Biological Vulnerabilities
  Bipolar disorder
  Substance use/disorder
  Shared
Age of Onset/Order of Onset
  Bipolar disorder
  Substance use/disorder
Other
  Aging-related physical changes
  Common medical comorbidities
  Gender

Bipolar Symptoms
Rapidity of cycling
Episode type

Alcohol/Drug Use Patterns and Symptoms

Bipolar Symptoms
Rapidity of cycling
Episode type

Alcohol/Drug Use Patterns and Symptoms

Social/Contextual Risk Factors
Family/Social Context Influences
  Stressors and supports
  Childhood Abuse History
Resources
  Insurance, treatment availability, transportation, functional mobility, etc.

Time

Fig. 8.1. Relations among individual and social/contextual risk factors and the course of bipolar symptoms and substance use.

"subthreshold" problematic use may become more common among older adults with bipolar disorder. There is a clear need for research that includes broader measures of substance use patterns and consequences common to older adulthood that could be used to estimate rates of problematic substance use among older adults with bipolar disorder.

Individuals with bipolar disorder and co-occurring disorders report poorer overall quality of life, in part due to the elevated levels of distress (Singh et al. 2005; Weiss et al. 2005). Increased levels of emotional distress along with the absence of effective coping strategies can cause some individuals to engage in extreme behaviors as an attempt to manage their emotional discomfort. One such extreme behavior is suicide. Risk of suicide is increased among individuals diagnosed with BPD-SUD. In one study, a group of patients with both disorders had a lifetime rate of 38% for attempted suicide, compared with 22% for a group without SUD (Potash et al. 2000). Individuals with bipolar disorder who are experiencing substance use–related symptoms have higher rates of recent suicide crises (OR = 3.1) (Comtois et al. 2004). This is an issue of significant concern, given that rates of suicide increase with age, particularly among white males. Older adults who frequently experience suicidal ideation are more likely to be male, be divorced or widowed, and have physical illness (Carney et al. 1999; Dorpat et al. 1968; U.S. Department of Health and Human Services 1999). As noted, older patients with bipolar disorder and co-occurring substance use problems are likely to be male, without a partner, and experiencing physical illness. This means that three high-risk conditions for suicide are extremely common in this population: having bipolar illness, having a substance use problem, and being older than 65.

Not surprisingly, lifetime substance use by individuals with bipolar disorder is associated with increased utilization of health services, including visits to emergency rooms and hospitalizations (Brady et al. 1991; Cassidy et al. 2001; Goldberg et al. 1999). Comparing use of health care among groups with bipolar disorder alone, substance use alone, and co-occurring illness, Verduin and colleagues (2005) reported that the group with co-occurring illness had a lower use of psychiatric services than the group with bipolar illness only, but the groups did not differ significantly in use of other services, such as case management, inpatient admission, primary care, and specialty care visits.

IMPLICATIONS FOR TREATMENT

Although very few, if any, studies have focused on the treatment of older adults with co-occurring bipolar and substance use disorders, we can highlight some important treatment-related issues based on studies of treatment for bipolar disorder, substance use disorders, and comorbid psychiatric and substance use disorders, and of elderly individuals with either substance use or mental health problems. Given that the number of older adults with BPD-SUD is expected to rise, it is important to understand how the pharmacotherapy and psychotherapy associated with treatment might need to change to better address the specific symptoms and problems in this population.

Substance use is associated with poorer adherence to medications and treatment (Keck et al. 1998), as well as poorer treatment outcomes (Salloum and Thase 2000). In a follow-up study of 134 patients after hospitalization for a manic/mixed episode, Keck and colleagues (1998) found that only substance use was predictive of nonadherence to treatment. In bipolar disorder, the primary goal of treatment is the effective management of symptoms. The scientific literature supports the long-term effectiveness of lithium in controlling these symptoms (Tondo et al. 1998), but poor responses to lithium have been reported in patients with BPD-SUD (Bowden, 1995; O'Connel et al. 1991). One report notes that patients with co-occurring bipolar and substance use disorder are less likely to adhere to lithium treatment (21%) than valproate treatment (50%) (Weiss et al. 1998). Valproate carries a risk of hepatoxicity (increasing the risk of adverse outcomes in a population at risk for liver disease). In a double-blind, placebo-controlled study on the use of valproate in a population with bipolar disorder and comorbid alcohol dependence, valproate use was associated with decreased heavy drinking — beyond its effect on mood (Le Fauve et al. 2004). These findings highlight the added complexity of treating bipolar disorder in elderly patients who also have SUD.

In addition to pharmacotherapy, psychotherapy is known to be effective for individuals with BPD-SUD (Levin and Hennessy 2004). However, there are few reports on the delivery of standard psychotherapy treatments to this patient population. One study compared a group receiving manual-based cognitive-behavioral therapy (CBT) with a group receiving medication management only, finding greater retention rates, increased adherence to medication regimens, and improved mood in the CBT intervention group (Schmitz et al. 2002). No differences were found in substance use outcomes between the two groups. In contrast, Weiss and colleagues (2000) reported that their manual-based CBT did result in greater abstinence from substance use in the intervention group versus the control group. We know that older adults who misuse substances frequently do not receive treatment for this problem (Curtis et al. 1989), despite the evidence that treatment is effective for this population (Barry et al. 2001).

Research indicates that integrating treatment for both the substance use and the psychiatric disorder is associated with better outcomes for both disorders (Drake et

al. 2004). A review of studies on the effect of integrated services for individuals
with comorbid substance use and mental health disorders found that the integration
of services helped patients reduce substance use, achieve remission, and improve
their emotional functioning (Drake et al. 1998). In fact, integrated treatment of co-
occurring disorders is currently accepted as an essential evidence-based practice
(Drake et al. 2001).

Despite this evidence and expert consensus supporting integrated treatment for
individuals with co-occurring psychiatric and substance use disorders, problems remain in the availability and accessibility of such services and in linking individuals
to appropriate care (Bartels et al. 2004; Mojtabai 2004). In a mixed-age sample of individuals with SUD alone and individuals with BPD-SUD, 92% of those with SUD
alone were referred to SUD treatment, compared with 41% of those with a co-
occurring bipolar illness (Verduin et al. 2005). It is unclear whether the differential
referral and treatment rates for those with and without SUD were a reflection of limited treatment resources (lack of available programs for those with co-occurring disorders), providers' perceptions about appropriate treatment (e.g., even though SUD
was present, SUD treatment settings were not perceived as indicated in the presence
of bipolar disorder), or patients' preferences (e.g., individuals with bipolar disorder
did not view their substance use as in need of intervention).

Treatment access, availability of integrated programming, and patients' engagement and retention in treatment are important because such factors support sustained remission from SUD, which is associated with improved functioning for individuals with bipolar disorder (Drake et al. 2004; Weiss et al. 2005). Realistically,
however, recovery and improved functioning can be intermittent in this population
(Drake et al. 2004; Weiss et al. 2005; Winokur et al. 1995). Drake and colleagues
(2004) followed up on an outpatient treatment sample of individuals with BPD-SUD
for three years. Although 73% reached full remission of their substance use disorder,
36% of these relapsed within a year of remission. Ongoing prevention of relapse and
continuing accessibility of services are an important part of treatment for this population.

We have alluded to the issues of availability and access to appropriate treatment
interventions as notable challenges for older adults with BPD-SUD. Currently, as is
the case for younger adults, there is a limited availability of integrated, empirically
informed services that target comorbid psychiatric and substance use problems for
older adults. Older adults with such comorbidities who receive treatment generally
do not receive integrated treatment or even simultaneous treatment of both their
bipolar and substance use problems. Several steps are needed to expand the availability of such services, including additional research to better identify the preva-

lence of BPD-SUD in older adults and the unique treatment needs of these individuals, as well as an increased emphasis in the behavioral health care fields (psychiatry, psychology, social work, addiction medicine) on training in empirically supported or informed treatments for patients with psychiatric problems or substance use problems or both.

Further, for older adults with comorbid bipolar (or other psychiatric) disorder and substance use problems, there may need to be a "paradigm shift" in the means of identifying, engaging, and retaining individuals in need of treatment services. Such a shift should include a move toward screening and assessment of the substance use patterns and consequences more common among older adults and of bipolar symptoms as they manifest in later life. In terms of treatment engagement and retention, older adults with BPD-SUD face some substantial barriers to treatment. These can include factors specifically associated with aging, such as increased difficulties with functional mobility and driving/transportation, other physical and cognitive limitations, and cohort-related stigma about mental health and substance use issues. Further, there may be a misattribution of symptoms by providers or patients (e.g., attributing symptoms of mania to old age or cognitive dysfunction; attributing mood variations to substance use or old age; lack of awareness or insight about how alcohol/substance use may interfere with medications or worsen mood and cognitive symptoms), and "noncompliance," which is relatively common among individuals with BPD-SUD. The lack of treatment programs specifically aimed at elderly persons can also be a barrier for older adults who do desire treatment, given the evidence that older adults often feel they do not fit in well with younger persons seeking treatment and tend to respond better to treatment that targets their age group (Barry et al. 2001; Blow 1998; Kofoed et al. 1987).

To better facilitate treatment for older adults with co-occurring bipolar and substance use disorders, it may be necessary to develop and implement treatment-linkage interventions to address psychological, physical, and other tangible barriers to treatment. Such interventions could include psychoeducation for providers, family/caregivers, and patients; assistance with transportation to treatment services; case management; and perhaps motivational enhancement strategies to address issues of problem recognition and motivation for treatment. And, because of some tangible barriers to attending frequent treatment appointments, case-management services, family involvement, residential services, and in-home and/or telephone-based supportive monitoring and intervention all may be necessary for delivering integrated treatment services.

CONCLUSIONS

Examining substance misuse among individuals with bipolar disorder is clinically important, as this comorbidity is associated with poor treatment outcomes, decreased functioning, and increased mortality. Substance use adversely affects the course and prognosis of bipolar disorder (Sonne and Brady 2002) and is associated with more frequent hospitalizations, more rapid cycling, and more mixed mania (Sonne et al. 1994), as well as higher rates of impulsivity and aggression (Salloum et al. 2002b). Higher rates of suicide have also been identified for individuals with both substance misuse and bipolar illness (Feinman and Dunner 1996): these individuals have a 2.3-fold greater risk of attempting suicide than those without a co-occurring substance use disorder (Potash et al. 2000). Finally, higher rates of medication and treatment noncompliance are a common problem in this group (Goldberg et al. 1999).

The impact of aging on persons with bipolar disorder and co-occurring substance use disorder is the central question addressed here. The effect of a co-occurring SUD on bipolar disorder seems to be additive, in that shared symptom clusters are more severe in individuals with both disorders than in those with either one alone. Adding the aging process to these co-occurring conditions is likely to compound the problems, resulting in even greater emotional distress, disability, and mortality. Further study is required to examine the possibility that there are not only additive effects but also some interaction effects among the three domains — age, substance use, and bipolar illness.

Given the very few studies that have focused on comorbid bipolar and substance use disorders in older adults, many areas are in need of additional research and clinical attention. These include (1) the cross-sectional and longitudinal relations between type and patterns of substance use, medication effects (both therapeutic and side effects), and bipolar symptoms; (2) the temporal sequencing of substance use and mood symptoms; (3) the identification of optimal pharmacological and psychological interventions; (4) diagnostic and etiological issues for late-onset bipolar disorder combined with substance use (e.g., differential diagnosis issues); (5) the availability of needed services; (6) means of training in, disseminating, and implementing best practices; (7) overcoming barriers to patients' engagement and retention in treatment; and (8) the use of alternative treatment- delivery strategies (e.g., alternative settings and in-home care).

REFERENCES

Adams, W. L., Yuan, Z., Barboriak, J. J., et al. 1993. Alcohol-related hospitalizations in elderly people: prevalence and geographic variation in the United States. *JAMA* 270:1222–1225.

Adams, W. L., Barry, K. L., and Fleming, M. F. 1996. Screening for problem drinking in older primary care patients. *JAMA* 276:1964–1967.

Ameblas, A. 1987. Life events and mania. *Br J Psychiatry* 150:235–240.

American Psychiatric Association. 2002. Practice guidelines for the treatment of patients with bipolar disorder (revision). *Am J Psychiatry* 159:1–50.

Angst, J. 1980. Clinical typology of bipolar illness. In Belmaker, R. H., and van Praag, H. M. (eds.), *Mania: an evolving concept* (pp. 61–76). Lancaster, England: MTP Press.

Baron, M., Mendlewicz, J., and Klotz, J. 1981. Age-of-onset and genetic transmission in affective disorders. *Acta Psychiatr Scand* 64:373–380.

Barry, K. L., Oslin, D. W., and Blow, F. C. 2001. *Alcohol problems in older adults: prevention and management.* New York: Springer.

Bartels, S. J., Coakley, E. H., Zubritsky, C., et al. 2004. Improving access to geriatric mental health services: a randomized trial comparing treatment engagement with integrated versus enhanced referral care for depression, anxiety, and at-risk alcohol use. *Am J Psychiatry* 8:1455–1462.

Bauer, M. S., Altshuler, L., Evans, D. R., et al. 2005. Prevalence and distinct correlates of anxiety, substance, and combined comorbidity in a multi-site public sector sample with bipolar disorder. *J Affect Disord* 85:301–315.

Bebbington, P., and Ramana, R. 1995. The epidemiology of bipolar affective disorder. *Soc Psychiatry Psychiatr Epidemiol* 30:279–292.

Blow, F. C. 1998. *Substance abuse among older adults.* Department of Health and Human Services pub. no. (SMA) 983179. Rockville, MD: U.S. Department of Health and Human Services.

Bowden, C. L. 1995. Predictors of response to divalproex and lithium. *J Clin Psychiatry* 56(suppl. 3):25–30.

Brady, K. T., Casto, S., Lydiard, R. B., et al. 1991. Substance abuse in an inpatient sample. *Am J Drug Alcohol Abuse* 17:389–397.

Brown, G. R., McBride, L., Bauer, M. S., et al. 2005. Impact of childhood abuse on the course of bipolar disorder: a replication study in U.S. veterans. *J Affect Disord* 89:57–67.

Carney, S. S., Rich, C. L., Burke, P. A., et al. 1999. Suicide over 60: the San Diego study. *J Am Geriatr Soc* 42:174–180.

Cassano, G. B., McElroy, S. L., Brady, K., et al. 2000. Current issues in the identification and management of bipolar spectrum disorder in "special populations." *J Affect Disord* 59:S69–S79.

Cassidy, F., Ahearn, E. P., and Carrol, B. J. 2001. Substance abuse in bipolar disorder. *Bipolar Disord* 3:181–188.

Chen, S., Altshuler, L., and Spar, J. 1998. Bipolar in late life: a review. *J Geriatr Psychiatry Neurol* 11:29–45.

Comtois, K. A., Russo, J. E., Roy-Byrne, P., et al. 2004. Clinician's assessments of bipolar disorder and substance abuse as predictors of suicidal behavior in acutely hospitalized psychiatric inpatients. *Biol Psychiatry* 56:757–763.

Criqui, M. H., Wallace, R. B., Mishkel, M., et al. 1981. Alcohol consumption and blood pressure: the lipid research clinics prevalence study. *Hypertension* 3:557–565.

Curtis, J. R., Geller, G., Stokes, E. J., et al. 1989. Characteristics, diagnosis, and treatment of alcoholism in elderly patients. *J Am Geriatr Soc* 37:310–316.

Day, J. C. 1996. *Population projections of the United States by age, sex, race, and Hispanic origin: 1995 to 2050.* Report no. P251130, U.S. Current Population Report. Last revised April 13, 1999. Washington, DC: U.S. Bureau of the Census. www.census.gov/prod/1/pop/p251130/

Depp, C. A., and Jeste, D. V. 2004. Bipolar disorder in older adults: a critical review. *Bipolar Disord* 6:434–367.

Dhingra, U., and Rabins, P. V. 1991. Mania in the elderly: a 5-year follow-up. *J Am Geriatr Soc* 39:581–583.

Dorpat, T. L., Anderson, W. F., and Ripley, H. S. 1968. The relationship of physical illness to suicide. In Resnik, H. P. (ed.), *Suicide behaviors: diagnosis and management* (pp. 209–219). Boston: Little, Brown.

Drake, R. E., Mercer-McFadden, C., Mueser, K. T., et al. 1998. Review of integrated mental health and substance abuse treatment for patients with co-occurring disorders. *Schizophr Bull* 24:589–608.

Drake, R. E., Goldman, H. H., Leff, H. S., et al. 2001. Implementing evidence-based practices in routine mental health service settings. *Psychiatr Serv* 52:179–182.

Drake, R. E., Xie, H., McHugo, G. J., et al. 2004. Three-year outcomes of long-term patients with co-occurring bipolar and substance use disorders. *Biol Psychiatry* 56:749–756.

DuFour, M. C., Archer, L., and Gordis, E. 1992. Alcohol in the elderly. *Clin Geriatr Med* 8:127–141.

Etminan, M., Hemmelgarn, B., Delaney, J. A., et al. 2004. Use of lithium and the risk of injurious motor vehicle crash in elderly adults: case-control study nested within a cohort. *BMJ* 328:558–559.

Feinman, J. A., and Dunner, D. L. 1996. The effect of alcohol and substance abuse on the course of bipolar affective disorder. *J Affect Disord* 37:43–49.

Gawin, F., and Kleber, H. 1986. Pharmacological treatments of cocaine abuse. *Psychiatr Clin North Am* 9:573–583.

Gfroerer, J., Penne, M., Pemberton, M., et al. 2002. Substance abuse treatment need among older adults in 2020: the impact of the aging baby-boom cohort. *Drug Alcohol Depend* 69:127–135.

Glynn, R. J., Bouchard, G. R., LoCastro, J. S., et al. 1985. Aging and generational effects on drinking behaviors in men: results from the normative aging study. *Am J Public Health* 75:1413–1419.

Goldberg, J. F., Garno, J. L., Leon, A. C., et al. 1999. A history of substance abuse complicates remission from acute mania in bipolar disorder. *J Clin Psychiatry* 60:733–740.

Hasegawa, K., Mukasa, H., Nakazawa, Y., et al. 1990. Primary and secondary depression in alcoholism — clinical features and family history. *Drug Alcohol Depend* 27:275–281.

Hays, J. C., Ranga, K., Frishnan, R., et al. 1998. Age of first onset of bipolar disorder: demographic, family history, and psychosocial correlates. *Depress Anxiety* 7:76–82.

Himmelhoch, J. M., Mulla, D., Neil, J. F., et al. 1976. Incidence and significance of mixed affective states in a bipolar population. *Arch Gen Psychiatry* 33:1062–1066.

Hirschfeld, R. M. A., Calalbrese, J. R., Weissman, M. M., et al. 2003. Screening for bipolar disorder in the community. *J Clin Psychiatry* 64:53–59.

James, N. M. 1977. Early and late onset bipolar affective disorder: a genetic study *Arch Gen Psychiatry* 34:715–717.

Keck, P. E., McElroy, S. L., and Strakowski, S. M. 1998. Anticonvulsants and antipsychotics in the treatment of bipolar disorder. *J Clin Psychiatry* 59 (suppl. 6):74–81.

Kessler, R. C., McGonagle, K. A., Zhao, S., et al. 1994. Lifetime and 12-month prevalence of DSM-III-R psychiatric disorders in the United States: results from the National Comorbidity Survey. *Arch Gen Psychiatry* 51:8–19.

Kessler, R. C., Nelson, C. B., McGonagle, K. A., et al. 1996. The epidemiology of co-occurring addictive and mental disorders: implications for prevention and service utilization. *Am J Orthopsychiatry* 66:17–31.

Kofoed, L. L., Tolson, R. L., Atkinson, R. M., et al. 1987. Treatment compliance of older alcoholics: an elder-specific approach is superior to "mainstreaming." *J Stud Alcohol* 48:47–51.

Korrapati, M. R., and Vestal, R. E. 1995. Alcohol and medications in the elderly: complex interactions. In Beresford, T. P., and Gomberg, E. (eds.), *Alcohol and ageing* (pp. 42–69). New York: Oxford University Press.

Le Fauve, C. E., Litten, R. Z., Randall, C. L., et al. 2004. Pharmacological treatment of alcohol abuse/dependence with psychiatric comorbidity. *Alcohol Clin Exp Res* 28:302–312.

Levin, F. R., and Hennessy, G. 2004. Bipolar disorder and substance abuse. *Biol Psychiatry* 56:738–748.

McDonald, W. M. 2000. Epidemiology, etiology, and treatment of geriatric mania. *J Clin Psychiatry* 61(suppl. 13):3–11.

McElroy, S. L., Altshuler, L. L., Suppes, T., et al. 2001. Axis I psychiatric comorbidity and its relationship to historical illness variables in 288 patients with bipolar disorder. *Am J Psychiatry* 158:420–426.

McKowen, J. W., Frye, M. A., Altshuler, L. L., et al. 2005. Patterns of alcohol consumption in bipolar patients comorbid for alcohol abuse or dependence. *Bipolar Disord* 7:377–381.

Meeks, S. 1999. Bipolar disorder in the latter half of life: symptom presentation, global functioning and age of onset. *J Affect Disord* 52:161–167.

Mojtabai, R. 2004. Which substance abuse treatment facilities offer dual diagnosis programs? *Am J Drug Alcohol Abuse* 30:525–536.

National Institute on Alcohol Abuse and Alcoholism. 1988. *Alcohol and aging.* Alcohol Alert no. 2. Rockville, MD: National Institute on Alcohol Abuse and Alcoholism.

National Institute on Alcohol Abuse and Alcoholism. 1995. *The physicians guide to helping patients with alcohol problems.* National Institutes of Health pub. no. 953769. Rockville, MD: National Institute on Alcohol Abuse and Alcoholism.

National Institute on Alcohol Abuse and Alcoholism. 2000. *10th special report to the U.S. Con-*

gress on alcohol and health. National Institutes of Health pub. no. 001583. Washington, DC: U.S. Department of Health and Human Services.

Neil, W., Curran, S., and Wattis, J. 2003. Antipsychotic prescribing in older people. *Age Ageing* 32:475–483.

O'Connel, R. A., Mayo, J. A., Flatow, L., et al. 1991. Outcomes of bipolar disorder on long-term treatment with lithium. *Br J Psychiatry* 159:123–129.

Pfefferbaum, A., Sullivan, E. V., Mathalon, D. H., et al. 1997. Frontal lobe volume loss observed with magnetic resonance imaging in older chronic alcoholics. *Alcohol Clin Exp Res* 21:521–529.

Ponce, H., Kunik, M., Molinari, V., et al. 1999. Divalproex sodium treatment in elderly male bipolar patients. *J Geriatr Drug Treat* 12:55–63.

Potash, J. B., Kane, H. S., Chiu, Y. F., et al. 2000. Attempted suicide and alcoholism in bipolar disorder: clinical and familial relationships. *Am J Psychiatry* 157:2048–2050.

Regier, D. A., Farmer, M. E., Rae, D. S., et al. 1990. Comorbidity of mental disorders with alcohol and drug abuse. *JAMA* 264:2511–2518.

Sajatovic, M., Popli, A., and Semple, W. 1996. Ten year use of hospital-based services by geriatric veterans with schizophrenia and bipolar disorder. *Psychiatr Serv* 47:961–965.

Sajatovic, M., Blow, F. C., Ignacio, R. V., et al. 2004. Bipolar disorder in the Veterans Health Administration: age related modifiers of clinical presentation and health services use. *Psychiatr Serv* 55:1014–1021.

Sajatovic, M., Blow, F. C., Ignacio, R. V., et al. 2005. New onset bipolar disorder in late life. *Am J Geriatr Psychiatry* 13:282–289.

Salloum, I. M., Cornelius, J. R., Daley, D. C., et al. 2002a. Efficacy of valproate maintenance in patients with bipolar disorder and alcoholism: a double-blind placebo-controlled study. *Arch Gen Psychiatry* 62:37–45.

Salloum, I. M., Cornelius, J. R., Mezzich, J. E., et al. 2002b. Impact of concurrent alcohol misuse on symptoms presentation of acute mania at initial evaluation. *Bipolar Disord* 4:418–421.

Salloum, I. M., Cornelius, J. R., Douaihy, A., et al. 2005. Patient characteristics and treatment implications of marijuana abuse among bipolar alcoholics: results from a double-blind, placebo-controlled study. *Addict Behav* 30:1702–1708.

Salloum, I. M., and Thase, M. E. 2000. Impact of substance abuse on the course and treatment of bipolar disorder. *Bipolar Disord* 2(3, pt. 2):269–280.

Saunders, P. A. 1994. Epidemiology of alcohol problems and drinking patterns. In John, R. M., Copeland, M. T., Aboou-Saleh, M. T., et al. (eds.), *Principles and practice of geriatric psychiatry* (pp. 801–805). New York: Wiley.

Sbrana, A., Bizzarri, J. V., Rucci, P., et al. 2005. The spectrum of substance use in mood and anxiety disorders. *Compr Psychiatry* 46:6–13.

Schmitz, J. M., Averill, P., Sayre, S., et al. 2002. Cognitive-behavioral treatment of bipolar disorder and substance abuse: a preliminary randomized study. *Addict Disord Treat* 1:17–24.

Schuckit, M. A., Tipp, J. E., Bergman, M., et al. 1997. Comparison of induced and independent major depression disorders in 2,945 alcoholics. *Am J Psychiatry* 154:948–957.

Schuckit, M. A., Smith, T. L., and Kalmijn, J. 2004. The search for genes contributing to the low level of response to alcohol: patterns of finding across studies. *Alcohol Clin Exp Res* 28:1449–1458.

Shulman, K. 1994. Mania in late life: conceptual and clinical issues. In Chiu, E., and Ames, D. (eds.), *Functional psychiatric disorders of the elderly* (pp. 212–220). Cambridge: Cambridge University Press.

Shulman, K. 1997. Neurologic comorbidity and mania in old age. *Clin Neurosci* 4:37–40.

Shulman, K., and Post, F. 1980. Bipolar affective disorder in old age. *Br J Psychiatry* 136:26–32.

Shulman, K. I., and Tohen, M. 1994. Unipolar mania reconsidered: evidence from an elderly cohort. *Br J Psychiatry* 164:547–549.

Singh, J., Mattoo, S. K., Sharon, P., et al. 2005. Quality of life and its correlates in patients with dual diagnosis of bipolar affective disorder and substance dependence. *Bipolar Disord* 7:187–191.

Snowden, J. A. 1991. A retrospective case note study of bipolar disorder in old age. *Br J Psychiatry* 158:485–490.

Sonne, S. C., and Brady, K. T. 2002. Bipolar disorder and alcoholism. *Alcohol Res Health* 26:103–108.

Sonne, S. C., Brady, K. T., and Morton, W. A. 1994. Substance abuse and bipolar affective disorder. *J Nerv Ment Dis* 182:349–352.

Stone, K. 1989. Mania in the elderly. *Br J Psychiatry* 155:220–224.

Strakowski, S. M., DelBello, M. P., Fleck, D. E., et al. 2005. Effects of co-occurring alcohol abuse on the course of bipolar disorder following a first hospitalization for mania. *Arch Gen Psychiatry* 62:851–858.

Substance Abuse and Mental Health Services Administration, Office of Applied Studies. 1996. *Preliminary estimates from the 1995 National Household Survey on Drug Abuse.* Department of Health and Human Services pub. no. SMA 963107, advance report no. 18. Rockville, MD: Substance Abuse and Mental Health Services Administration.

Substance Abuse and Mental Health Services Administration, Office of Applied Studies. 2000. *Summary of findings from the 1999 National Household Survey on Drug Abuse.* Department of Health and Human Services pub. no. SMA 003466, NHSDA ser. H-12. Rockville, MD: Substance Abuse and Mental Health Services Administration.

Taylor, M., and Abrams, R. 1973. Manic states: a genetic study of early and late onset affective disorders. *Arch Gen Psychiatry* 28:656–658.

Tondo, L., Baldessarini, R. J., Hennen, J., et al. 1998. Lithium maintenance treatment of depression and mania in bipolar I and bipolar II disorders. *Am J Psychiatry* 155:638–645.

Tsuang, D., Cowley, D., Ries, R., et al. 1995. The effects of substance use disorder on the clinical presentation of anxiety and depression in an outpatient psychiatric clinic. *J Clin Psychiatry* 56:549–555.

Umbricht-Schneiter, A., Santora, P., and Moore, R. D. 1991. Impact of alcohol-associated morbidity in hospitalized patients. *Subst Abuse* 12:145–155.

U.S. Department of Health and Human Services. 1999. *The Surgeon General's call to action to prevent suicide.* Washington, DC: Department of Health and Human Services. www.surgeongeneral.gov/library/calltoaction/default.htm

Verduin, M. L., Carter, R. E., Brady, K. T., et al. 2005. Health services use among persons with comorbid bipolar and substance use disorders. *Psychiatr Serv* 56:475–480.

Weiss, R. D., Greenfield, S. F., Najavits, L. M., et a. 1998. Medication compliance among patients with bipolar disorder and substance use disorder. *J Clin Psychiatry* 59:172–174.

Weiss, R. D., Griffin, M. L., Greenfield, S. F., et al. 2000. Group therapy for patients with bipolar and substance dependence: results of a pilot study. *J Clin Psychiatry* 61:361–367.

Weiss, R. D., Ostacher, M. J., Otto, M. W., et al. 2005. Does recovery from substance use disorder matter in patients with bipolar disorder? *J Clin Psychiatry* 66:730–735.

Weissman, M. M., Leaf, P. J., Tischler, G. L., et al. 1988. Affective disorders in five United States communities. *Psychol Med* 18:141–153.

Weissman, M. M., Bruce, M. L., Leak, P. J., et al. 1991. Affective disorders. In Robins, L. N., and Regier, D. A. (eds.), *Psychiatric disorders in America: the Epidemiological Catchment Area Study* (pp. 33–52). New York: Free Press.

Winokur, G., Coryell, W., Akiskal, H. S., et al. 1995. Alcoholism in manic-depression (bipolar) illness: familial illness, course of illness, and the primary-secondary distinction. *Am J Psychiatry* 152:365–372.

Yassa, R., Nair, V., Nastase, C., et al. 1988. Prevalence of bipolar disorder in a psychogeriatric population. *J Affect Disord* 14:197–201.

Young, R. 1997. Bipolar mood disorder in the elderly. *Psychiatr Clin North Am* 20:121–137.

Young, R. C., and Falk, N. R. 1989. Age, manic psychopathology and treatment response. *Int J Geriatr Psychiatry* 4:73–78.

CHAPTER NINE

Medical Comorbidity in Late-Life Bipolar Disorder

HELEN C. KALES, M.D.

Mr. P. is an 80-year-old man with a 50-year history of bipolar disorder. The disorder was diagnosed in 1955, when, at age 29, he had his first manic episode. During his younger adulthood he had several manic and depressive episodes, questionable adherence to his prescribed medication, and alcohol abuse. In his fifties, he stopped using alcohol and was maintained on lithium at 1,200 mg/day, with good results. Then, in 1995, during hospitalization for resection of a benign rectal tumor, Mr. P. became manic after reduction of his lithium dose. Surgery staff noted that he had an elevated mood, labile emotions, and hypersexuality. His mania abated with the resumption of his usual dose of lithium and with the addition of thiothixene; however, one month later he developed symptoms of a severe major depression and received electroconvulsive therapy (ECT) treatments as an inpatient. When Mr. P was discharged he was taking risperidone, which was tapered and discontinued while he was an outpatient; he eventually began taking lithium again, at 900 mg/day.

Mr. P. developed non-insulin-dependent diabetes mellitus in 1997, but he was psychiatrically stable until 1998, when he had an episode of lithium toxicity precipitated by addition of an angiotensin-converting enzyme (ACE) inhibitor to his antihypertensive regimen. Mr. P. restarted lithium at a dose of 600 mg/day, and his mood remained stable. In 2001 he developed memory problems, and following a cognitive workup that included magnetic resonance imaging (MRI) and neuropsychological testing, he was diagnosed with vascular dementia in the context of his diabetes. Mr. P. continued to live in a senior apartment, but because of his memory problems, he began to have difficulty adhering to his medication regimen. This resulted in an episode of severe mania with psychosis and three psychiatric hospitalizations. Because his difficulties with memory were contributing to his mood destabilization, and given the lack of family involvement, Mr. P. was eventually placed in a community nursing home.

Medical comorbidity frequently accompanies late-life bipolar disorder and often may complicate its treatment and course. The case of Mr. P. illustrates several themes to be discussed in this chapter: (1) common comorbidities in late-life bipolar disorder, including the connection between late-life mania and dementia syndromes; (2) medical disorders related to the pharmacological treatment of bipolar disorder; (3) medication interactions and changes in medication dosing required to address comorbidities; and (4) changes in care management necessitated by the co-occurrence of bipolar disorder and medical illnesses.

Medical, predominantly neurological, disorders also cause secondary or new-onset mania in late life. In these cases, the psychiatric disorder is not comorbid with the medical disorder but a manifestation of it (Krishnan 2005). Secondary mania is thus not a focus of this chapter; it is discussed in detail in chapter 4.

COMMON COMORBIDITIES IN LATE-LIFE BIPOLAR DISORDER

Medical illnesses accompany bipolar disorder at rates greater than that predicted by chance. In one study, 20% of older patients with bipolar disorder had seven or more co-occurring medical illnesses, a higher prevalence than in patients with schizophrenia (Brown 2001). Comorbidity takes on special significance in bipolar disorder. This disorder is among the illnesses associated with the largest suicide risk in older adults, and a study found strong associations between the cumulative number of illnesses and the estimated relative risk of suicide (Juurlink et al. 2004). In the latter study, patients with five illnesses were found to have a fivefold increase in suicide risk. As Krishnan (2005) noted, it is often not clear whether medical disorders among individuals with bipolar disorder are truly comorbid or are a consequence of treatment, or a combination of both.

Diabetes

A good example of the possibly bidirectional relation between bipolar disorder and some medical illnesses in late life is the link between bipolar illness, diabetes, and obesity (McElroy et al. 2002). The prevalence of diabetes in persons with bipolar disorder is significantly higher than that in the general population: the prevalence was found to be between 12% and 26% of mixed-age samples of patients with bipolar illness in various studies (Regenold et al. 2002; Ruzickova et al. 2003). Further, the prevalence of diabetes in hospitalized patients with bipolar illness was found to be approximately three times the national average (Cassidy and Carroll 2002).

The mechanisms of this comorbidity are not yet clear. As with the better-studied depression–diabetes connection (Lustman et al. 2000), the relation between diabetes and bipolar disorder may be bidirectional, and investigators have suggested that the following mechanisms may be involved: (1) underlying overlapping genetic connections; (2) hypothalamic suprachiasmatic nucleus dysfunction (noted in both diabetes and bipolar disorder), resulting in a disruption of circadian rhythms that leads to disturbances in sleep-wake cycles and glucose handling; (3) abnormal counter-regulatory hormone (cortisol, epinephrine, etc.) homeostasis; (4) release of proinflammatory cytokines in persons with affective disorders; (5) diabetic vascular lesions contributing to mania; and (6) effects of psychotropic medications with associated weight gain (Kupka et al. 2002a; McIntyre and Konarski 2005; Vanina et al. 2002). Patients more likely to develop treatment-emergent diabetes are those with baseline risk factors, including family history, race/ethnicity, increasing age, central obesity, physical inactivity, low high-density lipoprotein / high triglycerides, fasting glucose of 110 mg/dl or greater, history of gestational diabetes, hypertension, and polycystic ovary syndrome (McLaren and Marangell 2004; Sowell et al. 2002).

Cardiovascular Disorders

As noted above, persons with bipolar disorder have a higher prevalence of cardiac risk factors, such as dyslipidemia, glucose dysregulation, and obesity. The fat-patterning in individuals with bipolar disorder may lead to central adiposity, which is an independent risk factor for coronary artery disease (Elmslie et al. 2001; Poirier and Despres 2003). A recent study among a national mixed-age sample of Veterans Health Administration (VHA) patients found that hypertension was the most prevalent co-occurring condition, affecting one-third of those with bipolar disorder, followed by hyperlipidemia and diabetes — reflecting the substantial burden of vascular disease in persons with bipolar disorder (Kilbourne et al. 2004). Cardiovascular diseases and hypertension were also the most common diseases in a mixed-age outpatient population with bipolar illness (Beyer et al. 2005), occurring in 11% of the sample. Another study specifically involving older VHA patients with serious mental illness, including bipolar disorder, found that cardiovascular disorders were among the most common conditions, present in almost half of those older than 60 years (Kilbourne et al. 2005). Thus, it is not unexpected that individuals with bipolar disorder also have greater mortality from cardiovascular disease than the general population (Sharma and Markar 1994).

Dementia

There is some evidence that individuals with bipolar disorder develop dementia at a higher than expected rate (Berrios and Bakshi 1991; Dhingra and Rabins 1991; Kessing and Nilsson 2003), but not all studies support this (Lyketsos et al. 1995). A recent study found that elderly patients with bipolar disorder had more cognitive and functional impairment than younger patients (Depp et al. 2005). Cognitive dysfunction related to the hippocampus occurs in bipolar disorder and may be present even in euthymic states; such impairment is associated with the number of previous mood episodes, suggesting that progressive neural changes may occur over the course of the illness (Martinez-Aran et al. 2004). A recent study in Denmark of older patients with unipolar and bipolar disorders found that the risk of dementia was significantly increased with increasing number of prior affective episodes (Kessing and Andersen 2004).

Just as studies have suggested a bidirectional relation between depression and vascular disease, forming the basis of the "vascular depression" hypothesis (Alexopoulos et al. 1997), a similar relation may exist with bipolar disorder. Individuals with bipolar disorder may be at higher risk of cerebrovascular injury leading to vascular dementia. As with late-life depression, a higher prevalence of white matter hyperintensities is found on brain MRI in subjects with bipolar disorder than in controls (Ahn et al. 2004). Similarly, late-onset mania is associated with vascular risk factors such as smoking, hypertension, diabetes, coronary artery disease, and atrial fibrillation (Cassidy and Carroll 2002). Thus, a vascular mania subtype has also been proposed (Steffens and Krishnan 1998). Another possible mechanism linking bipolar disorder and dementia is cortisol-induced neurotoxicity and hypothalamic-pituitary-adrenal axis dysregulation (Watson et al. 2004).

MEDICAL DISORDERS RELATED TO THE PHARMACOLOGICAL TREATMENT OF BIPOLAR DISORDER
The Metabolic Syndrome

Metabolic syndrome is a term coined to describe the recognized clustering of metabolic and cardiovascular abnormalities such as obesity, dyslipidemia, and abnormalities of glucose homeostasis (Toalson et al. 2004). One cause of the metabolic syndrome in patients with bipolar disorder is the pharmacological treatment of the disorder itself. Many medications used in the treatment of bipolar disorder are associated with weight gain, which in turn is associated with the development of metabolic disturbances such as diabetes. These medications include lithium (Baptista et al. 1995), valproic acid (valproate) and carbamazepine (Swann 2001), and atypical antipsychotic agents (Allison and Casey 2001; Kato and Goodnick 2001; Lindenmayer et al. 2003).

The association between atypical antipsychotic agents and diabetes is the best studied link, and consensus panels currently recommend diabetic screening for patients treated with these agents. Diabetic screening recommendations for atypical antipsychotics are presented in table 9.1 (American Diabetes Association et al. 2004). If baseline physician assessments determine that a patient is overweight or obese (body mass index [BMI] 25–29.9 or ≥30, respectively), has pre-diabetes (fasting

TABLE 9.1
Recommendations for diabetic screening of patients receiving atypical antipsychotic treatment

Initiation of treatment	History
	Personal/family history of obesity diabetes, dyslipidemia, hypertension, cardiovascular disease
	Measurements
	Weight (BMI)
	Waist circumference
	Blood pressure
	Baseline lab tests
	Fasting glucose
	Fasting lipid profile
Treatment weeks 4 and 8	Measurements
	Weight (BMI)
Treatment week 12	Measurements
	Weight (BMI)
	Blood pressure
	Monitoring lab tests
	Fasting glucose
	Fasting lipid profile
Quarterly	Measurements
	Weight (BMI)
Annually	History
	Signs and symptoms of obesity, diabetes, dyslipidemia, hypertension, cardiovascular disease
	Measurements
	Waist circumference
	Blood pressure
	Monitoring lab tests
	Fasting glucose
Every 5 years (more frequently if clinically indicated)	Monitoring lab tests
	Fasting lipid profile

Source: Adapted from American Diabetes Association et al. 2004.
Abbreviations: BMI, body mass index.

plasma glucose 100–125 mg/dl) or diabetes (fasting glucose ≥126 mg/dl), has hypertension (blood pressure >140/90 mm Hg), or has dyslipidemia, appropriate treatment or referrals should be initiated. In terms of follow-up monitoring, if a patient (1) gains 5% or more of his or her initial weight at any time during therapy or (2) develops worsening glycemia or dyslipidemia, switching or discontinuing atypical agents should be considered. Immediate care or consultation should be requested for patients with symptomatic or severe hyperglycemia (glucose >300 mg/dl) or symptoms of hypoglycemia or diabetic ketoacidosis.

One study of patients with bipolar disorder followed up over a 10 year period found that weight gain primarily occurred in individuals who were not overweight at baseline, and it tended to occur early in the course of treatment (Fagiolini et al. 2002). Baseline depression rating was positively related to weight gain, leading the investigators to suggest that the relation between bipolar episodes and weight gain is influenced both by medication treatment (longer and more aggressive treatment exposure during depressive episodes) and by changes in mood-influenced variables such as appetite, diet, and energy expenditure. It is also noted that patients with mood and psychotic disorders have a cluster of risk factors for overweight (Keck et al. 2003; Malhotra and McElroy 2002; McIntyre et al. 2001), such as sedentary lifestyles, binge-eating disorders, and pharmacological-associated weight gain, which predispose to obesity and are in turn associated with disorders of glucose metabolism (McIntyre and Konarski 2005).

Thyroid Abnormalities

Lithium has been found to inhibit the processes involved in thyroid hormone secretion, causing hypothyroidism in 5%–10% of patients taking lithium (Laurberg et al. 2005). A recent Canadian population-based study of older adults newly prescribed lithium or valproate found that the risk of thyroid supplementation (as a proxy for hypothyroidism) was significantly greater in lithium users (Shulman et al. 2005).

Lithium-induced hypothyroidism is more common in individuals with circulating thyroid antibodies (Lazarus 1998). An important finding is that autoimmune hypothyroidism seems to be more common in women and older adults (Johnston and Eagles 1999; Kleiner et al. 1999). In a study by Kupka and colleagues (2002b), circulating thyroid antibodies were found in 28% of patients with bipolar disorder and were correlated with thyroid failure (found in 17% of patients) but not with age, gender, mood state, rapid cycling, or lithium exposure. Thyroid failure was more common in women. The authors concluded that lithium treatment does not play an etiological role in the high prevalence of thyroid autoimmunity in individuals with bipolar illness but that, nevertheless, when treated with lithium, these patients are at risk of developing hypothyroidism through other mechanisms. Thus, thyroid auto-immunity and lithium exposure may be two independent but synergistic risk factors for hypothyroidism in individuals with bipolar disorder.

Nephrotoxicity

The prevalence of chronic renal disease is on the rise, and in 2003 was estimated at 11% of the U.S. population (Coresh et al. 2003). Lithium is a cause of renal toxicity. Lithium competes with magnesium in the kidney and thus inhibits the magnesium-dependent proteins responsible for activating vasopressin-sensitive adenyl cyclase (Timmer and Sands 1999). Markowitz and colleagues (2000) divided lithium neph-rotoxicity into three main categories: (1) nephrogenic diabetes insipidus (NDI), (2) acute intoxication, and (3) chronic renal disease. These authors noted that NDI is the most common renal side effect of lithium therapy leading to polyuria and poly-dipsia, resulting from a urinary concentrating defect.

Acute intoxication is most commonly due to lithium overdose, though the frequency of toxicity is greater in elderly patients, for whom it may occur even at therapeutic doses (Sproule et al. 2000). One study found the frequency of lithium toxicity in older patients ranged from 11% to 23% (Foster 1992). The risk of lithium toxicity also climbs with comorbidity; in a sample of medically ill patients with bipolar disorder, 76% of patients (13 of 17) taking lithium experienced adverse effects (Stoudemire et al. 1998).

The predominant form of chronic renal disease associated with lithium treatment is chronic tubulointerstitial nephropathy, a harbinger of which is renal insufficiency (with little or no proteinuria) in the setting of chronic NDI (Markowitz et al. 2000). Most studies show relatively infrequent, mild renal insufficiency attributable to lithium therapy (Boton et al. 1987).

COMORBIDITY COMPLICATING THE MEDICAL MANAGEMENT OF BIPOLAR DISORDER

Age-related physiological changes that influence lithium pharmacokinetics, such as reduced renal clearance, are well documented. Less well described are the effects of co-occurring medical conditions on the pharmacokinetics of agents used to treat bipolar disorder (Sproule et al. 2000). Table 9.2 summarizes significant treatment considerations for older patients with bipolar disorder and medical comorbidities complicating pharmacological treatment of mania.

Reduced Renal Clearance

Although lithium is contraindicated in acute renal failure, *chronic* renal failure is not an absolute contraindication (McLaren and Marangell 2004). In the latter case, close monitoring is warranted, with blood lithium levels maintained between 0.6 and 0.8 mEq/L (DasGupta and Jefferson 1990). Lithium has also been used successfully for patients receiving hemodialysis, by administration of a single post-dialysis dose of 300–600 mg and monitoring of lithium levels both pre-dialysis and two to three hours post-dialysis (McLaren and Marangell 2004). The clearance of gabapentin also correlates with creatinine clearance, and the dose should be decreased accordingly for patients with renal insufficiency (Bernus et al. 1997). Dosage adjustment of risperidone is also recommended in renal disease and for elderly individuals, given the decreased clearance and increased half-life in these patients (Physicians' Desk Reference 2005b). One study found that the half-life of risperidone was 19 hours in younger adults versus 25 hours in elderly adults and in patients with renal disease (Snoeck et al. 1995). The pharmacokinetics of olanzapine, quetiapine, and oral ziprasidone are not altered in patients with renal disease (Aweeka et al. 2000; Ereshefsky 1996); however, as one of the agents used to solubilize intramuscular ziprasidone is cleared by renal filtration, this medication should be administered with caution to patients with impaired renal function (Physicians' Desk Reference 2005a).

Renal function in elderly persons is also affected by hypertension, atherosclerosis, and congestive heart failure (Fliser et al. 1997). Because decreased renal blood flow results in slowed clearance, patients with congestive heart failure may need lithium dose reductions of 50% (Benowitz 1984). Obese patients may require *larger* maintenance doses of lithium, because of an increased renal clearance (Reiss et al. 1994).

Reduced Liver Function

Given the increased rates of alcohol use found in mixed-age samples with bipolar disorder, especially among men (Kawa et al. 2005), as well as the increased rates of hepatitis C (Kilbourne et al. 2004), liver function may be a concern in this population. In patients with hepatic insufficiency, blood levels of most psychotropics except lithium and gabapentin are increased. Mechanisms include decreased oxidative metabolism; reduction of conjugation pathways; decreased hepatic blood flow due to portocaval shunting; decreased quantity and affinity of plasma proteins, re-

TABLE 9.2

Significant treatment considerations for older patients with bipolar disorder and medical comorbidities

Drug	Renal clearance reduced	Hepatic clearance reduced	Cardiovascular disease	Dementia	Drug-drug interactions
Lithium	Contraindicated in acute renal failure Adjust dosing in chronic renal failure and hemodialysis	May need to increase dose (fluid shifts in ascites)	May cause sinus node dysfunction at therapeutic levels Arrhythmias at toxic levels May exacerbate CHF; monitor level (fluid and electrolyte changes)	May be poorly tolerated Reduce dose and monitor closely for worsened cognition and other side effects	Increased risk of arrhythmia when combined with ACE inhibitors Levels affected by ACE inhibitors, thiazide diuretics, and NSAIDs (increased); and theophylline (decreased)
Valproate	None	Reduce dose with elevated transaminases	May need decreased dose in CHF	Patients may be more prone to adverse events such as sedation	Risk of liver injury with lipid-lowering agents Increased risk of bleeding with antiplatelet agents, warfarin, niacin

Drug					
Carbamazepine	May need to reduce dose (reduced clearance of toxic metabolite)	Reduce dose with elevated transaminases	Increased risk of complete heart block (quinidine-like) May need decreased dose in CHF	Patients may be more prone to adverse events such as ataxia and diplopia	Increased metabolism of some anti-coagulant and cardiovascular drugs via induction of CYP3A4
Gabapentin	May need to reduce dose	None	None	CNS side effects (somnolence, dizziness, ataxia) in some patients	Cimetidine may reduce clearance Antacids reduce bioavailability
Atypical antipsychotics	May need to reduce dose of risperidone by 50%–60% (decreased clearance); caution with intramuscular ziprasidone	May need to reduce dose	Ziprasidone: QT prolongation/risk of torsade de pointes (avoid post-MI) May need decreased dose in CHF Orthostatic hypotension with risperidone and quetiapine Increases in cardiac risk factors (weight gain, metabolic changes, hyperlipidemia)	Increased risk of mortality in analysis of pooled data from elderly patients with dementia-related behavioral disorders	CYP inhibitors or inducers may alter plasma concentrations

Abbreviations: CHF, congestive heart failure; ACE, angiotensin-converting enzyme; NSAID, nonsteroidal anti-inflammatory drug; CYP, cytochrome P450; CNS, central nervous system; MI, myocardial infarction.

sulting in increased free-drug levels; and increased volume of distribution in patients with ascites (Leipzig 1990). While doses of most psychotropics consequently need to be reduced for patients with comorbid liver disease, lithium doses may actually need to be increased when ascites is present (McLaren and Marangell 2004).

Reduced liver function associated with aging may also affect the elimination of antiepileptic drugs metabolized by oxidative mechanisms. In older adults, the capacity to eliminate valproate from the body is reduced compared with that in younger adults (Sajatovic et al. 2005). Monitoring for early signs of hepatic toxicity (apathy, malaise, decreased appetite, nausea and vomiting) and regular checking of aminotransferase levels are recommended to help identify patients with early or silent hepatotoxicity (Swann 2001).

Cardiovascular Disease

Many of the medications used to treat bipolar disorder may have cardiac side effects or toxicity; underlying cardiac disease may also affect the pharmacokinetics of psychotropic agents (McLaren and Marangell 2004). Lithium at therapeutic levels has been associated with sinus node dysfunction and, in toxicity, with atrioventricular block and dissociation, sinoatrial block, bradyarrhythmias, ventricular tachycardia, and ventricular fibrillation (DasGupta and Jefferson 1990). However, Glassman (2005) has noted that direct cardiovascular side effects of lithium tend to be rare and that most lithium-related cardiac symptoms are related to drug-drug interactions.

Carbamazepine is the antiepileptic mood stabilizer with the most recognized cardiovascular risk, associated with (1) increases in serum lipid levels and (2) complete heart block in patients with preexisting intraventricular conduction delays, due to carbamazepine's quinidine-like properties (Glassman 2005; Kasarkis et al. 1992). Atypical antipsychotics that antagonize alpha-1 receptors (quetiapine > risperidone > olanzapine and ziprasidone) increase the risk of orthostatic hypotension in patients with congestive heart failure (Carruthers 1994). QT interval prolongation is a concern with ziprasidone; although, theoretically, this drug increases the risk of torsade de pointes, ziprasidone has now been used in more than 600,000 patients with no reported cases (Glassman 2005).

Dementia

Comorbid dementia may confer added vulnerability to the neurocognitive side effects of medications used in the treatment of late-life bipolar disorder (Young et al. 2004). One study found lithium was poorly tolerated by patients with dementia or parkinsonian features (Himmelhoch et al. 1980). Caution should be exercised with lithium dosing, and patients should be monitored closely for worsened cognitive status and other side effects. Benzodiazepines can decrease memory consolidation and worsen cognitive impairment (Pomara et al. 1998). In a placebo-controlled trial of valproate in older patients with dementia and manic features, there was a 22% rate of valproate discontinuation due to adverse events, primarily sedation (Tariot et al. 2001). Another trial of carbamazepine noted diplopia and/or ataxia as side effects in 23% of patients with dementia (Smith and Perry 1992). However, as noted by Young and colleagues (2004), such reports of medication side effects in dementia have not included patients *without* dementia, which would allow a comparison of adverse event rates.

Executive impairment related to frontostriatal dysfunction may be associated with an attenuated antimanic response to lithium (Young et al. 2001) and valproate (Tariot et al. 2001). As in patients with depression and pseudodementia, acute treatment can improve cognitive performance for some patients with bipolar disorder (Wylie et al. 1999), but as with depression, cognitive impairments associated with mania may be persistent (Ferrier and Thompson 2002). A recent study reported that patients with bipolar disorder had functional disturbances in frontosubcortical structures, the cerebellum, and the limbic system (Benabarre et al. 2005).

The U.S. Food and Drug Administration (2005) has recently issued a public health advisory to warn health care providers, patients, and caregivers about the off-label use of atypical antipsychotic agents for the treatment of dementia-related behavioral disorders in the elderly. The warning was prompted by a concern for increased mortality detected in a pooled analysis of data from 17 placebo-controlled trials. These data showed that the use of olanzapine, aripiprazole, risperidone, and quetiapine by more than 5,000 elderly patients with dementia-related behavioral disorders was associated with an increased risk of mortality compared with placebo (4.5% vs. 2.6%). Most deaths seemed to be related to cardiovascular events (sudden death, heart failure) or infectious causes. Because the increased mortality risk was associated with medications from all three chemical classes of atypical antipsychotics, the FDA considers this to be a common pharmacological effect of atypical antipsychotics. Older antipsychotics are similarly associated with increased mortality (Wang et al. 2005). Until this risk is clarified, physicians should carefully consider the use of antipsychotic medications for older patients with dementia-related behavioral disorders, weighing risks and benefits in discussion with patients and their caregivers.

Drug-Drug Interactions

For older patients with bipolar disorder, it is also important to consider that drugs commonly taken for comorbid medical illnesses and bipolar disorder can cause clinically significant pharmacokinetic drug interactions. Lithium levels are increased by ACE inhibitors, thiazide diuretics, and nonsteroidal anti-inflammatory drugs (Sproule et al. 2000). The risk of arrhythmias is also increased when lithium is used in combination with ACE inhibitors (Dewan et al. 2003). Dietary salt restriction to control hypertension or congestive heart failure can also lead to increased lithium levels (Glassman 2005). Theophylline can decrease lithium levels via increased renal clearance; dosages of lithium may need to be increased by as much as 60% (Anthenelli 2005). Valproate levels are increased by concomitant use of aspirin (Abbott et al. 1986). Valproate itself increases levels of lamotrigine (Calabrese et al. 2002), amitriptyline (Wong et al. 1996), and warfarin (Panjehshahin et al. 1991). There is an increased risk of bleeding when valproate is used in combination with antiplatelet agents, warfarin, and niacin, and liver injury may result when valproate is used with lipid-lowering agents (McLaren and Marangell 2004). Drugs with possible interactions with carbamazepine include calcium channel blockers, cimetidine, and erythromycin (Fuller and Sajatovic 2002). Carbamazepine increases the metabolism of some anticoagulant and cardiovascular medications via induction of the cytochrome P450 (CYP) 3A4 isoenzyme (McLaren and Marangell 2004). Gabapentin seems to have few clinically significant drug interactions, although cimetidine is reported to decrease gabapentin clearance and antacids reduce gabapentin's bioavailability (Busch et al. 1992; Richens 1993). Inhibitors or inducers of CYP may alter plasma concentrations of atypical antipsychotics. For example, ketoconazole may increase quetiapine concentrations fourfold via inhibition of CYP3A4; ciprofloxacin may double olanzapine concentrations via inhibition of CYP1A2; and phenytoin may decrease quetiapine concentrations by 80% via induction of CYP3A4 (Spina et al. 2003).

MEDICAL COMORBIDITY AND CARE MANAGEMENT

Medical illnesses co-occurring with bipolar disorder complicate the care management of older patients. In the case illustrated at the beginning of this chapter, Mr. P. had been stable for many years on his medication regimen. The critical factors that led to his destabilization and deterioration were not psychiatric but medical: (1) an episode of lithium toxicity precipitated by addition of a medication (ACE inhibitor) for cardiovascular disease and (2) a prolonged and severe episode of mania brought on by nonadherence to his medication regimen resulting from the development of memory problems.

Implications for Preventive Care

Given that older adults with bipolar disorder are at higher risk for certain medical comorbidities, strategies are needed that focus on improving access to and quality of general medical services for older patients, as well as coordinating general medical and psychiatric care for this group (Kilbourne et al. 2005). In addition, physicians should consider screening for the disorders commonly co-occurring with or consequent to bipolar disorder. This would include screening for diabetes (fasting blood glucose), even in patients not taking atypical antipsychotics. Mr. P. developed diabetes several years *after* he had discontinued risperidone; thus, the diabetes may have been related more to the underlying mood disorder than to its treatment. Given the risk of liver disease related to either hepatitis C or alcohol use in a subset of patients with bipolar illness, as well as the impact of hepatic insufficiency on the blood levels of many psychotropics, screening for liver disease (liver function tests) is useful. Similarly, with increasing rates of renal disease in older patients, age-related changes in renal clearance, and histories of lithium exposure in older patients with bipolar illness, checking renal function (blood urea nitrogen and creatinine) also has merit. Thyroid autoimmunity and lithium exposure may be two independent but synergistic risk factors for hypothyroidism in individuals with bipolar disorder; thus, thyroid function testing is worthwhile. A baseline electrocardiogram is likely to be advisable in many patients. Finally, given the associations between the development of dementia and recurrent mood episodes, physicians should consider screening for cognitive disorders with the Mini Mental State Examination. Close collaboration between primary care physicians and psychiatrists is needed for older patients, especially if any of the screening tests show reason for concern.

Adherence

In the case of Mr. P., cognitive impairment resulted in nonadherence to his lithium regimen, leading to an episode of severe mania. In addition, once Mr. P. became manic, he also began to take his other medications, including oral hypoglycemics, erratically. Even for individuals without dementia, nonadherence can lead to poor psychiatric and medical outcomes. Thus, appropriate interventions designed to alleviate mood symptoms by improving adherence are likely to minimize medical complications (e.g., elevated blood glucose or hypoglycemia). Further, given the association between recurrent mood episodes and dementia (Kessing and Andersen 2004), adherence to treatment for bipolar disorder could possibly lower the risk for the development of dementia.

The Role of Social Support

If Mr. P. had had more adequate social support, such as involved family or friends who could have assisted him in taking his medications appropriately, his multiple psychiatric hospitalizations and eventual placement in a nursing home might have been averted. The role of social support in late-life bipolar disorder itself is poorly understood. One study found that older patients with bipolar disorder were more likely to perceive their social support as inadequate than were older persons without this disorder (Beyer et al. 2003). It is also known that older patients with depression and impaired social support are more likely to be resistant to treatment and have increased hospitalizations and poorer outcomes (Blazer et al. 1992). A recent study found that older patients with bipolar disorder had significantly more functional and cognitive impairment than younger adult patients and were significantly more likely to require case management (Depp et al. 2005).

Even when social support is available, manic, high-risk behaviors are often more difficult for family members to cope with than depressive states. A recent study confirmed the finding that older patients' manic symptoms are more strongly linked to caregiver well-being and relationship satisfaction than are patients' depressive symptoms (Martire et al. 2004). The investigators also found that nonadherence to treatment was associated with higher family burden; they concluded that the difficulty of bipolar patients in adhering to treatment may become especially salient in late life, as patients are challenged by physical illnesses. The added influence of medical comorbidity on negative outcomes such as revolving hospitalizations and premature placement in a nursing home merits further study, as community-based interventions could be of significant benefit.

CONCLUSIONS

The management and treatment of late-life bipolar disorder are made more complex by the co-occurring medical illnesses commonly found in older adults. Common late-life comorbidities, including diabetes, cardiovascular disorders, and dementia, may have bidirectional relations with bipolar disorder. Older patients with bipolar disorder may also be predisposed to medical disorders caused by psychopharmacological treatment—such as hypothyroidism, nephrotoxicity, or the metabolic syndrome—because of underlying biological abnormalities or medical illnesses. As a result of these complexities, the integration of medical and psychiatric care is critical. Physicians treating older adults with bipolar disorder must be aware of medication interactions and of the changes in medication dosing and in care management that are required by the co-occurrence of bipolar disorder with medical illnesses.

REFERENCES

Abbott, F. S., Kassam, J., Orr, J. M., et al. 1986. The effect of aspirin on valproic acid metabolism. *Clin Pharmacol Ther* 40:94–100.
Ahn, K. H., Lyoo, I. K., Lee, H. K., et al. 2004. White matter hyperintensities in subjects with bipolar disorder. *Psychiatry Clin Neurosci* 58:516–521.
Alexopoulos, G. S., Meyers, B. S., Young, R. C., et al. 1997. "Vascular depression" hypothesis. *Arch Gen Psychiatry* 54:915–922.
Allison, D. B., and Casey, D. E. 2001. Antipsychotic-induced weight gain: a review of the literature. *J Clin Psychiatry* 62(suppl.):22–31.
American Diabetes Association, American Psychiatric Association, American Association of Clinical Endocrinologists, and North American Association for the Study of Obesity. 2004. Consensus development conference on antipsychotic drugs and obesity and diabetes. *Diabetes Care* 27:596–601.
Anthenelli, R. M. 2005. Treating patients with bipolar disorder and COPD or asthma. *Curr Psychiatry* 4(suppl.):34–42.
Aweeka, F., Jayesekara, D., Horton, M., et al. 2000. The pharmacokinetics of ziprasidone in subjects with normal and impaired renal function. *Br J Clin Pharmacol* 49(suppl. 1):27S–33S.
Baptista, T., Teneud, L., Contreras, Q., et al. 1995. Lithium and body weight gain. *Pharmacopsychiatry* 28:35–44.
Benabarre, A., Vieta, E., Martinez-Aran, A., et al. 2005. Neuropsychological disturbances and cerebral blood flow in bipolar disorder. *Aust N Z J Psychiatry* 39:227–234.
Benowitz, N. L. 1984. Effects of cardiac disease on pharmacokinetics: pathophysiologic considerations. In Benet, L. Z., Massoud, N., and Gambertoglio, J. G. (eds.), *Pharmacologic basis for drug treatment*. New York: Raven Press.
Bernus, I., Dickinson, R. G., Hooper, W. D., et al. 1997. Anticonvulsant therapy in aged patients: clinical pharmacokinetic considerations. *Drugs Aging* 10:278–289.
Berrios, G. E., and Bakshi, N. 1991. Manic and depressive symptoms in the elderly: their relationships to treatment outcome, cognition, and motor symptoms. *Psychopathology* 24:31–38.
Beyer, J. L., Kuchibhatla, M., Looney, C., et al. 2003. Social support in elderly patients with bipolar disorder. *Bipolar Disord* 5:22–27.
Beyer J., Kuchibhatla, M., Gersing, K., et al. 2005. Medical comorbidity in a bipolar outpatient clinical population. *Neuropsychopharmacology* 30:401–404.

Blazer, D., Hughes, D. C., and George, L. K. 1992. Age and impaired subjective support: predictors of depressive symptoms at one-year follow-up. *J Nerv Ment Dis* 180:172–178.

Boton, R., Gaviria, M., and Batlle, D. C. 1987. Prevalence, pathogenesis, and treatment of renal dysfunction associated with chronic lithium therapy. *Am J Kidney Dis* 10:329–345.

Brown, S. 2001. Variations in utilization and cost of inpatient psychiatric services among adults in Maryland. *Psychiatr Serv* 52:841–843.

Busch, J. A., Radulovic, L. L., Bockbrader, H. N., et al. 1992. Effect of Maalox TC on single-dose pharmacokinetics of gabapentin capsules in healthy subjects. *Pharm Res* 9(suppl.): 315S.

Calabrese, J. R., Shelton, M. D., Rapport, D. J., et al. 2002. Bipolar disorders and the effectiveness of novel anticonvulsants. *J Clin Psychiatry* 63(suppl. 3):5S–9S.

Carruthers, S. G. 1994. Adverse effects of alpha 1-adrenergic blocking drugs. *Drug Saf* 11:12–20.

Cassidy, F., Ahearn E., and Carroll, B. J. 1999. Elevated frequency of diabetes mellitus in hospitalized manic-depressive patients. *Am J Psychiatry* 156:1417–1420.

Cassidy, F., and Carroll, B. J. 2002. Vascular risk factors in late onset mania. *Psychol Med* 32:359–362.

Coresh, J., Astor, B. C., Greene, T., et al. 2003. Prevalence of chronic kidney disease and decreased kidney function in the adult US population: third national health and nutrition examination survey. *Am J Kidney Dis* 41:1–12.

DasGupta, K., and Jefferson, J. W. 1990. The use of lithium in the medically ill. *Gen Hosp Psychiatry* 12:83–97.

Depp, C. A., Lindamer, L. A., Folsom, D. P., et al. 2005. Differences in clinical features and mental health service use in bipolar disorder across the life span. *Am J Geriatr Psychiatry* 13:290–298.

Dewan, N. A., Suresh, D. P., and Blomklans, A. 2003. Selecting safe psychotropics for post-MI patients. *Curr Psychiatry* 2:14–21.

Dhingra, U., and Rabins, P. V. 1991. Mania in the elderly: a five-to-seven year follow-up. *J Am Geriatr Soc* 39:581–583.

Elmslie, J. L., Mann, J. I., Silverstone, J. T., et al. 2001. Determinants of overweight and obesity in patients with bipolar disorder. *J Clin Psychiatry* 62:486–491.

Ereshefsky, L. 1996. Pharmacokinetics and drug interactions: update for new antipsychotics. *J Clin Psychiatry* 57(suppl. 11):12–25.

Fagiolini, A., Frank, E., Houck, P. R., et al. 2002. Prevalence of obesity and weight change during treatment in patients with bipolar I disorder. *J Clin Psychiatry* 63:528–533.

Ferrier, I. N., and Thompson, J. M. 2002. Cognitive impairment in bipolar affective disorder: implications for the bipolar diathesis. *Br J Psychiatry* 180:293–295.

Fliser, D., Franek, E., Joest, M., et al. 1997. Renal function in the elderly: impact of hypertension and cardiac function. *Kidney Int* 51:1196–1204.

Foster, J. R. 1992. Use of lithium in elderly psychiatry patients: a review of the literature. *Lithium* 3:77–93.

Fuller, M., and Sajatovic, M. 2002. *Drug information handbook for psychiatry* (3rd ed). Cleveland, OH: Lexi-Comp.

Glassman, A. H. 2005. Treatment of patients with bipolar disorder and cardiovascular disease. *Curr Psychiatry* 4(suppl.):21–33.

Himmelhoch, J. M., Neil, J. F., May, S. J., et al. 1980. Age, dementia, dyskinesias, and lithium response. *Am J Psychiatry* 137:941–945.

Johnston, A. M., and Eagles, J. M. 1999. Lithium-associated clinical hypothyroidism: prevalence and risk factors. *Br J Psychiatry* 175:336–339.

Juurlink, D. N., Herrmann, N., Szalai, J. P., et al. 2004. Medical illness and the risk of suicide in the elderly. *Arch Intern Med* 164:1179–1184.

Kasarskis, E. J., Kuo, C. S., Berger, R., et al. 1992. Carbamazepine-induced cardiac dysfunction: characterization of two distinct clinical syndromes. *Arch Intern Med* 152:186–191.

Kato, M. M., and Goodnick, P. J. 2001. Antipsychotic medication: effects on regulation of glucose and lipids. *Expert Opin Pharmacother* 2:1571–1582.

Kawa, I., Carter, J. D., Joyce, P. R., et al. 2005. Gender differences in bipolar disorder: age of onset, course, comorbidity, and symptom presentation. *Bipolar Disord* 7:119–125.

Keck, P. E., Buse, J. B., Dagogo-Jack, S., et al. 2003. *Managing metabolic concerns in patients with severe mental illness.* Postgraduate medicine special report. Minneapolis: Healthcare Information Programs, McGraw-Hill Healthcare Informations Group.

Kessing, L. V., and Andersen, P. K. 2004. Does the risk of developing dementia increase with the number of episodes in patients with depressive disorder and in patients with bipolar disorder? *J Neurol Neurosurg Psychiatry* 75:1662–1666.

Kessing, L. V., and Nilsson, F. M. 2003. Increased risk of developing dementia in patients with major affective disorders compared to patients with other medical illnesses. *J Affect Disord* 73:261–269.

Kilbourne, A. M., Cornelius, J. R., Han, X., et al. 2004. Burden of general medical conditions among individuals with bipolar disorder. *Bipolar Disord* 6:368–373.

Kilbourne, A. M., Cornelius, J. R., Han, X., et al. 2005. General-medical conditions in older patients with serious mental illness. *Am J Geriatr Psychiatry* 13:250–254.

Kleiner, J., Altshuler, L., Hendrick, V., et al. 1999. Lithium-induced subclinical hypothyroidism: review of the literature and guidelines for treatment. *J Clin Psychiatry* 60:249–255.

Krishnan, K. R. 2005. Psychiatric and medical comorbidities of bipolar disorder. *Psychosom Med* 67:1–8.

Kupka, R. W., Breunis, M. N., Knijff, E., et al. 2002a. Immune activation, steroid resistance and bipolar disorder. *Bipolar Disord* 4(suppl.):73–74.

Kupka R. W., Nolen, W. A., Post, R. M., et al. 2002b. High rate of autoimmune thyroiditis in bipolar disorder: lack of association with lithium exposure. *Biol Psychiatry* 51:305–311.

Laurberg, P., Andersen, S., Bulow P. I., et al. 2005. Hypothyroidism in the elderly: pathophysiology, diagnosis, and treatment. *Drugs Aging* 22:23–38.

Lazarus, J. H. 1998. The effects of lithium therapy on thyroid and thyrotropin-releasing hormone. *Thyroid* 8:909–913.

Leipzig, R. M. 1990. Psychopharmacology in patients with hepatic and gastrointestinal disease. *Int J Psychiatry Med* 20:109–139.

Lindenmayer, J. P., Czobor, P., Volavka, J., et al. 2003. Changes in glucose and cholesterol levels in patients with schizophrenia treated with typical or atypical antipsychotics. *Am J Psychiatry* 160:290–296.

Lustman, P. J., Anderson, R. J., Freedland, K. E., et al. 2000. Depression and poor glycemic control: a meta-analytic review of the literature. *Diabetes Care* 23:934–942.

Lyketsos, C. G., Corazzinini, K., and Steele, C. 1995. Mania in Alzheimer's disease. *J Neurol Clin Neurosci* 7:350–352.

Malhotra, S., and McElroy, S. L. 2002. Medical management of obesity associated with mental disorders. *J Clin Psychiatry* 63(suppl. 4):24–32.

Markowitz, G. S., Radhakrishnan, J., Kambham, N., et al. 2000. Lithium nephrotoxicity: a progressive combined glomerular and tubulointerstitial nephropathy. *J Am Soc Nephrol* 11:1439–1448.

Martinez-Aran, A., Vieta, E., Colom, F., et al. 2004. Cognitive impairment in euthymic bipolar patients: implications for clinical and functional outcome. *Bipolar Disord* 6:224–232.

Martire, L. M., Schulz, R., Mulsant, B. H., et al. 2004 Family caregiver functioning in late-life bipolar disorder. *Am J Geriatr Psychiatry* 12:335–336.

McElroy, S. L., Frye, M. A., Suppes, T., et al. 2002. Correlates of overweight and obesity in 644 patients with bipolar disorder. *J Clin Psychiatry* 63:207–213.

McIntyre, R. S., and Konarski, J. Z. 2005. Bipolar disorder, overweight/obesity, and disorders of glucose metabolism. *Curr Psychiatry* 4(suppl.):11–20.

McIntyre, R. S., McCann, S. M., and Kennedy, S. H., 2001. Antipsychotic metabolic effects: weight gain, diabetes mellitus, and lipid abnormalities. *Can J Psychiatry* 46:273–281.

McLaren, K. D., and Marangell, L. B. 2004. Special considerations in the treatment of patients with bipolar disorder and medical comorbidities. *Ann Gen Hosp Psychiatry* 3:7.

Panjehshahin, M. R., Bowman, C. J., and Yates, M. S. 1991. Effect of valproic acid, its unsaturated metabolites and some structurally related fatty acids on the binding of warfarin and dansylsacrosine to human albumin. *Biochem Pharmacol* 41:1227–1233.

Physicians' Desk Reference. 2005a. Geodon for injection. *Physicians' desk reference* (59th ed.) Montvale, NJ: Thomson.

Physicians' Desk Reference. 2005b. Risperidone. *Physicians' desk reference* (59th ed.) Montvale, NJ: Thomson.

Poirier, P., and Despres, J. P. 2003. Waist circumference, visceral obesity, and cardiovascular risk. *J Cardiopulm Rehabil* 23:161–169.

Pomara, N., Tun, H., DaSilva, D., et al. 1998. The acute and chronic performance effects of alprazolam and lorazepam in the elderly: relationship to duration of treatment and self-rated sedation. *Psychopharmacol Bull* 34:139–153.

Regenold, W. T., Thapar, R. K., Maran, C., et al. 2002. Increased prevalence of type 2 diabetes mellitus among psychiatric inpatients with bipolar I affective and schizoaffective disorders independent of psychotropic drug use. *J Affect Disord* 70:19–26.

Reiss, R. A., Haas, C. E., Karki, S. D., et al. 1994. Lithium pharmacokinetics in the obese. *Clin Pharmacol Ther* 55:392–398.

Richens, A. 1993. Clinical pharmacokinetics of gabapentin. In Chadwick, D. (ed.), *New trends in epilepsy management: the role of gabapentin* (pp. 41–46). London: Royal Society of Medicine.

Ruzickova, M., Slaney, C., Garnham, J., et al. 2003. Clinical features of bipolar disorder with and without comorbid diabetes. *Can J Psychiatry* 48:458–461.

Sajatovic, M., Madhusoodanan, S., and Coconcea, N. 2005. Managing bipolar disorder in the elderly: defining the role of the newer agents. *Drugs Aging* 22:39–54.

Sharma, R., and Markar, H. R. 1994. Mortality in affective disorder. *J Affect Disord* 31:91–96.

Shulman, K. I., Sykora, K., Gill, S. S., et al. 2005. New thyroxine treatment in older adults beginning lithium therapy. *Am J Geriatr Psychiatry* 13:299–304.

Smith, D. A., and Perry, P. J. 1992. Nonneuroleptic treatment of disruptive behavior in organic mental syndromes. *Ann Pharmacother* 26:1400–1408.

Snoeck, E., Van Peer, A., Sack, M., et al. 1995. Influence of age, renal and liver impairment on the pharmacokinetics of risperidone in man. *Psychopharmacology* 122:223–229.

Sowell, M. O., Mukhopadhyay, N., Cavazzoni, P., et al. 2002. Hyperglycemic clamp assessment of insulin secretory responses in normal subjects treated with olanzapine, risperidone, or placebo. *J Clin Endocrinol Metab* 87:2918–2923.

Spina, E., Scordo, M. G., and D'Arrigo, C. 2003. Metabolic drug interactions with new psychotropic agents. *Fundam Clin Pharmacol* 17:517–538.

Sproule, B. A., Hardy, B. G., and Shulman, K. I. 2000. Differential pharmacokinetics of lithium in elderly patients. *Drugs Aging* 16:165–177.

Steffens, D. C., and Krishnan, K. R. 1998. Structural neuroimaging and mood disorders: recent findings, implications for classification, and future directions. *Biol Psychiatry* 43:705–712.

Stoudemire, A., Hill, C. D., Lewison, B. J., et al. 1998. Lithium intolerance in a medical-psychiatric population. *Gen Hosp Psychiatry* 20:85–90.

Swann, A. C. 2001. Major system toxicities and side effects of anticonvulsants. *J Clin Psychiatry* 62(suppl. 14):16–21.

Tariot, P. N., Schneider, L. S., Mintzer, J. E., et al. 2001. Safety and tolerability of divalproex sodium in the treatment of signs and symptoms of mania in elderly patients with dementia: results of a double-blind, placebo-controlled trial. *Curr Ther Res* 62:51–67.

Timmer, R. T., and Sands, J. M. 1999. Lithium intoxication. *J Am Soc Nephrol* 10:666–674.

Toalson, P., Ahmed, S., Hardy, T., et al. 2004. The metabolic syndrome in patients with severe mental illnesses. *Prim Care Companion J Clin Psychiatry* 6:152–158.

U.S. Food and Drug Administration. 2005. Public health advisory: deaths with antipsychotics in elderly patients with behavioral disturbances. April 11. www.fda.gov/cder/drug/advisory/antipsychotics.htm

Vanina, Y., Podolskaya, A., Sedky, K., et al. 2002. Body weight changes associated with psychopharmacology. *Psychiatr Serv* 53:842–847.

Wang, P.S., Schneeweiss, S., Avorn, J., et al. 2005. Risk of death in elderly users of conventional vs. atypical antipsychotic medications. *N Engl J Med* 353:2335–2241.

Watson, S., Gallagher, P., Ritchie, J. C., et al. 2004. Hypothalamic-pituitary-adrenal axis function in patients with bipolar disorder. *Br J Psychiatry* 184:496–502.

Wong, S. L., Cavanaugh, J., Shi, H., et al. 1996. Effects of divalproex sodium on amitriptyline and nortriptyline pharmacokinetics. *Clin Pharmacol Ther* 60:48–53.

Wylie, M. E., Mulsant, B. H., Pollock, B. G., et al. 1999. Age at onset in geriatric bipolar disorder: effects on clinical presentation and treatment outcomes in an inpatient sample. *Am J Geriatr Psychiatry* 7:77–83.

Young, R. C., Murphy, C. F., and DeAsis, J. M. 2001. Executive dysfunction and treatment outcome in geriatric mania. Presented at Annual Meeting, American Psychiatric Association, New Research.

Young, R. C., Gyulai, L., Mulsant, B. H., et al. 2004. Pharmacotherapy of bipolar disorder in old age: review and recommendations. *Am J Geriatr Psychiatry* 12:342–357.

CHAPTER TEN

Cultural Issues in the Diagnosis and Treatment of Bipolar Disorder

SANA LOUE, J.D., PH.D., M.P.H.

Culture has been defined as "a common heritage or set of beliefs, norms, and values" (U.S. Department of Health and Human Services 1999). Such a definition gives the impression that culture is something that is static and that resides in the individual, however common the particular values may be. Kleinman (1996) defined culture as follows:

> Culture is constituted by, and in turn constitutes, local worlds of everyday experience. That is to say, culture is built up ("realized") out of the everyday patterns of daily life activities — common sense, communication with others, and the routine rhythms and rituals of community life that are taken for granted — which reciprocally reflect the patterning downward of social relations by shared symbolic apparatuses — language, aesthetic sensibility, and core value orientations conveyed by master metaphors. In these local worlds, experience is an interpersonal flow of communication, interaction, and negotiation — that is, it is social, not individual — which centers on agreement and contestation about what is most at stake and how that which is at stake is to be sought and gained. Gender, age cohort, social role and status, and personal desire all inflect this small universe in different ways. The upshot is culture in the making, in the processes that generate action and that justify practices. Thus the locus of culture is not the mind of the isolated person, but the interconnected body/self of groups: families, work settings, networks, whole communities. (16)

This definition underscores both that culture is a system and that it is shared by members of a defined group.

How individuals come to be considered part of a specific group varies. Individuals may identify with a particular culture and look to that culture for relevant standards of behavior (C. R. Cooper and Denner 1998). Indeed, individuals may self-identify as a member of several cultures simultaneously and may have a composite self-identity. For instance, someone may self-identify as a member of the Irish, Catholic, white, and American cultures.

The concept of *race* has often been used to explain differences in appearance and in behavior across individuals and groups of individuals and, as a consequence, race is often mistakenly equated with culture (Gaines 1994). This frequently leads to an incorrect assumption that all individuals of a particular race share a common culture. Although race is frequently conceived of as a biological category that is assessed on the basis of the color of someone's skin or other physical attributes (Boas 1940; Gould 1981; Montagu 1964), research has demonstrated that racial categories are socially constructed and vary over time, place, and purpose. How race is defined in a particular place at a particular time is often reflective of culture. As an example, before 1989, a child born to a "white" father and a Japanese mother in the United States was classified as Japanese on his or her birth certificate. In pre-1985 Japan, however, the same child would have been classified as white on his or her birth certificate (LaVeist 1994). What this means is that, depending on the society and the era, older and younger individuals who are seemingly in the same circumstances may be classified differently with respect to race.

In contrast, *ethnicity* has been defined as a common heritage that is shared by members of a particular group (Zenner 1996). Three elements have been identified that are critical to the formation of an ethnic group: (1) the perception by other members of the society of differences between the group members and others with respect to certain traits, such as language, religion, race, or homeland; (2) the perception of these same differences by the group members; and (3) the participation of group members in shared activities that are founded on their perceived heritage or culture (Yinger 1994).

Culture affects mental illness in a number of ways: in how individuals express or present their symptoms (Kleinman 1977, 1988); in the meaning they ascribe to their illness in an attempt to make sense of their experience (Kleinman 1988); in how individuals and their families communicate about the problem or the symptom(s) (Tseng 1975); in whether, how, and from whom individuals seek treatment; in how they address the consequences of their illness (U.S. Department of Health and Human Services 2001); in how the problem or the symptom is understood and perceived by the clinician (Tseng et al. 1982); and in how the clinician classifies the disorder for clinical usage (J. E. Cooper et al. 1969; Tseng et al. 1992a, 1992b). Older and, perhaps, more traditional individuals may express their concerns differently than younger individuals and may even experience their illness differently. For instance, in this age of television dramas and Internet chat rooms, younger persons may be less reticent to speak about their symptoms, because of the attention now given to mental illness. Older individuals may be more reluctant to disclose symptoms, because of the shame and stigma more strongly associated with mental illness during their earlier years.

BIPOLAR DISORDER AND CULTURE

The lifetime prevalence of bipolar disorder is relatively consistent across parts of Asia, Europe, and North America, ranging from 0.3% in Taiwan to 1.5% in New Zealand (Weissman et al. 1996). Incidence, although difficult to determine because of the need for longitudinal assessment, has been found to range from 2.4 per 100,000 individuals in London, England, and Aarhus, Denmark (Leff et al. 1976), to 32.5 cases per 100,000 females in some Scandinavian locations (Boyd and Weissman 1981). These data, together with data derived from family and molecular genetic studies, have led some investigators to conclude that bipolar disorder has a high degree of heritability (National Institute of Mental Health 1998) and that cultural and societal factors play a secondary role in its causation (U.S. Department of Health and Human Services 2001). Investigators of a Finnish twin study, for instance, found from their analysis of data from 25 pairs of same-sex twins that the variance in liability for bipolar I disease was best explained by a model that included both genetic and specific environmental factors, with high heritability being demonstrated (Kieseppa et al. 2004). A recent review of family, twin, and adoption studies reached a similar conclusion (Shih et al. 2004).

Nevertheless, culture remains relevant to the experience and meaning of illness, including the shaping of symptoms; the management of illness episodes, including healing activities; and the management of outcomes. As an example, investigators have attempted to identify the gene or genes responsible for bipolar disorder through research conducted with the Amish community in Pennsylvania, believing that the relatively closed nature of the community would provide insights into the heritability of the disorder. One research group reported a link between chromosome 11 and a dominant gene that they thought conferred a predisposition to bipolar disorder (Egeland et al. 1987). An investigative team in Israel reported possible linkage of bipolar disorder to the X chromosome (Baron et al. 1987). These findings linking the disorder to chromosome 11 and the X chromosome have since been called into question (Hodgkinson et al. 1987). However, these investigations did reveal that a substantial proportion of individuals who carry the gene(s) for bipolar disorder will never develop the disease, indicating that there may be significant interplay between genetic predisposition and the physical and psychological environment.

In another study, investigators examining the prevalence of bipolar disorder and other bipolar spectrum disorders in various countries found that differences in prevalence seemed to be related to the lifelong ingestion of seafood (Noaghiul and Hibbeln 2003). They concluded that the consumption of omega-3 fatty acids, found in seafood, may be protective against the development of bipolar disorder. This further suggests that various environmental and cultural factors, such as dietary patterns, may be implicated in the development of bipolar disorder. Unfortunately, as will be seen below, relatively little research has focused on the interplay between culture and these dimensions of experience in the context of bipolar disorder. And even the relatively few studies that have examined bipolar disorder in the context of culture have often failed to consider how the cultural experience and expression of the disorder might vary across age groups.

THE EXPERIENCE, MEANING, AND PRESENTATION OF BIPOLAR ILLNESS

Relatively few studies have examined how symptoms indicative of bipolar disorder are experienced and expressed across cultures, although published studies suggest that the experience and expression do vary across cultures. One study of 134 individuals under the age of 55 of three ethnic groups living in the United Kingdom, all of whom were taking lithium prophylaxis, found that of patients who had been diagnosed with bipolar I disorder, those of African origin were significantly more likely than the white British patients to display symptoms of mania, while the African Caribbean patients were more likely to experience mood-incongruent delusions (Kirov and Murray 1999). The investigators were unable to explain the underlying reasons for this difference in the expression of the disorder. Other researchers have similarly reported a greater tendency for African Caribbean immigrants in the United Kingdom to present with manic symptoms compared with similarly diagnosed whites (van Os et al. 1996).

An investigation of first manic episode in bipolar disorder I among African Caribbean, African, and white European individuals in the United Kingdom found that the African Caribbean and African individuals were significantly less likely to have experienced a depressive episode before the onset of the first episode of mania (Kennedy et al. 2004). This finding persisted even after controlling for differences across the groups in sex, occupational category, educational level, and use of substances. The investigators hypothesized that this finding could be related to decreased access to treatment for depression among the African Caribbean and African patients and a resulting absence of depression in a patient's history, or to cultural beliefs about the unacceptability of depression or treatment of depression, or both.

Both the African Caribbean and African groups in this study had experienced an earlier onset of mania and bipolar disorder compared with the group of European whites, which the authors attributed to differences in population distribution (Kennedy et al. 2004). The African Caribbean and African groups were more likely to display symptoms of psychosis at the occurrence of first mania, including persecutory delusions, delusions of influence, and auditory hallucinations. The authors were unable to account for this finding, but they surmised that this severe clinical presentation might explain the overdiagnosis of schizophrenia that has been noted among African American patients (Strakowski et al. 2003).

A study of individuals with bipolar disorder in Israel noted the predominance of manic episodes over time (Osher et al. 2000), in contrast to the pattern of predominantly depressive episodes noted among European patients with bipolar disorder (Angst 1986; Judd et al. 2002). Two studies of the presentation and course of bipolar disorder in Nigeria also found that a unipolar manic course was most common (Makanjuola 1982, 1985). All of these studies taken together suggest that the clinical presentation of bipolar disorder may vary across cultures, for a variety of reasons.

There may be significant dissonance in the interpretation of symptoms of bipolar disorder between the patient and the care provider. In a study involving 147 patients diagnosed with bipolar disorder, investigators found that 19% had received conflicting advice from their physicians and their spiritual advisers; this was particularly true for patients who adhered to an evangelical faith (Mitchell and Romans 2003). Fully one-third of the conflicts involved instances in which the spiritual advisers had told the patients that they did not need their medications because they had been healed spiritually. Individuals who practiced their faith more frequently and who placed greater emphasis on the importance of prayer were more likely to experience conflict between the advice of their medical care provider and that of their spiritual leader. In general, older individuals were more likely to endorse the importance of spirituality in their lives.

Even the definition of what constitutes a symptom, or the classification of specified behaviors as symptoms, may require reformulation in the context of the local culture. For instance, in the study of bipolar disorder among the Amish people referred to above, researchers reinterpreted the behaviors indicative of symptoms of bipolar disorder to reflect the nature of the Amish culture. Accordingly, the diagnostic criterion of "excessive involvement in activities," which often encompasses sexual indiscretions, buying sprees, and ill-advised business ventures and indicates the presence of mania, was reformulated to refer to such things as "racing one's horse and carriage too hard or driving a car (recklessness not implied), buying or using machinery or worldly items forbidden by church rules (e.g., dressing up in worldly clothes), flirting with a married person (indeed any overt sexuality), treating livestock too roughly, excessive use of the public telephones (telephones are forbidden in homes), going on a smoking binge, and desiring to give gifts or planning vacations during the wrong season (because the agrarian principle and frugality confine these activities to a given time and place)" (Egeland et al. 1983, 68). However, just as it is important to consider culture in the formulation of diagnostic criteria, it is equally critical that clinicians and investigators avoid the assumption that specific cultural features must necessarily be displayed by each and every individual and that there is homogeneity across all individuals within a specified cultural community (Floersch et al. 1997). What may be considered appropriate for younger individuals, for example, may be considered entirely inappropriate for older persons.

MANAGING THE ILLNESS

Some differences in the management of bipolar disorder seem to be related to race and/or ethnicity and the characteristics attributed to specific race/ethnicity. A study of the psychopharmacological management of bipolar disorder found that African American teenagers diagnosed with the disorder and hospitalized were twice as likely as whites with the same diagnosis to receive antipsychotics, despite similarities in age, co-occurring diagnoses, length of hospitalization, and number of episodes of seclusion or restraint (Delbello et al. 2000). The authors hypothesized that this difference in illness management might be a result of a perception by the clinicians, all of whom were white, of greater disruptiveness among the African American adolescents than among the white adolescents. They also suggested that the different treatment provided to the African American adolescents might be linked to a misinterpretation of African Americans' culturally based paranoia as a psychotic symptom. Previous research findings suggest that mild forms of paranoia may be more common among African Americans than whites (Whaley 1998).

A study involving 42 African American and 80 white patients hospitalized for treatment of bipolar disorder examined the coping resources within each group. Individuals were between the ages of 18 and 65 (mean age 35.4 years). African American individuals received significantly higher scores on the Coping Resources Inventory than their white counterparts. They also scored significantly higher on the cognitive, emotional, and spiritual-philosophical scales, which refer to internal resources (Pollack et al. 2000). The investigators could not find any difference in the demographic or psychiatric backgrounds of the two groups and ultimately concluded that these differences in the use of internal coping mechanisms most likely resulted from "cultural orientations influencing personal life philosophies" (1311). The authors hypothesized that "because of having overcome many obstacles in life in the past, the African-Americans perceived themselves more as having an internal strength, a positive outlook, and more resources with which to cope than did the white participants. The strong spiritual foundation that is part of the upbringing of many African Americans may instill powerful internal resources that persist into adulthood" (1311–1312).

In a study of individuals diagnosed with bipolar disorder in Morocco, researchers hypothesized that the relapse experienced by patients whose disease had been stabilized with lithium treatment was attributable to fasting and changes in routine during the period of Ramadan (Moussaoui and Kadri 2002). The literature does not indicate whether this pattern has been investigated or detected in persons with bipolar disorder in similarly observant cultures located elsewhere.

An understanding of how patients construct their illness is critical in understanding how they will manage illness episodes and which activities they will select to promote healing. In the study of 147 patients with bipolar disorder described above (Mitchell and Romans 2003), the investigators concluded that meditation, group prayer, and physical actions helped some individuals in the management of their illness. Individuals who held strong religious beliefs were significantly more likely than others to engage in prayer. Those who belonged to evangelical denominations were more likely than those who were members of conservative, traditional, or liberal denominations to practice their faith more often and to be aware of a "power's influence" on their ability to cope. Individuals who had been more unwell during the previous five years were more likely to report that their beliefs had not helped them in the management of their illness.

In the United States, the Internet has become a resource for the exchange of information between individuals diagnosed with bipolar disorder (e.g., www.bipolar .about.com). Web postings may focus on topics such as relationships, support networks, self-perceptions, and adherence to medication regimens. It is unclear to what extent anonymous access to others with similar diagnoses via chat rooms and web postings may assist individuals in managing their illness, or to what extent this mechanism is used outside western cultures. This mechanism may be particularly important for individuals who lack transportation to attend support groups, for individuals who are homebound because of the severity of their symptoms, and for aging individuals who are homebound or confined to care settings because of comorbidities. However, elderly individuals may be less likely to use the Internet than younger persons.

The following postings from one website dedicated to bipolar disorder reveal how some individuals have chosen to manage their illness (posted on www.bipolar.about.com):

> I have [stopped meds] many times and recently have because I feel I am gaining weight either depressed on them or the pills are doing it. (Katem21)

> In 15 years I've probably quit my meds at least 6 or 7 times . . . I just have this feeling that I am "less than" because I have these meds and what if long-term use causes problems down the road (i.e., Alzheimer's) . . . Friends indicate that I was using meds as a crutch. (Tina)

These postings suggest, but obviously cannot confirm, the influence of U.S. culture on the way these persons manage their illness. The first individual is concerned with her weight; we do not know whether this is because of her weight itself posing a threat to good health, or because of self-perceptions related to body image, which may be associated with cultural dictates relating to women's bodies. The second posting underscores the importance of friends' opinions, raising the issue of the generalizability of this sentiment in U.S. culture and its relevance to cultures that may emphasize the greater importance of family.

CONCLUSIONS

A significant number of questions of critical importance in the diagnosis and management of bipolar disorder remain uninvestigated. Consider, for instance, the following:

—At what point do individuals recognize their experience as something requiring evaluation? Does this realization occur only as the result of serious, adverse effects of the illness (e.g., loss of employment or relationship)? Or are there other signs that assist an individual in recognizing that he or she is ill?

—At what point do individuals who interpret their situation as out of the ordinary seek assistance? What types of assistance and in what hierarchy of use? What barriers exist to seeking and using services?

—Does the epidemiological profile of bipolar disorder differ across ethnic and cultural groups?

— Are there differences in the clinical presentation of bipolar disorder across age, gender, socioeconomic status, educational level, religion, race, ethnicity, and/ or culture?

— How do individuals resolve external conflict in the interpretation of their behaviors/situation (e.g., diversity of opinions among family members and friends, conflict between health care provider and spiritual advisor)? And how does that resolution affect their access to and willingness to use care and to adhere to recommended medication regimens?

— Are there differences in the experience and management of illness that are related to sex, age, socioeconomic status, educational level, ethnicity, cultural background, and so forth?

Unfortunately, relatively little attention has been paid to these research areas. The answers to these and other questions may be critical to informing clinical practice in the diagnosis and management of bipolar disorder.

REFERENCES

Angst, J. 1986. The course of affective disorders. *Psychopathology* 19:47–52.

Baron, M., Risch, N., Hamburger, R., et al. 1987. Genetic linkage between X-chromosome markers and bipolar affective illness. *Nature* 326:289–292.

Boas, F. 1940. *Race, language, and culture.* New York: Free Press.

Boyd, J. H., and Weissman, M. M. 1981. Epidemiology of affective disorders: a re-examination and future directions. *Arch Gen Psychiatry* 38:1039–1046.

Cooper, C. R., and Denner, J. 1998. Theories linking culture and psychopathology: universal and community-specific processes. *Annu Rev Psychol* 49:559–584.

Cooper, J. E., Kendal, R. E., Gurland, B. J., et al. 1969. Cross-national study of diagnosing the mental disorders: some results from the first comparative investigation. *Am J Psychiatry* 125(suppl.):21–29.

Delbello, M. P., Soutullo, C. A., and Strakowski, S. M. 2000. Racial differences in the treatment of adolescents with bipolar disorder. *Am J Psychiatry* 157:837–838.

Egeland, J. A., Hostetter, A. M., and Eshleman, S. K. 1983. Amish study: III. The impact of cultural factors on diagnosis of bipolar illness. *Am J Psychiatry* 140:67–71.

Egeland, J. A., Gerhard, D. S., Pauls, D. L., et al. 1987. Bipolar affective disorders linked to DNA markers on chromosome 11. *Nature* 325:783–787.

Floersch, J., Longhofer, J., and Latta, K. 1997. Writing Amish culture into genes: biological reductionism in a study of manic depression. *Cult Med Psychiatry* 21:137–159.

Gaines, A. D. 1994. Race and racism. In Reich, W. (ed.), *Encyclopedia of bioethics.* New York: Macmillan.

Gould, S. J. 1981. *The mismeasure of man.* New York: W. W. Norton.

Hodgkinson, S., Sherrington, R., Gurling, H., et al. 1987. Molecular genetic evidence for heterogeneity in manic depression. *Nature* 325:805–806.

Judd, L. L., Akiskal, H. S., Schettler, P. J., et al. 2002. The long-term natural history of the weekly symptom atic status of bipolar I disorder. *Arch Gen Psychiatry* 59:530–537.

Kennedy, N., Boydell, J., van Os, J., et al. 2004. Ethnic differences in first clinical presentation of bipolar disorder: results from an epidemiological study. *J Affect Disord* 83:161–168.

Kieseppa, T., Partonen, T., Haukka, J., et al. 2004. High concordance of bipolar I disorder in a nationwide sample of twins. *Am J Psychiatry* 161:1814–1821.

Kirov, G., and Murray, R. M. 1999. Ethnic differences in the presentation of bipolar affective disorder. *Eur Psychiatry* 14:199–204. ·

Kleinman, A. 1977. Depression, somatization, and the "new cross-cultural psychiatry." *Soc Sci Med* 11:3–10.

Kleinman, A. 1988. *Rethinking psychiatry: from cultural category to personal experience*. New York: Free Press.

Kleinman, A. 1996. How is culture important for DSM-IV? In Mezzich, J. E., Kleinman, A., Fabrega, H. Jr., et al. (eds.), *Culture and psychiatric diagnosis: a DSM-IV perspective*. Washington, DC: American Psychiatric Press.

LaVeist, T. A. 1994. Beyond dummy variables and sample selection: what health services researchers ought to know about race as a variable. *Health Serv Res* 29(1):1–16.

Leff, J. P., Fischer, M., and Bertelsen, A. 1976. A cross-national epidemiological study of mania. *Br J Psychiatry* 129:428–442.

Makanjuola, R. O. A. 1982. Manic disorder in Nigerians. *Br J Psychiatry* 141:459–463.

Makanjuola, R. O. A. 1985. Recurrent unipolar manic disorder in the Yoruba Nigerian: further evidence. *Br J Psychiatry* 147:434–437.

Mitchell, L., and Romans, S. 2003. Spiritual beliefs in bipolar affective disorder: their relevance for illness management. *J Affect Disord* 75:247–257.

Montagu, A. 1964. *Man's most dangerous myth: the fallacy of race* (4th ed.). Cleveland, OH: World.

Moussaoui, D., and Kadri, N. 2002. Culture matters too in bipolar disorder. In Maj, M., Akiskal, H. S., Lopez-Ibor, J. J., et al. (eds.), *Bipolar disorder* (pp. 355–359). Chichester, England: Wiley.

National Institute of Mental Health. 1998. *Genetics and mental disorders: report of the National Institute of Mental Health's genetics workgroup*. Rockville, MD: National Institute of Mental Health.

Noaghiul, S., and Hibbeln, J. R. 2003. Cross-national comparisons of seafood consumption and rates of bipolar disorders. *Am J Psychiatry* 160:2222–2227.

Osher, Y., Yaroslavsky, Y., el-Rom, R., et al. 2000. Predominant polarity of bipolar patients in Israel. *World J Biol Psychiatry* 1:187–189.

Pollack, L. E., Harvin, S., and Cramer, R. D. 2000. Coping resources of African-American and white patients hospitalized for bipolar disorder. *Psychiatr Serv* 51:1310–1312.

Shih, R. A., Belmonte, P. L., and Zandi, P. P. 2004. A review of the evidence from family, twin, and adoption studies for genetic contribution to adult psychiatric disorders. *Int Rev Psychiatry* 16:260–283.

Strakowski, S. M., Keck, P. E., Arnold, L. M., et al. 2003. Ethnicity and diagnosis in patients with affective disorders. *J Clin Psychiatry* 64:747–754.

Tseng, W. S. 1975. The nature of somatic complaints among psychiatric patients: the Chinese case. *Compr Psychiatry* 16:237–245.

Tseng, W. S., McDermott, J. F. Jr., Ogino, K., et al. 1982. Cross-cultural differences in parent-child assessment: USA and Japan. *Int J Soc Psychiatry* 18:305–317.

Tseng, W. S., Asai, M., Chita Nishi, K., et al. 1992a. Social phobia: diagnostic pattern in Tokyo and Hawaii. *J Nerv Ment Disord* 180:380–385.

Tseng, W. S., Mo, K. M., Li, L. S., et al. 1992b. Koro epidemic in Guangdong China: a questionnaire study. *J Nerv Ment Disord* 180:117–123.

U.S. Department of Health and Human Services. 1999. *Mental health: a report of the Surgeon General*. Rockville, MD: U.S. Department of Health and Human Services

U.S. Department of Health and Human Services. 2001. *Mental health: culture, race, and ethnicity — a supplement to Mental Health: A Report of the Surgeon General*. Rockville, MD: U.S. Department of Health and Human Services, Substance Abuse and Mental Health Services Administration, Center for Mental Health Services.

van Os, J., Takei, N., Castle, D. J., et al. 1996. The incidence of mania: time trends in relation to gender and ethnicity. *Soc Psychiatry Psychiatr Epidemiol* 31(3–4):129–136.

Weissman, M. M., Bland, R. C., Canino, G. J., et al. 1996. Cross-national epidemiology of major depression and bipolar disorder. *JAMA* 276:293–299.

Whaley, A. L. 1998. Cross-cultural perspective on paranoia: a focus on the black American experience. *Psychiatry* 69:325–343.

Yinger, J. 1994. *Ethnicity: source of strength? Source of conflict?* Albany: State University of New York Press.

Zenner, W. 1996. Ethnicity. In Levinson, D., and Ember, M. (eds.), *Encyclopedia of cultural anthropology* (pp. 393–395). New York: Holt.

PART FOUR

Specialized Care Delivery and Research

CHAPTER ELEVEN

Specialized Care Delivery for the Older Adult

Quality of Care

AMY M. KILBOURNE, PH.D., M.P.H.,

AND HAROLD A. PINCUS, M.D.

Despite the existence of clinical practice guidelines, the quality of care and subsequent outcomes for older persons with bipolar disorder remain suboptimal (Bauer et al. 2002; Kilbourne 2005a). Moreover, patients with bipolar disorder are more likely to have medical comorbidities than the general patient population (Kilbourne et al. 2004a), and subsequent medical and preventive care may be lacking as well (Druss et al. 2001). In this chapter we review the current knowledge on the quality of psychiatric care for older patients with bipolar disorder. We then propose a new paradigm in thinking about the quality of care and quality improvement for these older patients. This new approach involves (1) assessing the quality of care, using performance measures; (2) adapting guideline-based treatment models designed to reduce system-level barriers to appropriate care; and (3) translating and implementing such models into "real-world" settings. Ultimately, measuring quality is the foundation for improving quality, as the monitoring of performance is a key tool in evaluating quality improvement initiatives. Performance measures also provide the means by which good quality of care for older patients with bipolar disorder can be "indexed" as an important benchmark for which health care providers and other administrators can strive.

QUALITY OF CARE FOR OLDER PERSONS WITH BIPOLAR DISORDER: CURRENT EVIDENCE

Outcomes for older persons with bipolar disorder remain suboptimal (Bauer et al. 2001a), even with the availability of efficacious pharmacotherapy (Suppes et al. 2001; Wyatt et al. 2001) and practice guidelines (American Psychiatric Association 1994, 2002; Bauer et al. 1999; Goodwin 2003; Suppes et al. 2001). Without adequate treatment, a 25-year-old person with bipolar disorder can expect to lose 14 years of major effective activity and 9 years of life (Bauer et al. 2002; U.S. Department of Health, Education, and Welfare 1979). The Donabedian quality-of-care model describes a framework in which health care structural, or system, factors influence the processes of care (which typically constitute measures of "quality of care"), which, in turn, influence patients' health outcomes (Donabedian et al. 1982). Hence, improving quality, especially processes of care, for older individuals with bipolar disorder should be a key focus of treatment. In the findings described below, "older age" was defined as 50 years or older, in part because of the potential years of life lost resulting from the destructive effects (e.g., suicide) of inadequately treated bipolar disorder (Bauer et al. 2002; Kilbourne et al. 2004a).

Quality of Care Is Suboptimal

Recent evidence suggests that older patients with bipolar disorder are less likely than younger patients to receive adequate quality of care. In a recently completed study of Department of Veterans Affairs (VA) patients from the mid-Atlantic region, the quality of care for older versus younger patients with bipolar disorder was evaluated using indicators of the minimum necessary standard of care (Kilbourne 2005a). These quality indicators included adequate pharmacotherapy (i.e., prescription of a mood stabilizer within the same year as the bipolar disorder diagnosis), outpatient follow-up care (receipt of an outpatient visit ≤490 days from a previous visit), and adequate post-hospitalization care (receipt of an outpatient follow-up visit ≤430 days after discharge), all of which represent appropriate care based on American Psychiatric Association and VA practice guidelines for the vast majority of patients diagnosed with bipolar disorder, regardless of current mood state (American Psychiatric Association 1994, 2002; Bauer et al. 1999). Overall, of 2,958 patients in the VA sample, 70.9% received a first-line mood stabilizer (lithium, divalproex / valproic acid, carbamazepine, or lamotrigine) and 65.8% received an outpatient mental health visit within 90 days. Of the 2,958 patients, 629 had a psychiatric hospitalization, and of those, 53.1% received an outpatient visit on or within 30 days of discharge. Older patients (=50 years) were less likely than their younger counterparts to receive a mood stabilizer and less likely to receive outpatient care within 90 days, after controlling for patient factors and comorbidity. There was no difference in post-hospitalization follow-up care by age. Nonetheless, these results suggest that older patients are not receiving adequate pharmacotherapy or follow-up care for bipolar disorder.

Guidelines and Measurement of Quality Are Unclear

One of the key barriers to improving quality of care for older patients is that current knowledge about appropriate pharmacotherapy and management strategies for bipolar disorder in later life is somewhat limited. In the aforementioned VA study, measurement of quality of pharmacotherapy was limited to one measure for mood-stabilizer use, in part because of the dearth of information on appropriate use of specific medications or use of multiple medications. Many pharmacotherapy options and practice guidelines for the management of bipolar disorder in general (American Psychiatric Association 1994, 2002) have not been tailored for older adults in particular. The current guidelines reviewed by Young and colleagues (2004) still recommend lithium as the first-line treatment for mania, followed by divalproex/valproic acid and carbamazepine. For antipsychotic medications, further research is needed on their efficacy and safety for older adults with bipolar disorder (Neil et al. 2003). Experts in geriatric psychiatry and related fields recommend that antipsychotics in combination with a mood stabilizer are appropriate for older patients with psychotic or severe nonpsychotic mania (Alexopoulos et al. 2004; U.S. Food and Drug Administration 2005). However, experts caution that there are risks associated with some of the atypical antipsychotics, including an increased risk of diabetes and other metabolic syndromes (Alexopoulos et al. 2004). Young and colleagues (2004) were less certain about appropriate antipsychotic use for the treatment of mania in older adults, given that the side effects may be even more damaging for older than for younger patients. Additional evidence suggests that atypical antipsychotics may cause delirium in geriatric patients (Neil et al. 2003). Moreover, there are no indicators for when polypharmacy is appropriate for older persons with bipolar disorder (given that few randomized controlled trials have evaluated polypharmacy). Constructing more age-specific quality indicators for antipsychotic use thus requires additional research on the efficacy and long-term effects of these medications, as well as considerations about their safety for older patients. Given concerns related to the use of atypical antipsychotics and the changes in drug metabolism that accompany aging (Alexopoulos et al. 2004), quality indicators are needed that encompass routine checking for side effects and toxicity to monitor the quality of care for older patients with bipolar disorder who are taking mood stabilizers and/or antipsychotic medications.

Optimizing Quality of Care Is a Multidisciplinary Process

For older patients with bipolar disorder, optimizing the quality of care involves not only guideline-concordant pharmacotherapy for the disorder but adequate follow-up services and care for coexisting medical conditions that may impede the response to psychotropic treatment. Medical comorbidities further complicate quality improvement efforts for treating bipolar disorder in older adults (Kilbourne et al. 2004a). It is well known that persons with bipolar disorder are more likely than the general population to have a substance use disorder (SUD) (Regier et al. 1990; Strakowski et al. 2000; Weiss and Mirin 1986), and recent evidence suggests that older patients with bipolar disorder experience more general medical comorbidities than the general population of older patients (Kilbourne et al. 2004a). The burden of medical comorbidity is also greater among older than among younger patients with bipolar disorder. In a recent analysis, the burden of medical comorbidity was compared between older and younger adults in a mid-Atlantic VA health care network who had either one inpatient or two separate outpatient International Classification of Diseases–Ninth Revision (ICD-9) diagnoses of bipolar disorder (defined as ICD-9 codes 296.0–296.16, 296.4–296.89, or 301.13) in fiscal year 2001 (Unützer et al. 2000). The sample consisted of 2,958 patients so diagnosed. Using data from the VA National Patient Care Database, investigators identified comorbidities with ICD-9 codes by using the Agency for Healthcare Research and Quality Clinical Classification Software (Yu et al. 2003). Of the 2,958 patients, 55% (n = 1,625) were aged 50 years or older and 11% (n = 314) were women. Younger (<50 years old) patients were more likely than older patients to have a SUD (table 11.1). However, older patients were more likely to have medical comorbidities, and, in particular, at least half had a diagnosis of a cardiovascular or metabolic condition.

Older individuals with bipolar disorder are especially prone to the adverse effects of medical comorbidity, because of aging, the inherent instability and "wear and tear" on the body caused by alternating periods of mania and depression over the lifespan (Baldessarini 2002), and use of multiple medications (e.g., anticonvulsants, antipsychotics, antidepressants) with their associated toxic effects (Caykoylu et al. 2002; Masand and Gupta 2002; Peipho 2002). For example, the potential for atypical antipsychotics to increase the risk of diabetes and other metabolic syndromes has received much attention (American Diabetes Association et al. 2004; Peipho 2002).

TABLE 11.1
Burden of medical comorbidity among older and younger persons with bipolar disorder
(N = 2,958)

Comorbid conditions*	Age <50 (n = 133)		Age ≥50 (n = 1,625)		χ^2 (df)	p-value
	n	%	n	%		
Cardiovascular disease	327	24.5	871	53.6	256.78 (1)	<.0001
Metabolic disease	404	30.3	817	50.3	120.47 (1)	<.0001
Musculoskeletal conditions	347	26.0	429	26.4	0.07 (1)	.79
Alcohol or drug use	575	43.1	367	22.6	141.54 (1)	<.0001
Pulmonary conditions	125	9.4	307	18.9	53.16 (1)	<.0001
Accidents or injuries	192	14.4	197	12.1	3.52 (1)	.06
Hepatic conditions	142	10.7	88	5.4	28.01 (1)	<.0001
Cancers (excluding skin)	16	1.2	89	5.5	39.12 (1)	<.0001

*Based on ICD-9 codes from the Agency for Healthcare Research and Quality clinical classifications software.

Hence, the complexities of comorbid conditions can contribute to poor adherence to medication regimens and an unstable treatment course, resulting in suboptimal outcomes.

GAPS IN QUALITY OF GENERAL MEDICAL CARE

Evidence suggests that medical comorbidity among older patients with mental disorders, including bipolar disorder, is underdetected and inadequately treated. Primary care for these patients remains suboptimal for, in particular, cardiovascular disease (Druss et al. 2000), diabetes (Desai et al. 2002), and preventive services (Druss et al. 2002). In a study of older patients with bipolar disorder (248 patients ≥50 years old), only 25% received a flu vaccination, 30% received colorectal cancer screening, 59% of those taking lithium received a thyroid function test, and 33% of those taking divalproex received a hepatic function test. In addition, only half of those diagnosed with hypertension or hyperlipidemia received an antihypertensive medication or statin, respectively (Kilbourne 2005a).

Poor quality of care for medical conditions may be primarily due to the inherent separation of "physical" and "mental" health care (Pincus 2003). Because bipolar disorder is a serious mental illness, patients are often treated in the mental health setting (Druss and Rosenheck 2000). Medical conditions that a general internist would typically screen for may be underdetected in psychiatric facilities (Faulkner et al. 1986; Koran et al. 1989), and mental health practitioners often lack the time to care for coexisting medical conditions (Faulkner et al. 1986). Furthermore, chronic medical conditions in older individuals with bipolar disorder are often missed, for several reasons: patients may receive care in multiple settings, they may fail to recall medical symptoms, or their medical illnesses may be overlooked (Redelmeier et al. 1998; Rost et al. 2000). In the treatment of bipolar disorder, the introduction of medications that are sometimes associated with metabolic syndromes has enhanced the recognition of risk factors for medical complications. As a result, quality-improvement efforts are needed that promote collaborative care between general medical and mental health providers.

MEASURING QUALITY: BENCHMARKING PERFORMANCE AND DETECTING GAPS IN CARE

Potential disparities in quality of care for older persons with bipolar disorder cannot be addressed without quantitative information on the quality gap, and where such gaps might exist (e.g., in pharmacotherapy, follow-up care, or preventive care). That is, to improve care, one must be able to measure how well care is delivered in the first place (i.e., measure performance).

One of the more significant impediments to improving the quality of care for older persons with bipolar disorder is the lack of comprehensive performance data on both medical and psychiatric care for these patients. Potential users of information (e.g., researchers, practitioners, health care organizations, and advocacy organizations) want a "bottom line" conclusion about overall quality of care to help identify older patients who might be experiencing gaps in care and to help clarify decisions about resource priorities and provision of services. Developing and refining measures of use and quality of care is one of the first steps in improving efficiencies and patients' outcomes.

Performance measures can be used to benchmark trends in quality of care at the system and national levels, and can ultimately inform interventions to reduce costs and adverse outcomes for older patients with bipolar disorder. Performance data can also be used to assist providers in identifying patients at risk of poor outcomes and to evaluate the success (or failure) of quality improvement interventions across different health care practices.

Selecting Quality Indicators for Older Patients with Bipolar Disorder

Because of the persisting potential for gaps in quality of care for older persons with bipolar disorder, efforts are needed to promote the validation and application of performance measures to monitor efforts to improve quality for these patients. In doing so, researchers are encouraged to look beyond simply measuring the quality of psychiatric care and to focus on measures of drug safety/toxicity and medical co-

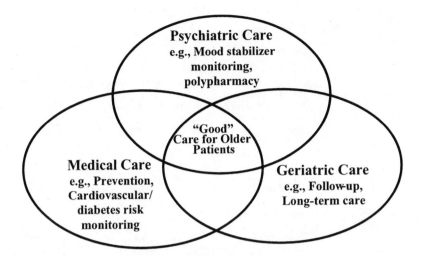

Fig. 11.1. The universe of performance measures (quality indicators) pertaining to the comprehensive care of older persons with bipolar disorder. Researchers should consider combining quality indicators relevant to psychiatric, general medical, and geriatric care to develop and implement an "index of good care" that is appropriate for these patients.

morbidity, to obtain a comprehensive picture of quality of care for older patients with this condition (fig. 11.1). Examples of key measures are provided in table 11.2. They encompass psychiatric care, care for common medical conditions, preventive care, and adequate outpatient follow-up care.

One of the first steps in measuring quality of care is to derive quantifiable indicators, based on clinical practice guidelines, that can be used to assess quality for older patients with bipolar disorder. Ideally, quality indicators should be valid, feasible to measure, and clinically meaningful to providers. Valid quality indicators should be based on current practice guidelines. When the guidelines are not fully clear or are not consistent, then an expert panel should be used to obtain consensus on the guidelines and subsequent indicators (Kilbourne and Pincus 2004). Selected indicators should also be feasible to ascertain, such as those based on administrative data, to be practical across multiple health care settings. Quality indicators based on administrative data are preferred mainly because those based on chart-review data can be costly and time-consuming (i.e., they require patient's consent in some cases and adequate clinical expertise to review charts). In addition, while chart-review data can contain additional information on a provider's effort in treating patients, such information, especially if obtained implicitly, can be unreliable (Kilbourne 2005b).

Clinically meaningful measures are those that reflect what providers can control

TABLE 11.2
Examples of quality indicators customized for older persons with bipolar disorder

Category	Indicator description	Reference
Mood stabilizers	Drug-level monitoring for lithium and anticonvulsants	APA 1994, 2002
	Thyroid function test every 6 months if patient is taking lithium	APA 1994, 2002
	Hematological and hepatic function tests if patient taking divalproex or valproic acid	APA 1994, 2002
	Olanzapine, clozapine, or conventional antipsychotics not recommended if patient has uncontrolled diabetes, dyslipidemia, or obesity	Alexopoulos et al. 2004
	Avoidance of antidepressant monotherapy	APA 1994, 2002
CHD/diabetes risk monitoring	Blood pressure check, BMI screening, fasting glucose test, and/or lipid panel (<65 years old) every year for patients taking atypical antipsychotics	USPSTF ADA et al. 2004
General medical disease prevention	Pneumococcal vaccine	USPSTF
	Influenza vaccine every year for patients not known to have allergy to eggs or influenza vaccine	USPSTF
	Colorectal cancer screening	USPSTF
	Alcohol disorders screening (assessment, lab test)	Garnick et al. 2003
Post-hospitalization follow-up	Outpatient visit <30 days from discharge date	Unutzer et al. 2000

Abbreviations: APA, American Psychiatric Association; USPS TF, U.S. Preventive Task Force guidelines (www.ahrq.gov/clinic/uspstfix.htm); ADA, American Diabetes Association; CHD, coronary heart disease; BMI, body mass index.

in providing patient care. For example, providers have more control over prescribing statins than over patients' serum cholesterol levels, so indicators should focus on actions that providers can take to improve care, such as prescribing statins for patients with low-density lipoprotein (LDL) exceeding 120 mg/dl. Also, providers are more likely to accept performance measures if such measures are within their "sphere of influence" (Valenstein et al. 2004). In developing a comprehensive index of quality-of-care measures for older patients with bipolar disorder, measures of processes of care are ideal, as they do not require risk adjustment. In contrast, outcomes-based indicators (e.g., functional status, LDL levels) depend on the severity of disease and are prone to "gaming" by providers, who may improve their quality scores by selecting out sicker patients (Werner and Asch 2005).

Methodological Challenges in Measuring Quality

The growing need to measure and improve quality of care for older persons with bipolar disorder has led to an increased reliance on administrative databases to assess trends in care and use of such data to assess whether patients are receiving appropriate care. Use of administrative data from health care organizations (e.g., the

VA, Medicare, private health plans) can be a cost-efficient alternative to primary data collection for identifying large numbers of patients with rare conditions. Findings from administrative data are also potentially more generalizable, because the data are population-based and reflect routine (real-world) care.

However, there are some disadvantages to using administrative data to measure the quality of care. Foremost is that not all health systems include comprehensive information on care received by their patients. Many older patients receive care from multiple providers (e.g., Medicare, private health plans), so their utilization information may be recorded in two or more databases. While the VA provides some of the most comprehensive datasets on a "captive" audience of patients, a not insignificant number of veterans receive care from providers outside the VA, and such care may not be recorded in the VA administrative data.

In addition, administrative datasets primarily contain diagnostic data based on ICD-9 codes, which may be recorded by different providers and professional coders for the same patient over time. ICD-9 codes give very little information about a patient's clinical status, thereby limiting the ability of investigators to assess appropriate care for a given episode. In addition, administrative data often contain multiple psychiatric diagnoses. For example, a recent analysis of VA administrative data found that more than a third of patients diagnosed with bipolar disorder also received concurrent (i.e., within the same year) diagnoses of schizophrenia — though these are considered mutually exclusive diagnoses (Kilbourne et al. 2004b). Older African Americans diagnosed with bipolar disorder were the most likely to have a concurrent diagnosis of schizophrenia. Perhaps some apparently high rates of multiple diagnoses are attributable to the "carrying forward" of old diagnoses from past encounters into current history forms, which then appear in administrative records; or perhaps patients are not receiving adequate follow-up care to confirm diagnoses (Kilbourne et al. 2004b). Researchers need to find indicators that are treatment-based rather than diagnosis-based and are independent of bipolar subdiagnoses — such as the receipt of drug-level monitoring tests. Moreover, treatment-related administrative data such as lab and pharmacy data have their limitations. For example, it can be difficult to discern medications that have been discontinued or switched by providers.

Administrative databases, then, while convenient and cost-efficient, are not designed for research, hence investigators need to carefully consider the limitations of the data from administrative sources. One potential solution when relying on administrative data is to validate ICD-9 codes by comparing them with a provider's report or formal diagnostic assessment. Specific algorithms based on ICD-9 codes that maximize the validity can then be evaluated, such as the identification of patients with two or more diagnoses from separate encounters. Improving the accuracy and validity of ICD-9 codes for psychiatric diagnoses is an important next step in research on bipolar disorder in late life, especially as investigators increasingly rely on large administrative databases to conduct their research (Bryant-Comstock et al. 2002; Unützer et al. 2000).

Researchers should interpret quality scores based on administrative data with caution, as lack of receipt of care may reflect patients' preferences or poor adherence to treatment. For example, patients not receiving follow-up visits or lab tests may have failed to appear at a scheduled appointment. This is especially likely for older patients, who often lack adequate transportation. Similarly, inadequate pharmacotherapy may be a reflection of a patient's nonadherence to treatment (e.g., failure to refill medications) rather than a provider's lack of adherence to guidelines. Furthermore, many practitioners might be providing good care to their older patients with bipolar disorder, yet must choose the timing of such care in response to a patient's emotional state or comorbid substance use. For example, many providers, in reaction to a patient's "crisis visit," might choose to treat the comorbid substance use first, to stabilize the patient before initiating a guideline-concordant mood stabilizer. There is little way of distinguishing these unscheduled "crisis visits" in administrative datasets or even in chart reviews. Still, the provider has some responsibility to encourage adequate adherence and to work with the patient to ensure adequate follow-up care. Researchers should determine to what extent these extraneous circumstances occur and factor this information into their benchmark for "good care" (e.g., achieving an 80% rate on an indicator, given that up to 20% of the patient population will refuse treatment or that the indicator may not apply to special cases).

MONITORING QUALITY: ACCOUNTABILITY

Monitoring quality of care can be successful only if there is a clear sense of who is accountable when gaps in care are found for older patients with bipolar disorder. The separation of physical and mental health services has impeded the translation of evidence-based general medical and psychiatric care into real care for patients with bipolar disorder. This results in part from a lack of standards for holding different providers accountable for the medical, psychiatric, and geriatric care of these patients. That is, if older patients with bipolar disorder are not undergoing lab tests for drug level and toxicity, or are not being monitored for diabetes risk factors, who is responsible for improving the quality of these services?

The separation of physical and mental health care further complicates efforts to improve quality, because communication and coordination of care are inhibited between providers, each perceiving that the other practitioner is responsible for drug-level monitoring, diabetes risk assessments, and so forth. Therefore, measurements of quality need to be implemented beyond the provider and should involve health care payers and plans that oversee different provider specialties. For example, a group of health care policymakers, researchers, and managed-care representatives in the Washington, DC, area who were interested in improving the quality of care for people with SUDs convened to establish guideline-based indicators for adequate follow-up treatment based on administrative data, as a means to monitor quality across different practice settings (Garnick et al. 2002).

These measures can ultimately be used by health care purchasers to identify health plans that encompass both medical and psychiatric care and to ensure that all are providing the best care for, say, SUDs. Additional efforts to integrate care across different entities treating older patients with bipolar disorder are essential in order to encourage collaboration across providers and thus improve care for these patients.

FROM MEASURING TO IMPROVING QUALITY: EMERGING TREATMENT MODELS

Despite the separation of physical and mental health services, health care organizations are increasingly being held accountable for improving quality across all of their providers. This is illustrated in a report by the Institute of Medicine, *Crossing the Quality Chasm* (2001), which concluded that barriers at the level of the health care system are contributing to gaps in quality of care. The National Committee on Quality Assurance (2005), one of the pioneering organizations that has implemented quality-of-care performance measures to benchmark health plans and provider groups on the quality of care, has beta-tested performance measures for monitoring medication toxicity that will be used to compare health plans on how they manage the treatment of older patients. However, evidence suggests that performance monitoring alone, while an essential tool for quality improvement, may not be sufficient to improve quality of care overall (Balas et al. 1996; Kiefe et al. 1995).

The gaps in quality of care for older patients with bipolar disorder, as well as the significant burden of medical comorbidity in this patient population, suggest the need for a more systematic strategy for improving the quality of care. That is, given that gaps in quality of care exist beyond psychiatric care to include general medical and continuity-of-care services, treatment strategies and models for older patients with bipolar disorder should be designed to promote changes at the health system level, to provide coordinated medical, psychiatric, and social services.

Treatment Models Based on Quality Improvement:
The Chronic Care Model

Treatment models such as the Wagner chronic care model (CCM; Wagner et al. 1996), which involve organizational changes in health care delivery from an acute to a chronic disease-management focus, improve coordination of care across medical and psychiatric providers for older patients with unipolar depression receiving care in general medical settings (Bruce et al. 2004) and, more recently, for adult patients with bipolar disorder (Bauer et al. 2006; Simon et al. 2002). The Wagner CCM is one of the most widely adopted frameworks for improving care for chronic illness. This is primarily because of its focus on organizational change and patient-activation strategies that facilitate the coordination of care across existing providers (e.g., primary care providers, mental health specialists), minimizing the marginal costs of its implementation (Shortell 2000). The CCM's core components are (1) *decision support*: the systematic incorporation of evidence-based guidelines; (2) *delivery system design*: the use of nonphysician staff (i.e., care managers) to coordinate services; (3) *clinical information system*: the use of clinical and population-based data in monitoring quality of care; and (4) *self-management support*: fostering patients' self-management skills. Together, these components can improve coordinated care and subsequent outcomes for older patients with bipolar disorder, who often receive care in multiple settings (Kilbourne et al. 2004c).

The advantage of the CCM over other approaches is that it is versatile and easily translatable into routine care (Wagner et al. 2001). That is, the CCM is a "manual-based" treatment model (requiring limited training to implement) as opposed to more intensive case-management models (which require hiring new teams of personnel). The manual-based framework of the CCM allows its customization and adaptability to a range of settings and populations, because personnel from a variety of backgrounds (e.g., nurses [RNs], social workers [MSWs]) can be trained to implement the model (Bauer et al. 2006). The emphasis of the CCM on guidelines, information systems, and support of patients' self-management make this model applicable across patients with differing severities of illness and levels of need. Manual-based models are also best suited for coordinating care across providers that already exist, thus precluding the high start-up costs of hiring additional personnel (Kilbourne et al. 2004c).

Several more intensive treatment models are available within mental health settings—such as Assertive Community Treatment (Drake et al. 1998) and similar intensive case-management models (Burns et al. 1999)—that could be applicable for older patients with bipolar disorder, but these models were primarily designed for treatment of uncontrolled SUDs. They were not designed for treating the vast majority of patients with bipolar disorder with medical comorbidity, many of whom are able to function more independently. Moreover, the high start-up costs of hiring additional personnel preclude the dissemination of these models into routine care (Quinlivan et al. 1995). In contrast, CCM-based treatment models have proved cost-effective when applied to unipolar depression and other chronic illnesses (Lave et al. 1998).

In addition, although other approaches to improving general medical care for patients with mental disorders do exist (table 11.3) — such as training psychiatrists in the management of general medical conditions (Carney et al. 1998; Golomb et al. 2000) — ample evidence suggests that psychiatrists often lack the time, resources, and incentives to treat their patients' medical conditions (Faulkner et al. 1986). Another integrated care model, which involves the placement of a general medical physician in a mental health clinic (Druss et al. 2001), may be feasible for staff-model health care systems, in which the health plan and the general medical and mental health provider groups are within the same entity (e.g., the VA, Kaiser Permanente health plan). However, this model may not be cost-efficient for the majority of patients who receive care in network health systems. Network health systems in the United States face unique challenges, most notably the lack of a centralized source of data and multiple provider groups and health plans. A CCM-based model in which a physician extender (e.g., an RN) provides care management across existing providers may be more desirable and cost-efficient for these network health plans (Kilbourne et al. 2004c).

TABLE 11.3

Treatment models for providing coordinated medical and psychiatric care for persons with serious mental illness (e.g., bipolar disorder)

Model	Key advantage	Key disadvantage
Psychiatrist provides medical care, with some supervision	"One-stop shopping" for patient	Lack of time, competing needs, supervision
Physician double-boarded in general and internal medicine and psychiatry	Consultation with general medical provider not required; "one-stop shopping" for patient	Unable to bill for both services in most health plans; scarcity of double-boarded practitioners
PCPs in mental health clinic	Patient can be seen by both psychiatrist and PCP in same clinic	Costly, with multiple sites, personnel
"Manual-based" via Chronic Care Model	Care manager (nurse) more cost-efficient than PCP; can work across multiple clinics	Requires rapport building with PCP to foster access to more complex medical care

Abbreviation: PCP, primary care provider.

TABLE 11.4
Adapting the Chronic Care Model (CCM) to improve quality of care for older persons with bipolar disorder

	Decision support	Delivery system design	Clinical information system	Self-management support
General features of CCM	Clinical practice guidelines	Roles, responsibilities, and accountability of CM and other providers	Registry provides information flow from CM to MHS and PCP; Registry tracks visits, patient progress; updated by CM; Monitors quality of care at the population level	CM trained in brief counseling techniques; serves as advocate and lifeline for patients
Specific features				
Improving access to general medical and preventive health care visits	General medical and behavioral health plans agree on protocol to facilitate PCP access	CM procedures to communicate with PCP, arrange appointments; CM takes patient to appointment if needed	Tracks completion of visits, prevention screening, evaluation for cardiovascular and diabetes risk factor	Brief counseling by CM focused on reducing medical risk factors (CVD); Helps patients navigate through medical care by counseling on PCP communication, diaries; CM arranges transportation to appointment if needed
Improving care for bipolar disorder	Guideline-based clinical reminders for MHS; Response protocol for suicidal ideation	Manual-based procedures for CM to coordinate care with MHS; 24/7 coverage to handle manic symptoms, suicidal ideation	Tracks follow-up visits, medication use (e.g., to avoid multiple medications, duplicate prescriptions), serum drug monitoring and other lab tests	Brief counseling program by CM focused on improving adherence (e.g., medication, clinic visits); Support for patients in manic phase/suicidal
Improving care for complex cases	Referral guidelines for active SUD and social service needs	CM refers patients to ACT, intensive case management, social services agency	CM tracks completion of referral visits	CM educates patient on accessing available social services, SUD treatment

Abbreviations: CM, care manager; PCP, primary care provider; MHS, mental health specialist (i.e., psychiatrist); CVD, cardiovascular disease; SUD, substance use disorder; ACT, assertive community treatment (or other intensive case-management program).

However, while the CCM has recently been adapted to improve psychiatric care for adult patients with bipolar disorder (Bauer et al. 2006; Simon et al. 2002), it has not been customized to the needs of older adults (e.g., to include increased medical and social support services). Subsequent adaptations of the CCM or similar treatment models to improve coordinated care for patients with later-life bipolar disorder should take into consideration the unique needs of these older individuals, including sensitivity to side effects from mood stabilizers and antipsychotics, an increased risk of medical comorbidity and cognitive impairment, and an increased need for social support and long-term care. An example of how the four core components of the CCM could be adapted for older patients with bipolar disorder is described below and summarized in table 11.4. These elements, in combination, could enhance linkages between general medical, mental health, and social services for these older patients.

Components of the CCM Adapted to Older Patients with Bipolar Disorder

Decision Support Decision support includes the operationalization of clinical practice guidelines to routine care to cover care for medical conditions — in particular, preventive services and evaluation of cardiovascular and diabetes risk factors. Decision support materials are often flow sheets, which are convenient for the provider and outline protocols for identifying and referring patients for more intensive treatment, especially for bipolar disorder and/or active SUDs. The materials can also be tailored to the needs of general medical providers who see older patients with bipolar disorder, by outlining guidance in working with these patients such as knowing the warning signs of a manic episode and understanding the consequences of manic episodes and subsequent risk factors (e.g., sexual indiscretions and the need for HIV risk counseling; counseling on adherence to treatment when patients are reluctant to continue medications). Decision support also involves guidelines on the sharing of patients' information between primary care providers and mental health specialists, which can be used to develop a common protocol for handling private health information (e.g., dual release forms for both the health plan and the mental health provider carve-out plans).

Delivery System Design The CCM emphasizes a delivery system design that promotes a coordinated and integrated approach to managing treatment for patients with chronic illness. A care manager (i.e., a physician extender such as an RN) collaborates with psychiatrists and other health care providers to ensure the patient receives adequate treatment and follow-up care. The ultimate goal is to delineate the lines of responsibility and authority among providers so that there is a clear sense of who is accountable for which aspect of the patient's care. For example, the care manager's primary goal is to refer patients to medical care providers and to follow up with those providers through phone calls and e-mails, to remind them when patients are due for preventive check-ups or chronic care management. Thus, the care manager's communication with providers and patients should be ongoing, not just limited to referrals. Coordination of care can also occur through regular phone calls with mental health and primary care providers to discuss the patient's progress. The care manager should also be in regular contact with patients by phone or in person (or both) to remind them of upcoming appointments and to provide guidance on medical care management (e.g., monitoring of side effects, adherence counseling), and should track patients' progress, providers' communications, and clinical reminders.

Clinical Information System One of the most important aspects of the CCM is the development of a system to collect and share information among providers on patients' treatment and health status. The care manager can use a patients' "registry" to track patients' care over the course of their treatment. Registries are specific databases containing information on a cohort of patients undergoing follow-up and treatment management, and are designed to provide timely and accurate information about patients — including their treatment, utilization, and outcomes — to care managers and providers. Baumgardner and Hindmarsh (2003) recommend that registries should be simple to develop and use, with minimal complexities. The registry can track a patient's current treatment (medical and psychiatric visits, medications, lab tests, and preventive care), side effects, follow-up visits, and other information pertinent to the management of care. A simple stand-alone database has been widely used by practices implementing the CCM and has proved effective in tracking care for depression and other chronic illnesses (Kilbourne et al. 2004c). Collected information on patients' health status in near-real time can also be used to enhance ongoing performance-measurement strategies, as described earlier.

Self-management Support The CCM also emphasizes a patient-centered approach to treatment that incorporates self-management strategies and promotion of overall health and well-being. Care managers can instruct older patients with bipolar disorder in self-management through brief counseling on adherence to treatment, communication with providers, and lifestyle changes. The goals of self-management approaches are to activate, educate, and support patients and families in the management of bipolar disorder. These techniques have been widely used in other CCM-based models for patients with mood disorders, including the Bauer model (Life Goals; Bauer et al. 2001b). Lifestyle changes pertinent to older patients with bipolar disorder include improving adherence to medication regimens and clinic visits, aging-related issues, and lifestyle improvements (diet, exercise) to reduce cardiovascular and diabetes risk factors.

Given the challenges of coordinating care across multiple entities (e.g., medical, psychiatric, and geriatric services), further research is needed to adapt and implement CCM-based treatment models for older patients with bipolar disorder in routine care settings. It is well known that treatment models proven to be efficacious in tightly controlled settings are rarely translated effectively into routine care in a timely manner (Kilbourne et al. 2004c). Some strategies are available for closing the gap between efficacy and effectiveness research, as described below.

IMPLEMENTING EVIDENCE-BASED TREATMENT MODELS INTO ROUTINE CARE

Researchers are increasingly being called upon to engage community-based providers outside the academic realm to ensure a more rapid translation and implementation and, ultimately, a greater sustainability of evidence-based treatment models in settings that benefit the majority of patients — those who do not seek care in academic settings (Kilbourne et al. 2004c). To implement treatment models into real-world, routine care settings, researchers must be cognizant of the priorities of health care managers and providers who are not in the realm of academic medicine. In many cases, health care leaders are concerned about the bottom line and ensuring that all their patients can take advantage of new treatment models. More importantly, many treatment models and the tools used to evaluate patients (e.g., structured psychiatric assessments, lengthy patient surveys) cannot be implemented in routine care because they were originally developed in tightly controlled settings with ample resources. Consequently, at the outset, researchers must obtain buy-in and input from health care leaders and front-line providers and must be prepared to tailor treatment models to routine care settings.

Applications of Management Theory and Participatory Management

In the light of these challenges, another aspect of this new paradigm of quality of care for older patients with bipolar disorder involves the translation and implementation of treatment models into real-world settings. Researchers have adopted strategies used in business and management to better engage health care leaders and providers in implementing evidence-based treatment models in the real world. Management theory approaches, such as total quality management (Schonberger 1992) and participatory management theory (Leana and Florkowski 1992; Miller and Monge 1986; Valentine 1996; Yukl and Fu 1999), take into consideration organizational theory and employee culture when implementing quality improvement strategies. Participatory management (PM) theory is an emerging strategy, widely adopted over several decades in the organizational effectiveness literature and in health care settings and other service sectors (Locke and Schweiger 1979; Valentine 1996; Walshe and Rundall 2001). PM theory is based on some of the same theories that arose from community-based participatory research (Agency for Healthcare Research and Quality 2005). It emphasizes the involvement of front-line employees (defined as those who are directly providing care for patients, including physicians, nurses, social workers, and other clinic staff) at different levels of the health care organization, and the involvement of patients/consumers, in developing, customizing, and standardizing a quality-improvement initiative. As a result, PM theory can promote sustainable quality improvement by involving providers and patients/consumers, at the outset, in the decision-making process of model development and implementation.

The goal of PM theory is to institute changes and improve quality of services by encouraging a shared decision-making process that engages front-line employees, and other individuals directly affected by the proposed changes, in providing input and participating in the design and implementation of the strategy. PM seeks to empower employees at all levels, by shifting the decision-making authority from leaders to staff members actually involved in the delivery of services and by providing an opportunity (e.g., through focus groups and a consensus panel) to garner their input and decide on improvement processes. Such input is needed to identify (1) potential barriers to implementing treatment models in routine care and (2) aspects of the model that need to be customized to, for example, the needs of older patients with bipolar disorder in a given treatment setting. The PM process can also enhance the motivation and commitment of front-line employees who will deliver the treatment model (e.g., CCM) by giving them a higher stake or sense of ownership in a program they helped design. By better integrating mental and physical health care for patients, the PM approach should enhance front-line employees' sense that they are carrying out a meaningful, complete set of tasks, which should in turn enhance staff motivation and decrease turnover. The advantage of PM theory over other management models such as total quality management (which involves setting up committees to work on improving discrete processes of care) is that PM theory is suited to settings with a multidisciplinary and diverse workforce (e.g., general medical providers and psychiatrists) whose members do not traditionally work together and who come from different organizational cultures.

Participatory Management Processes

Participatory management consists of four processes to ensure that front-line staff and stakeholder inputs are incorporated into the development of the treatment model: design, customization, evaluation and refinement, and implementation (fig. 11.2). Each process involves garnering input from different levels (e.g., providers and patients/consumers) in the development and implementation of the treatment model and, in turn, establishing consensus and obtaining buy-in; this ultimately leads to the successful pilot testing and implementation of the treatment model to improve continuity of care and patients' outcomes.

PM process 1, the design phase, establishes how to develop and customize the model and key evaluation measures. PM process 2 involves customization of the treatment model and relevant outcomes in the health care setting, usually through provider and leader focus groups. The third PM process, evaluation and refinement, involves outlining contingencies to the treatment model and potential solutions, as well as evaluating the PM process itself. Process 3 can be accomplished through additional focus groups or consensus panels of representatives of the health plan and providers.

Full Circle: Implementation and Monitoring Quality over Time

Process 4 of participatory management is implementation, including the pilot testing of the intervention, preparing for full implementation in the treatment setting, and evaluating the treatment model's effectiveness. Some of the best methods for evaluating the implementation of treatment models include the performance (quality) measures described above (table 11.2), in part because these measures can be collected without much provider or patient burden. Overall, the implementation of evidence-based treatment models goes hand-in-hand with continued efforts to monitor the quality of care for older patients with bipolar disorder, so that health care leaders can respond quickly to reduce gaps in care for these individuals. Ultimately, the sustainability of quality improvement strategies in routine care relies on the continued surveillance of the effectiveness of care over time, using quality indicators at the patient-population level, to ensure that the implementation of treatment models is effective in improving care and thus outcomes for older individuals with bipolar disorder.

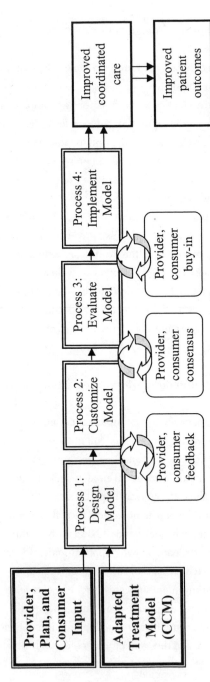

Fig. 11.2. A model of patient care based on participatory management theory. The model can be operationalized into four steps: (1) design the treatment model (e.g., chronic care model [CCM]) appropriate for older patients with bipolar disorder; (2) customize it to the particular treatment setting based on front-line provider and consumer input; (3) evaluate it through feedback and consensus of providers and consumers; and (4) implement and evaluate it in the treatment setting.

CONCLUSIONS

The current state of quality of care for bipolar disorder in later life suggests the need for more efforts to promote (1) quality-measurement initiatives, (2) quality improvement programs, and (3) strategies to implement and sustain such efforts in routine care settings. Efforts are needed to refine quality measures that are valid, feasible, and meaningful for assessing care for older persons with bipolar disorder across treatment settings, to benchmark trends in quality of care at the system and national levels. Treatment models designed to better integrate medical, psychiatric, and geriatric services for these older patients should also be tested and evaluated. For quality-of-care research to have an optimal effect in treating late-life bipolar disorder, researchers and health care leaders need to translate multidisciplinary treatment models that improve health outcomes into real-world settings and to continue evaluating these quality-improvement efforts so as to maximize their sustainability.

REFERENCES

Agency for Healthcare Research and Quality. 2005. *The role of community-based participatory research: creating partnerships, improving health.* AHRQ pub. no. 030037. Rockville, MD: Agency for Healthcare Research and Quality. www.ahrq.gov/research/cbprrole.htm

Alexopoulos, G. S., Streim, J., Carpenter, D., et al. 2004. Expert Consensus Panel for Using Antipsychotic Drugs in Older Patient. Re: using antipsychotic agents in older patients. *J Clin Psychiatry* 65:5–99

American Diabetes Association, American Psychiatric Association, American Association of Clinical Endocrinologists, North American Association for the Study of Obesity. 2004. Consensus development conference on antipsychotic drugs and obesity and diabetes. *J Clin Psychiatry* 65:267–272.

American Psychiatric Association. 1994. Guideline for the treatment of patients with bipolar disorder. *Am J Psychiatry* 151(Dec. suppl.).

American Psychiatric Association. 2002. Practice guideline for the treatment of patients with bipolar disorder (revision). *Am J Psychiatry* 159:S1–S50.

Balas, E. A., Boren, S. A., and Brown, G. D. 1996. Effect of physician profiling on utilization: metaanalysis of randomized clinical trials. *J Gen Intern Med* 11:584–590.

Baldessarini, R. J. 2002. Treatment research in bipolar disorder: issues and recommendations. *CNS Drugs* 16:721–729.

Bauer M. S., Callahan, A., and Jampala, M. 1999. Clinical practice guidelines for bipolar disorder from the Department of Veterans Affairs. *J Clin Psychiatry* 60:9–21.

Bauer, M. S., Kirk, G., Gavin, C., et al. 2001a. Correlates of functional and economic outcome in bipolar disorder: a prospective study. *J Affect Disord* 65:231–241.

Bauer, M. S., Williford, W., and Dawson, E. 2001b. Principles of effectiveness trials and their implementation in VA Cooperative Study #430, "Reducing the Efficacy-Effectiveness Gap in Bipolar Disorder." *J Affect Disord* 67:61–78.

Bauer, M., Unützer, J., Pincus, H. A., et al. 2002. Bipolar disorder. NIMH Affective Disorders Workgroup. *Ment Health Serv Res* 4:225–229

Bauer, M. S., McBride, L., Williford, W. O., et al. 2006. Collaborative care for bipolar disorder: part II. Impact on clinical outcome, function, and costs. *Psychiatr Serv* 57:937–945.

Baumgardner, G., and Hindmarsh, M. F. 2003. *Evaluate physician office registries special study*. Qualis Health doc. no. 7SOW-WA-OUTPT-0314. Washington, DC: Qualis Health.

Bruce, M., TenHave, T., Reynolds, C. F., et al. 2004. A randomized trial to reduce suicidal ideation and depressive symptoms in older primary care patients: the PROSPECT study. *JAMA* 291:1081–1091.

Bryant-Comstock, L., Stender, M., and Devercelli, G. 2002. Health care utilization and costs among privately insured patients with bipolar I disorder. *Bipolar Disord* 4:398–405.

Burns, T., Creed, F., Fahy, T., et al. 1999. Intensive versus standard case management for severe psychotic illness: a randomised trial. UK 700 Group. *Lancet* 353:2185–2189.

Carney, C. P., Yates, W. R., Goerdt, C. J., et al. 1998. Psychiatrists' and internists' knowledge and attitudes about delivery of clinical preventive medical services. *Psychiatr Serv* 49:1594–1600.

Caykoylu, A., Capoglu, I., Unuvar, N., et al. 2002. Thyroid abnormalities in lithium-treated patients with bipolar affective disorder. *J Int Med Res* 30:80–84.

Desai, M. M, Rosenheck, R. A., Druss, B. G., et al. 2002. Mental disorders and quality of diabetes care in the Veterans Health Administration. *Am J Psychiatry* 159:1584–1590.

Donabedian A., Wheeler, J. R., and Wyszewianski, L. 1982. Quality, cost, and health: an integrative model. *Med Care* 20:975–992.

Drake, R. E., McHugo, G. J., Clark, R. E., et al. 1998. Assertive community treatment for patients with co-occurring severe mental illness and substance use disorder: a clinical trial. *Am J Orthopsychiatry* 68:201–215.

Druss, B. G., Bradford, D. W., Rosenheck, R. A., et al. 2000. Mental disorders and use of cardiovascular procedures after myocardial infarction. *JAMA* 283:506–511.

Druss, B. G., Rohrbaugh, R. M., Levinson, C. M., et al. 2001 Integrated medical care for patients with serious psychiatric illness: a randomized trial. *Arch Gen Psychiatry* 58:861–868.

Druss, B. G., Rosenheck, R. A., Desai, M. M., et al. 2002. Quality of preventive medical care for patients with mental disorders. *Med Care* 40:129–136.

Druss, B. G., and Rosenheck, R. A. 2000. Locus of mental health treatment in an integrated service system. *Psychiatr Serv* 51:890–892.

Faulkner, L. R., Bloom, J. D., Bray, J. D., et al. 1986. Medical services in community mental health programs. *Hosp Community Psychiatry* 37:1045–1047.

Garnick, D. W., Lee, M. T., and Chalk, M. 2002. Establishing the feasibility of performance measures for alcohol and other drugs. *J Subst Use Treat* 23:375–385.

Golomb, B. A., Pyne, J. M., Wright, B., et al. 2000. The role of psychiatrists in primary care of patients with severe mental illness. *Psychiatr Serv* 51:766–773.

Goodwin, G. M. 2003. Evidence-based guidelines for treating bipolar disorder: recommendations from the British Association for Psychopharmacology. Consensus Group of the British Association for Psychopharmacology. *J Psychopharmacol* 17:149–173.

Institute of Medicine. 2001. *Crossing the quality chasm: a new health system for the 21st century.* Washington, DC: National Academy Press.

Kiefe, C. I., Allison, J. J., Williams, O. D., et al. 1995. Improving quality improvement using achievable benchmarks for physician feedback: a randomized controlled trial. *JAMA* 274:700–705.

Kilbourne, A. M. 2005a. Are older patients receiving adequate quality of care for bipolar disorder? Paper presented at Bipolar Disorder in Later Life, AAGP Symposium. March 4.

Kilbourne, A. M. 2005b. Bipolar disorder in late life: future directions in efficacy and effectiveness research. *Curr Psychiatry Rep* 7:10–17.

Kilbourne, A. M., and Pincus, H. A. 2004. Improving quality of care for bipolar disorder. *Curr Opin Psychiatry* 17:513–517.

Kilbourne, A. M., Cornelius, J. R., Han, X., et al. 2004a. Bur den of general medical conditions among individuals with bipolar disorder. *Bipolar Disord* 6:368–373.

Kilbourne, A. M., Haas, G. L., Mulsant, B., et al. 2004b. Concurrent psychiatric diagnoses by age and race among persons with bipolar disorder. *Psychiatr Serv* 55:931–933.

Kilbourne, A. M., Schulberg, H. C., Post, E. P., et al. 2004c. Translating evidence-based depression-management services to community-based primary care practices. *Milbank Q* 82:631–659.

Koran, L. M., Sox, H. C., and Marton, K. I. 1989. Medical evaluation of psychiatric patients: I. Results in a state mental health system. *Arch Gen Psychiatry* 46:733–740.

Lave, J. R, Frank, R. G., Schulberg, H. C., et al. 1998. Cost-effectiveness of treatments for major depression in primary care practice. *Arch Gen Psychiatry* 55:645–651.

Leana, C., and Florkowski, G. 1992. Employee involvement programs: implementing psychological theory and management practice. *Res Personnel Hum Resources Manage* 10:233–270.

Locke, E., and Schweiger, D. 1979. Participation in decision making: one more look. *Res Organ Behav* 1:265–339.

Masand, P. S., and Gupta, S. 2002. Long-term side effects of newer-generation antidepressants: SSRIs, venlafaxine, nefazodone, bupropion, and mirtazapine. *Ann Clin Psychiatry* 14:175–182.

Miller, K., and Monge, P. 1986. Participation, satisfaction and productivity: a meta-analytic review. *Acad Manage J* 29:727–753.

National Committee on Quality Assurance. 2005. The health plan and employer data information set 2005 measures. www.ncqa.org/Programs/HEDIS/Hedis%202004%20Summary%20Table.pdf

Neil, W., Curran, S., and Wattis, J. 2003. Antipsychotic prescribing in older people. *Age Ageing* 32:475–483.

Peipho, R. W. 2002. Cardiovascular effects of antipsychotics used in bipolar illness. *J Clin Psychiatry* 63(suppl. 4):20–23.

Pincus, H. A. 2003. The future of behavioral health and primary care: drowning in the mainstream or left on the bank? *Psychosomatics* 44:1–11.

Quinlivan, R., Hough, R., Crowell, A., et al. 1995. Service utilization and costs of care for severely mentally ill clients in an intensive case management program. *Psychiatr Serv* 46:365–371.

Redelmeier, D. A., Tan, S. H., and Booth, G. L. 1998. The treatment of unrelated disorders in patients with chronic medical diseases. *N Engl J Med* 338:1516–1520.

Regier, D. A., Farmer, M. E., and Rae, D. S. 1990. Comorbidity of mental disorders with alcohol and other drug abuse: results from the Epidemiologic Catchment Area (ECA) study. *JAMA* 264:2511–2518.

Rost, K., Nutting, P., Smith, J., et al. 2000. The role of competing demands in the treatment provided primary care patients with major depression. *Arch Fam Med* 9:150–154.

Samuels, S., and Fang, M. 2004. Olanzapine may cause delirium in geriatric patients. *J Clin Psychiatry* 65:582–583.

Schonberger, R. J. 1992. Total quality management cuts a broad swath: through manufacturing and beyond. *Organ Dynamics*, spring: 18.

Shortell, S. 2000. A model approach to chronic illness management. In Shortell, S. M., Gillies, R. R., Anderson, D. A., et al. (eds.), *Remaking health care in America: the evolution of organized delivery systems* (pp. 141–162). San Francisco: Jossey-Bass.

Simon, G. E., Ludman, E., Unützer, J., et al. 2002. Design and implementation of a randomized trial evaluating systematic care for bipolar disorder. *Bipolar Disord* 4:226–236.

Strakowski, S. M., DelBello, M. P., Fleck, D. E., et al. 2000. The impact of substance abuse on the course of bipolar disorder. *Biol Psychiatry* 48:477–485.

Suppes, T., Swann, A. C., and Dennehy, E. B. 2001. Texas medication algorithm project: development and feasibility testing of a treatment algorithm for patients with bipolar disorder. *J Clin Psychiatry* 62:439–447.

Unützer, J., Simon, G., Pabiniak, C., et al. 2000. The use of administrative data to assess quality of care for bipolar disorder in a large staff model HMO. *Gen Hosp Psychiatry* 22:1–10.

U.S. Department of Health, Education, and Welfare, Medical Practice Project. 1979. *A state-of-the-science report for the Office of the Assistant Secretary for the U.S. Department of Health, Education, and Welfare.* Baltimore, MD: Policy Research.

U.S. Food and Drug Administration. 2005. Public health advisory: deaths with antipsychotics in elderly patients with behavioral disturbances. April 11. www.fda.gov/cder/drug/advisory/antipsychotics.htm.

Valenstein, M., Mitchinson, A., Ronis, D. L., et al. 2004. Quality indicators and monitoring of mental health services: what do frontline providers think? *Am J Psychiatry* 161:146–153.

Valentine, N. M. 1996. A national model for participative management and policy development. *Nurs Adm Q* 21:24–34.

Wagner, E. H., Austin, B. T., and Von Korff, M. 1996. Organizing care for patients with chronic illness. *Milbank Q* 74:511–544.

Wagner, E. H., Austin, B. T., and Davis, C. 2001. Improving chronic illness care: translating evidence into action. *Health Aff (Millwood)* 20:64–78.

Walshe, K., and Rundall, T. G. 2001. Evidence-based management: from theory to practice in health care. *Milbank Q* 79:429–457.

Weiss, R. D., and Mirin, S. M. 1986. Subtypes of cocaine abusers. *Psychiatr Clin North Am* 9:491–501.

Werner, R. M., and Asch, D. A. 2005. The unintended consequences of publicly reporting quality information. *JAMA* 293:1239–1244.

Wyatt, R. J., Henter, I. D., and Jamison, J. C. 2001. Lithium revisited: savings brought about by the use of lithium, 1970–1991. *Psychiatr Q* 72:149–166.

Young, R. C., Gyulai, L., and Mulsant, B. H. 2004. Pharmacotherapy of bipolar disorder in old age: review and recommendations. *Am J Geriatr Psychiatry* 12:342–357.

Yu, W., Ravelo, A., and Wagner, T. H. 2003. Prevalence and costs of chronic conditions in the VA health care system. *Med Care Res Rev* 60: 146S–167S.

Yukl, G., and Fu, P. 1999. Determinants of delegation and consultation by managers. *J Organ Behav* 20:219–232.

CHAPTER TWELVE

Evidence-Based Medicine and the Treatment of Older Adults with Bipolar Disorder

STEPHEN J. BARTELS, M.D., M.S.,

AND ARICCA D. VAN CITTERS, M.S.

Evidence-based medicine (EBM) is the provision of health care that systematically integrates the best available research evidence with clinical expertise and a patient's unique values, preferences, and circumstances (Straus et al. 2005). In this chapter, we discuss the importance of EBM in the treatment of older adults with bipolar disorder, the rationale and methodology for the use of EBM in geriatric mental health practices, the evidence supporting the effective treatment of older adults with bipolar disorder, the barriers and approaches to implementing treatment in geriatric mental health care, and the limitations of EBM.

IMPORTANCE OF EVIDENCE-BASED MEDICINE FOR TREATING BIPOLAR DISORDER IN OLDER ADULTS

Approximately 5%–19% of older adults treated in inpatient mental health settings and 2%–8% of older adults treated in outpatient mental health settings are diagnosed with bipolar disorder (Depp and Jeste 2004). Although bipolar disorder is less prevalent in older than in younger age groups (Narrow et al. 2002), the projected increase in the number of older adults will pose challenges to providing effective treatment for this population (U.S. Census Bureau 2004). Compared with older persons with unipolar major depression, older adults with bipolar disorder have more severe symptoms, have more impaired community functioning, use almost four times the amount of mental health services, and are four times more likely to be psychiatrically hospitalized (Bartels et al. 2000).

Despite the substantial impact of bipolar disorder on functioning, quality of life, and health care costs for older persons, the empirical knowledge base of effective treatments for late-life bipolar disorder is limited. To date, treatment has been largely modeled from research studies and guidelines focusing on younger adults (Fountoulakis et al. 2005; Grunze et al. 2002, 2003, 2004). However, extrapolating research on younger populations to treatment recommendations for older adults may be problematic, given age-associated differences in cognition, physiological functioning, medical comorbidity, and response and tolerance to treatment (Depp et al. 2005; Snowdon 2000). Older people experience an increased sensitivity to medication and greater likelihood of side effects (Banerjee and Dickinson 1997); changes in the sensitivity of neurotransmitter receptors, general metabolism, and the potential for drug-drug interactions further complicate treatment. In addition, older adults with bipolar disorder and other serious mental illnesses are more likely than younger adults to have multiple co-occurring medical illnesses, including cardiovascular, endocrine, or pulmonary diseases (Kilbourne et al. 2005). The selection of appropriate and optimal treatments for older adults with bipolar disorder should accommodate these age-associated modifications and individual patient characteristics, while also reflecting a critical ascertainment of the evidence base.

EVIDENCE-BASED MEDICINE: RATIONALE AND PROCESS
Rationale

Sackett and colleagues (1996) defined evidence-based medicine as "the conscientious and judicious use of current best evidence from clinical care research in the management of individual patients." Over the past decade, EBM has been rapidly incorporated into the mainstream of contemporary medical care and has become a core component of medical student education (Claridge and Fabian 2005). In contrast to a tradition of clinical decisions based on professional experience, case anecdotes, and accumulated medical facts, EBM emphasizes a systematic approach to formulating and answering clinical questions by quickly finding and evaluating the current best evidence. In medical education, this has translated into training practitioners in the real-time use of technology to find the answers to clinical questions and to critically appraise the scientific evidence supporting the effectiveness of tests, treatments, and services.

Unfortunately, mental health practitioners have been slow to adopt EBM into training and clinical practice. Some of the impediments to adopting an EBM approach in mental health care may be due to differences in access to technology (e.g., routine use of computers, electronic medical records, web-based information, and personal digital assistants [PDAs] by clinicians in the practice setting) and more limited development of systematic evidence-based reviews and syntheses of the research literature. The adoption of an evidence-based approach in mental health care has also been challenged by misconceptions about the basic assumptions and practical application of EBM. For example, the lack of large, well-designed, randomized clinical trials in a particular area (e.g., pharmacological treatments for geriatric bipolar disorder) has been cited as a limitation in using an evidenced-based, data-driven approach to identifying the best treatment option. This objection misses the key point that EBM is a systematic approach to identifying and critically appraising the *best available evidence*. The research evidence is conceptualized along a hierarchy, from the highest levels of evidence (e.g., results from meta-analyses of multiple randomized clinical trials with similar methods and outcomes) to the lowest levels (e.g., quasi-experimental studies or pre- and post-treatment clinical case reports). In fact, it can be argued that a systematic evaluation of the literature is particularly critical when the research literature is not well described or when only a small number of studies are available to inform clinical decision-making.

Another common misconception about EBM is that it promotes a "cookbook" or "one-size-fits-all" approach to clinical situations, in a manner that devalues clinical expertise or the individual situation or preferences of the mental health patient/consumer. As described by Straus and colleagues (2005), the practice of EBM "requires the integration of the best research evidence with our clinical expertise and our patient's unique values and circumstances" (1). Clinical skills and past experience are crucial to identifying the specific health status, risks, benefits, and unique circumstances for each individual patient. This is especially important in the field of geriatrics, where the risk and potential benefits of an evidence-based treatment may vary substantially for a young adult with few medical problems and for a frail older person with multiple medical problems, concurrent treatments, and functional challenges.

Finally, some stakeholders in the mental health arena have expressed fears that evidence-based practices are too expensive to implement, favor a medical model that does not support the individual's personal recovery goals, and exclude the use of promising practices that lack research data but are widely perceived to have positive effects (Ganju 2003). To the contrary, the use of EBM may offset health care costs associated with underuse, overuse, or misuse of other services. EBM incorporates the unique values and preferences of the patient or health care consumer into the process of selecting treatments. The process of shared clinical decision-making thus includes both the patient and provider as consumers of information on the best evidence. Moreover, strategies have been developed for incorporating recovery-oriented programming and values into the development and implementation of evidence-based mental health practices (Farkas et al. 2005). Finally, identification of the evidence base is a dynamic process that must take into account priority areas that lack extensive research (Ganju 2003). In these instances, the best available evidence may be limited to extrapolation from related populations or early findings that are promising but do not meet the standards of a large randomized controlled trial. For instance, despite a paucity of rigorously controlled studies that evaluate the effectiveness of interventions for geriatric bipolar disorder, current practice should use principles from the best available evidence while constantly evolving to incorporate new findings.

Process

A three-step approach to EBM has been proposed that includes (1) formulating a well-developed clinical question using the "PICO" criteria (explained below), (2) evaluating available resources, and (3) assessing the quality of the available literature (Bartkowiak 2004, 2005a, 2005b). In this framework, the process of EBM begins with asking a well-developed answerable question that is appropriately formulated for a search of the literature (Straus et al. 2005). The well-designed clinical question can be either a general knowledge question or a specific question designed to inform a clinical decision. A general knowledge question considers topics such as prevalence, pathogenesis, therapeutics, or broad knowledge in a given area. For example, a general knowledge question might ask: "What are the most common causes of new-onset mania in people over age 65?" or "What are the most common side effects of lithium in older persons?" A specific well-designed clinical question includes a clearly identified patient situation or problem and an identified intervention. The acronym "PICO" has been proposed to help clinicians in formulating a well-designed clinical question based on four essential components: (1) Patient or population, (2) Intervention and exposure, (3) Comparisons, and (4) Outcomes (Bartkowiak 2004). For example, "For an adult with unstable bipolar disorder who is taking a mood stabilizer such as divalproex, would adding an atypical antipsychotic reduce rates of relapse enough over three to five years to be worth the side effects commonly associated with long-term treatment with atypical antipsychotics?"

Once a well-designed clinical question has been formulated, clinicians can use a variety of resources in seeking answers. The most efficient resources for busy practitioners are previously synthesized summaries of the research. For example, evidence-based treatment algorithms and practice guidelines can help guide decision-making without requiring the clinician to conduct a search of the primary research literature (Addis and Krasnow 2000). However, these guidelines and algorithms should clearly document a systematic review of evidence linking treatment options to outcomes, provide a discussion of relevant patient groups and preferences or values associated with the treatment recommendations, and clearly indicate the level of empirically based certainty for each recommendation (Guyatt and Rennie 2002). For example, well-designed evidence-based guidelines and treatment algorithms present objective ratings of the strength of the evidence for each specific recommendation, ranging from recommendations that are strongly supported by research from at least two randomized clinical trials to recommendations that are supported by expert opinion only and lack experimental evidence.

An example of an algorithmic approach to clinical decision-making in the treatment of bipolar disorder is provided by Sachs (2003). Although this algorithm does not specifically consider older adults, it provides a sample of an approach that could be adapted to help guide clinical practice for geriatric bipolar disorder. A decision tree is used to separate clinical presentations into broad categories, including new onset of an acute manic or mixed episode, new onset of acute bipolar depression, and entry into treatment between episodes. Thereafter, decisions are guided by several overarching treatment principles reflecting the current state of research knowledge. These include starting treatment with clearly proven interventions, using a mood stabilizer for every phase of the illness, and using a multiphase treatment strategy to link current assessment with an appropriate treatment plan. A grading system reflects the weight of evidence supporting the use of various options. For example, multiple well-designed studies support the use of lithium, divalproex (valproate), carbamazepine, olanzapine, and haloperidol as initial interventions for acute mania. In contrast, Sachs (2003) concludes that the evidence does not support the use of standard antidepressants as adding significant benefit beyond that provided by mood stabilizers alone. Finally, preliminary data that are suggestive of potential benefit are considered within the hierarchy of best available evidence, when proven approaches have not yielded clear benefit. For example, preliminary findings suggest the potential benefit of lamotrigine as a mood stabilizer, and divalproex and topiramate may have potential antidepressant benefits. It is important to underscore that optimal treatment algorithms or guidelines should clearly identify the level of evidence supporting each treatment decision at each particular decision node. To our knowledge, evidence-based algorithms and guidelines that meet this level of rigor have not yet been developed for geriatric bipolar disorder.

In the absence of evidence-based guidelines or algorithms, pre-filtered electronic databases offer an alternative approach to evaluating the evidence associated with a specific intervention or clinical practice. These sources synthesize and objectively evaluate the quality of research for the clinician. For example, the Cochrane Collaboration prepares, maintains, and provides quarterly updates of systematic reviews of many health care interventions. Other resources — such as Evidence Based Medicine, Evidence Based Mental Health, and the ACP (American College of Physicians) Journal Club — summarize, evaluate, and provide commentaries on original articles and reviews that have been published elsewhere and that meet basic methodological standards (Guyatt and Rennie 2002). These pre-filtered resources facilitate rapid evaluations of the evidence base by using transparent standards and well-established procedures. However, these resources are most likely to be available in clinical areas with extensive research. For example, systematic reviews exist for treatment of geriatric depression, yet other clinical conditions with a less extensive research literature (e.g., geriatric bipolar disorder) may require further development of the field before these pre-filtered resources become available.

For clinical questions that lack previously synthesized reviews of the literature, primary sources such as Medline offer a readily accessible database of the medical literature. The comprehensive nature of the Medline database requires a careful selection of search strategies and an understanding of the database structure. The clinician must efficiently search the literature, select the most relevant and valid studies, extract the clinical message, and apply it to the problem. Furthermore, evaluating the strength of the evidence for a particular clinical practice requires evaluations of the quality of the study, the effect on relevant outcomes (including magnitude of effect, sample size, power), and consistency across studies (West et al. 2002). EBM searches can also be conducted through the "clinical queries" component of Medline, and several recent publications propose strategies for improving the quality of Medline searches (Haynes et al. 2005; Montori et al. 2005; Wilczynski et al. 2004; Wong et al. 2004).

Although empirical data supporting the treatment of geriatric bipolar disorder are limited, an evaluation of the best available evidence can be used to guide evidence-based decision-making. The clinician can classify the evidence for effectiveness by following the hierarchy outlined in table 12.1 (Gray 1997).

A review of the empirical evidence supporting psychotherapy traditionally presents additional challenges. These challenges are heightened in the treatment of geriatric bipolar disorder, given the few studies that have evaluated these practices. However, guidelines suggest that the evaluation of psychosocial treatments should use the following organization. The highest support is given to interventions with ev-

TABLE 12.1
Hierarchical classification of evidence for effectiveness in research studies

1. A meta-analysis or systemic review of well-designed randomized controlled trials
2. A single properly designed randomized controlled trial
3. Studies with randomization (i.e., single group pre- and post-treatment, cohort, time-series, or matched case-control studies)
4. Other quasi-experimental studies from more than one center or research group
5. Expert reports and authorities' recommendations based on descriptive studies or clinical evidence

idence of efficacy (1) from at least two well-designed, prospective, randomized controlled studies by different investigators with clearly described interventions, or (2) from a large series (>9) of single-case-design experiments. Probable effectiveness is denoted (1) by two studies showing that the treatment was superior to nontreatment in a waiting-list control group, (2) by a small series (>3) of single-case-design experiments, or (3) by one or more studies that meet the criteria for the highest level of evidence but have not yet been replicated by other investigators (Chambless and Hollon 1998; Chambless and Ollendick 2001).

Research on the effectiveness of different approaches to the treatment of bipolar disorder in older adults is reviewed in detail elsewhere in this book; these reviews underscore both an emerging evidence base and a substantial array of future directions and unanswered research questions. For example, standard pharmacological approaches consisting of the use of lithium and divalproex by younger adults seem to be effective for older adults as well, though lower initial doses and close attention to the monitoring of serum levels are necessary. Aggregate results from four uncontrolled studies showed that two-thirds of older adults with manic bipolar disorder had improved outcomes following lithium treatment (Young et al. 2004). However, the use of lithium in older persons is complicated by lowered renal clearance and a longer elimination half-life compared with younger persons (Sajatovic 2002). Aggregate data from five studies evaluating the use of divalproex by older adults found that 59% improved following treatment (Young et al. 2004). As with lithium, the elimination half-life of divalproex is longer in older than in younger adults. To date, research is lacking on the comparative effectiveness of lithium and divalproex for older adults with bipolar disorder. The data supporting the use of other anticonvulsants and antipsychotic medications are also limited, as are data on the nonpharmacological and psychosocial treatment of bipolar disorder (Sajatovic 2002). Given the potential for medication side effects in older patients, clinicians should obtain a history of adverse medication responses and associated doses and concentrations, and the tolerability of specific agents should guide the selection and dosing of phar-macotherapy.

In contrast to the emerging literature on pharmacological treatments for geriatric bipolar disorder, there are few data on the effectiveness of psychosocial interventions and service models, though older adults with bipolar disorder frequently use these services. A study of older adults with bipolar disorder found that 73% used case-management services, 51% received psychotherapy or counseling services, and 32% received skills training (community living skills and illness-management skills) (Bartels et al. 2000).

IMPLEMENTATION OF EVIDENCE-BASED PRACTICES IN GERIATRIC MENTAL HEALTH CARE

A landmark report by the Institute of Medicine (2001) described a "quality chasm" in health care between research defining the most effective treatments and actual clinical practice in usual care. This lack of correspondence between research and practice is both qualitative and temporal. For example, estimates indicate that it takes well over a decade for research findings on effective treatments to be routinely implemented by health care providers (Lenfant 2003). Barriers to disseminating and implementing evidence-based practices across mental health settings include a lack of specific skills and knowledge among clinical staff, limited time available for training, and a lack of dedicated financing to support the implementation and sustainability of systems change (Corrigan et al. 2001).

Conventional approaches to improving quality of care, consisting of developing and disseminating guidelines, show only modest results in the absence of additional systems-change interventions (Callahan 2001). Even when the dissemination of guidelines is augmented by education, feedback, and use of reminders, the resulting improvement in quality of care is modest. A review of 235 studies evaluating approaches to dissemination and implementation of guidelines indicated a median 10% improvement across a spectrum of interventions (Grimshaw and Eccles 2004; Grimshaw et al. 2004). The most common dissemination strategies included reminder systems, followed (respectively) by multifaceted interventions involving educational outreach, dissemination of educational materials, and audit and feedback. Median improvement in performance across these interventions ranged from 14.1% for reminders, to 6% for multifaceted interventions involving educational outreach, 8.1% for dissemination of educational materials, and 7.0% for audit and feedback. While these findings support the position that dissemination and implementation of guidelines can improve the quality of care by modifying provider practices, improvements are small to moderate in size (Grimshaw and Eccles 2004; Grimshaw et al. 2004).

Implementation is aided by identifying champions of EBM, redefining clinicians' roles to include EBM activities, allocating time and money to the EBM process, and creating an organizational culture that fosters EBM. An evidence-based organizational culture should involve front-line care providers in initiating change, formulating clinical questions, and evaluating the evidence needed to answer those questions (Fineout-Overholt et al. 2004). In addition, specific strategies have been developed to assist in the translation and implementation of research findings into clinical practice. For instance, one recommended strategy includes the use of the RE-AIM (Reach, Efficacy/effectiveness, Adoption, Implementation, and Maintenance) framework. The RE-AIM framework provides research translation tools and support designed to help researchers, health care providers, and policymakers evaluate health behavior interventions and overcome barriers to implementation and dissemination (Dzewaltowski et al. 2004). In addition to changes that support the implementation of priority evidence-based practices, the change in culture includes equipping practitioners with the skills to ask and answer questions about the best evidence to support clinical decision-making for individual patients. This includes developing the skill set to identify relevant, evidence-based systematic reviews of the research literature at the point of care and to combine clinical evidence with patient-centered care (Slawson and Shaughnessy 2005). Novel strategies for teaching health care providers to apply these skills are being developed. For example, a recent report describes a two-year course for psychiatry residents that is designed to teach the skills necessary to incorporate evidence-based decision-making into routine practice. Modules provide case conferences followed by a literature review of related papers, as well as reviews of guidelines, algorithms, review articles, and research studies. Although psychiatry residents have shown improvements in knowledge and evaluation skills, this program has not yet been compared with other strategies (Osser et al. 2005).

Effective strategies for developing a culture of evidence-based practice will also need to complement systems changes with practical, easy-to-use information technology. For example, in a study evaluating the application of evidence-based practices by senior psychiatrists, Lawrie and colleagues (2000) found that 40% perceived their practices to be evidence-based, though the largest barrier to EBM was lack of time. Given this perceived lack of time, a question-answering service was considered to be a valuable resource for clinicians. Of note, two areas for which these psychiatrists most frequently requested additional evidence-based treatment information were identification of the relative efficacy of lithium and valproate and the relative efficacy of the combination of lithium and valproate versus monotherapy. Another survey of medical (nonpsychiatric) physicians noted that only 5% believed that learning identification and appraisal skills was the most effective way to move toward practicing EBM (McColl et al. 1998).

Finally, different practices and practitioners are at different levels of readiness to adopt EBM in day-to-day practice. Efficient approaches to targeting organizations and individual providers can be facilitated by multidimensional measures of clinicians' attitudes and readiness to adopt evidence-based practices. One such measure has characterized the general appeal of evidence-based practices, the likelihood of adopting an evidence-based practice when required to do so, clinicians' openness to the use of new or innovative practices, and the perceived divergence between usual care practices and academically developed or research-based interventions (Aarons 2004).

LIMITATIONS OF EVIDENCE-BASED MEDICINE

Several qualifications must be considered in applying EBM methodology to clinical care. First, decisions on the selection of treatments must incorporate evidence of effectiveness as well as patient-specific risk factors and preferences. For example, a discussion of treatment of bipolar disorder with olanzapine may differ substantially for a physically healthy 20-year-old man who is hoping to sleep better and for a 70-year-old woman who is obese, has diabetes, has experienced falls, and who wants to lose weight. Second, there is a shortage of consistent scientific evidence on the effectiveness of the treatment of geriatric bipolar disorder, and clinicians are likely to identify questions for which no direct evidence is available to guide treatment decisions. Third, data are largely based on conventional experimental designs that compare single interventions. Studies are unlikely to consider common comorbid disorders in medical decision-making and are often unable to inform complex clinical decision-making. In addition, the unique characteristics of specific patients challenge the generalizability and application of evidence.

Finally, the inclusion and exclusion criteria associated with randomized controlled trials limit the ability to generalize findings to typical patients. For example, a comparison of adults with bipolar disorder or schizophrenia who were included in and excluded from clinical research trials noted that the patients who were ineligible for inclusion had more comorbid conditions and were more likely to be white, female, and older than the patients included in the clinical trials (Zarin et al. 2005). Fifty-five percent of patients with bipolar disorder receiving treatment in routine practice settings would have been ineligible for participation in one study. Patients who were ineligible for participation in clinical trials had lower global functioning and greater medical comorbidity and were receiving more complex medication treatments. Patients' participation in research trials can be affected not only by protocol exclusion criteria but by other issues that affect the likelihood of participation, such as methods of recruitment, physicians' bias in referring patients, patients' access to research centers, patients' motivation, and patients' willingness to be randomized in the trial.

CONCLUSIONS

Translating research into clinical practice has been highlighted as one of the most important priorities in health care, in reports from the Institute of Medicine (2001) and the National Institute of Mental Health (1999). According to the NIMH report, "All too often, clinical practices and service system innovations that are validated by research are not fully adopted in treatment settings and service systems for individuals with mental illnesses." These reports noted that health care services can be continually improved by focusing on the transitions between basic science, the development of new treatments, clinical trials, and implementation into practice settings.

The NIMH Clinical Trials and Translation Workgroup defined five priority areas as part of the Strategic Plan for Mood Disorders Research. These priority areas are relevant to all age groups, though special note was made of the more limited availability of information pertinent to children and older adults. This work group also specifically identified the need for studying all aspects of geriatric bipolar disorder (Frank et al. 2002). The priority areas are (1) maximizing the effectiveness and cost-effectiveness of acute treatment across all populations and care settings; (2) identifying services that are most likely to reduce symptoms and improve functioning in treatment-resistant patients; (3) identifying cost-effective interventions for preventing relapse and maintaining optimal functioning during remission; (4) identifying markers for predicting treatment effectiveness, course of illness, and risk of adverse events and tolerability of medications; and (5) developing methodology associated with lower research costs and greater generalizability earlier in the development and testing of treatment.

A rigorous, systematic review of the current evidence base for interventions and services for geriatric bipolar disorder will be critical to further refining this research agenda. In addition to reviews of the current state of research included in this volume, attention is warranted to changing the practice culture and systems of care where older persons with bipolar disorder seek and receive services. Despite the current lack of an extensive empirical literature specific to older persons, with the rapid developments and emerging findings, providers and service organizations must be able to quickly incorporate findings from newly published and ongoing research. In this chapter we have described a systematic approach to identifying, evaluating, and implementing clinical decisions and practices through application of the principles of evidence-based medicine. This process will help facilitate the rapid incorporation of new findings into clinical practice by building bridges that span the gap between science and service.

REFERENCES

Aarons, G. A. 2004. Mental health provider attitudes toward adoption of evidence-based practice: the Evidence-Based Practice Attitude Scale (EBPAS). *Ment Health Serv Res* 6:61–74.

Addis, M. E., and Krasnow, A. D. 2000. A national survey of practicing psychologists' attitudes toward psychotherapy treatment manuals. *J Consult Clin Psychol* 68:331–339.

Banerjee, S., and Dickinson, E. 1997. Evidence based health care in old age psychiatry. *Int J Psychiatry Med* 27:283–292.

Bartels, S. J., Forester, B., Miles, K. M., et al. 2000. Mental health service use by elderly patients with bipolar disorder and unipolar major depression. *Am J Geriatr Psychiatry* 8:160–166.

Bartkowiak, B. A. 2004. Searching for evidence-based medicine in the literature: part 1. The start. *Clin Med Res* 2:254–255.

Bartkowiak, B. A. 2005a. Searching for evidence-based medicine in the literature: part 2. Resources. *Clin Med Res* 3:39–40.

Bartkowiak, B. A. 2005b. Searching for evidence-based medicine in the literature: part 3. Assessment. *Clin Med Res* 3:113–115.

Callahan, C. M. 2001. Quality improvement research on late life depression in primary care. *Med Care* 39:772–784.

Chambless, D. L., and Hollon, S. D. 1998. Defining empirically supported therapies. *J Consult Clin Psychol* 66:7–18.

Chambless, D. L., and Ollendick, T. H. 2001. Empirically supported psychological interventions: controversies and evidence. *Annu Rev Psychol* 52:685–716.

Claridge, J. A., and Fabian, T. C. 2005. History and development of evidence-based medicine. *World J Surg* 29:547–553.

Corrigan, P. W., Steiner, L., McCracken, S. G., et al. 2001. Strategies for disseminating evidence-based practices to staff who treat people with serious mental illness. *Psychiatr Serv* 52:1598–1606.

Depp, C. A., and Jeste, D. V. 2004. Bipolar disorder in older adults: a critical review. *Bipolar Disord* 6:343–367.

Depp, C. A., Lindamer, L. A., Folsom, D. P., et al. 2005. Differences in clinical features and mental health service use in bipolar disorder across the lifespan. *Am J Geriatr Psychiatry* 13:290–298.

Dzewaltowski, D. A., Glasgow, R. E., Klesges, L. M., et al. 2004. RE-AIM: evidence-based standards and a web resource to improve translation of research into practice. *Ann Behav Med* 28:75–80.

Farkas, M., Gagne, C., Anthony, W., et al. 2005. Implementing recovery oriented evidence based programs: identifying the critical dimensions. *Community Ment Health J* 41:141–158.

Fineout-Overholt, E., Levin, R. F., and Melnyk, B. M. 2004. Strategies for advancing evidence-based practice in clinical settings. *J N Y State Nurs Assoc* 35(2):28–32.

Fountoulakis, K. N., Vieta, E., Sanchez-Moreno, J., et al. 2005. Treatment guidelines for bipolar disorder: a critical review. *J Affect Disord* 86:1–10.

Frank, E., Rush, A. J., Blehar, M., et al. 2002. Skating to where the puck is going to be: a plan for clinical trials and translation research in mood disorders. *Biol Psychiatry* 52:631–654.

Ganju, V. 2003. Implementation of evidence-based practices in state mental health systems: implications for research and effectiveness studies. *Schizophr Bull* 29:125–131.

Gray, J. A. M. 1997. *Evidence-based healthcare: how to make health policy and management decisions.* New York: Churchill Livingston.

Grimshaw, J. M., and Eccles, M. P. 2004. Is evidence-based implementation of evidence-based care possible? *Med J Aust* 180(6 suppl.):S50–S51.

Grimshaw, J. M., Thomas, R. E., MacLennan, G., et al. 2004. Effectiveness and efficiency of guideline dissemination and implementation strategies. *Health Technol Assess* 8(6):iii–iv, 1–72.

Grunze, H., Kasper, S., Goodwin, G., et al. 2002. World Federation of Societies of Biological Psychiatry (WFSBP) guidelines for biological treatment of bipolar disorders: part I. Treatment of bipolar depression. *World J Biol Psychiatry* 3:115–124.

Grunze, H., Kasper, S., Goodwin, G., et al. 2003. The World Federation of Societies of Biological Psychiatry (WFSBP) guidelines for the biological treatment of bipolar disorders: part II. Treatment of mania. *World J Biol Psychiatry* 4:5–13.

Grunze, H., Kasper, S., Goodwin, G., et al. 2004. The World Federation of Societies of Biological Psychiatry (WFSBP) guidelines for the biological treatment of bipolar disorders: part III. Maintenance treatment. *World J Biol Psychiatry* 5:120–135.

Guyatt, G. H., and Rennie, D. 2002. *Users' guides to the medical literature: a manual for evidence-based clinical practice.* Chicago: American Medical Association Press.

Haynes, R. B., McKibbon, K. A., Wilczynski, N. L., et al. 2005. Optimal search strategies for retrieving scientifically strong studies of treatment from Medline: analytical survey. *BMJ* 330:1179–1184.

Institute of Medicine. 2001. *Crossing the quality chasm: a new health system for the 21st century.* Washington, DC: Institute of Medicine.

Kilbourne, A. M., Cornelius, J. R., Han, X., et al. 2005. General-medical conditions in older patients with serious mental illness. *Am J Geriatr Psychiatry* 13:250–254.

Lawrie, S. M., Scott, A. I., and Sharpe, M. C. 2000. Evidence-based psychiatry — do psychiatrists want it and can they do it? *Health Bull* 58:25–33.

Lenfant, C. 2003. Shattuck lecture — clinical research to clinical practice — lost in translation? *N Engl J Med* 349:868–874.

McColl, A., Smith, H., White, P., et al. 1998. General practitioner's perceptions of the route to evidence based medicine: a questionnaire survey. *BMJ* 316:361–365.

Montori, V. M., Wilczynski, N. L., Morgan, D., et al. 2005. Optimal search strategies for retrieving systematic reviews from Medline: analytical survey. *BMJ* 330:68–73.

Narrow, W. E., Rae, D. S., Robins, L. N. et al. 2002. Revised prevalence estimates of mental disorders in the United States: using a clinical significance criterion to reconcile 2 survey's estimates. *Arch Gen Psychiatry* 59:115–123.

National Institute of Mental Health. 1999. *Bridging science and service*. Pub. no. 99-4353. Rockville, MD: National Institute of Mental Health.

Osser, D. N., Patterson, R. D., and Levitt, J. J. 2005. Guidelines, algorithms, and evidence-based psychopharmacology training for psychiatric residents. *Acad Psychiatry* 29:180–186.

Sachs, G. S. 2003. Decision tree for the treatment of bipolar disorder. *J Clin Psychiatry* 64(suppl. 8):35–40.

Sackett, D. L., Rosenberg, W. M., Gray, J. A., et al. 1996. Evidence based medicine: what it is and what it isn't. *BMJ* 312:71–72.

Sajatovic, M. 2002. Treatment of bipolar disorder in older adults. *Int J Geriatr Psychiatry* 17:865–873.

Slawson, D. C., and Shaughnessy, A. F. 2005. Teaching evidence-based medicine: should we be teaching information management instead? *Acad Med* 80:685–689.

Snowdon, J. 2000. The relevance of guidelines for treatment of mania in old age. *Int J Geriatr Psychiatry* 15:779–783.

Straus, S. E., Richardson, W. S., Glasziou, P., et al. 2005. *Evidence-based medicine: how to practice and teach EBM* (3rd ed.). Edinburgh: Churchill Livingstone.

U.S. Census Bureau. 2004. U.S. interim projections by age, sex, race, and Hispanic origin: table 2a. Projected population of the United States, by age and sex: 2000 to 2050. www .census.gov/ipc/www/usinterimproj/

West, S., King, V., Carey, T. S., et al. 2002. *Systems to rate the strength of scientific evidence: evidence report/technology assessment no. 47*. AHRQ pub. no. 02-E016. Prepared by the Research Triangle Institute–University of North Carolina Evidence-Based Practice Center under contract no. 290970011. Rockville, MD: Agency for Healthcare Research and Quality.

Wilczynski, N. L., Haynes, R. B., Lavis, J. N., et al. 2004. Optimal search strategies for detecting health services research studies in Medline. *CMAJ* 171:1179–1185.

Wong, S. S., Wilczynski, N. L., and Haynes, R. B. 2004. Developing optimal search strategies for detecting clinically relevant qualitative studies in Medline. *Medinfo* 11:311–316.

Young, R. C., Gyulai, L., Mulsant, B. H., et al. 2004. Pharmacotherapy of bipolar disorder in old age: review and recommendations. *Am J Geriatr Psychiatry* 12:342–357.

Zarin, D. A., Young, J. L., and West, J. C. 2005. Challenges to evidence-based medicine: a comparison of patients and treatments in randomized controlled trials with patients and treatments in a practice research network. *Soc Psychiatry Psychiatr Epidemiol* 40:27–35.

CHAPTER THIRTEEN

Legal and Ethical Issues in Bipolar Disorder Research Involving Older Adults

SANA LOUE, J.D., PH.D., M.P.H.

Research with participants who have been diagnosed with bipolar disorder entails significant legal and ethical issues. Many of these issues relate to the informed consent process, such as the capacity of the prospective research participant to provide or withhold his or her consent to participation, the ability of the individual to understand the information provided by the research team, the designation of a surrogate for consent to participate and the standard to be used by the surrogate in providing or withholding that consent, and the standard by which to assess and balance the risks and benefits that may result from participation. The resolution of these issues in a specific context may be rendered even more difficult as individuals with bipolar disorder age and develop additional conditions that may affect their ability to understand and process information, such as stroke, dementia, hearing loss, and vision loss or encounter circumstances, such as placement in a nursing home or an assisted living situation, that reduce their actual or perceived ability to participate in research free of coercion or duress.

Conducting research with individuals who have bipolar disorder is critical if we are to improve our understanding of the causes of this disorder, our ability to assess individuals' capabilities, and our ability to develop and implement more effective and supportive interventions. Yet past history demonstrates the vulnerability of persons who are cognitively impaired, mentally ill, or institutionalized to abuse in research (Advisory Committee on Human Radiation Experiments 1996; Bein 1991; Garnett 1996; *Kaimowitz v. Michigan Department of Mental Health* 1973; Lubasch 1982; Rothman 1991; *Scott v. Casey* 1983; *Valenti v. Prudden* 1977). An outright prohibition against the participation of individuals with bipolar disorder in research would shield them from the potential for such abuse, but would also result in a loss of their individual autonomy and possibly exacerbate their societal isolation and stigmatization. Such a prohibition would also deprive future generations of important scientific knowledge critical to the amelioration or prevention of the disease and improvements in care. Consequently, individuals with mental illness, including bipolar disorder, may face the twin dangers of exploitation and overprotection; our challenge is to foster such research while simultaneously protecting research participants from potential exploitation and abuse.

THE REQUIREMENT OF INFORMED CONSENT

Ethically and legally, researchers are required to obtain the informed consent of an individual in order to enroll that individual into a study. This ethical requirement derives from several international documents, including the Nuremberg Code and the Helsinki Declaration, and has been integrated into U.S. law by federal regulations. These federal regulations state that "no investigator may involve a human being as a subject in research . . . unless the investigator has obtained the legally effective informed consent of the subject or the subject's legally authorized representative" (Code of Federal Regulations 2005).

The federal regulations, however, do not provide specific guidance to researchers who wish to conduct studies with cognitively impaired individuals, including those whose decision-making abilities are diminished by mental illness. Regulations applicable to all research participants mandate the presence of four elements in a valid informed consent process: (1) the individual from whom consent is to be obtained must be given the information necessary to make a decision; (2) the individual must understand the information; (3) the individual must have the capacity to consent; and (4) the consent of the individual to participate must be voluntary (Faden and Beauchamp 1986; Meisel et al. 1977). It cannot be emphasized enough that informed consent is a process that continues from the time of recruitment and enrollment throughout the study; it is not and should not be construed as the mere signing of a document by the prospective research participant.

Enhanced procedures during this informed consent process may be ethically required to ensure that research participants who have been diagnosed with a mental illness are able to provide valid informed consent. Still other enhancements may be required to protect those who have cognitive impairment due to mental illness, dementia, or age-related processes that result in their heightened vulnerability. Vulnerable participants are those individuals with "insufficient power, prowess, intelligence, resources, strength or other needed attributes to protect their own interests through negotiations for informed consent" (Levine 1988, 72). However, the mere fact of having been diagnosed with a mental illness, such as bipolar disorder, should not serve as the basis for automatically assuming that the individual lacks capacity (National Bioethics Advisory Commission 1998). These additional enhancements and protections are discussed below in the context of maximizing understanding, assessing capacity, balancing the risks and benefits of participation, and specifying the mechanisms for indicating consent.

Assessing Capacity to Consent

The terms *capacity* and *competence* are often used synonymously, but they actually represent distinct concepts. The term *capacity* is used here to refer to an individual's decision-making ability. In contrast, the term *competence* reflects a legal judgment that an individual has a minimal level of mental, cognitive, or behavioral functioning to perform or assume a specified legal role (Bisbing et al. 1995; Loue 2001). It is important to recognize that being diagnosed with a particular condition is "relevant to, but not determinative of, incapacity for informed consent" (High et al. 1994). For instance, the course of bipolar disorder may fluctuate, so there may be periods of time during which an individual is able to understand and to give legally valid consent. Additionally, the course of bipolar disorder may change over time, and older persons may be more impaired than younger persons.

In general, it is presumed at the commencement of research studies that a prospective participant has the capacity to consent, unless there is some reason to believe that he or she does not or that the capacity to give consent may be limited in some way. However, if a study focuses on a disorder involving either permanent cognitive impairment (such as mental retardation), or progressive impairment (such as Alzheimer disease), or fluctuating impairment (such as bipolar disorder), an assessment of capacity should be conducted at the commencement of participation. Longitudinal studies with participants with bipolar disorder may find two or more forms of impairment even within the same individual. For instance, individuals may experience fluctuating impairment due to the progression of their bipolar disorder, but, as they age, they may develop Alzheimer disease or other neurological illness, resulting in additional levels of progressive impairment. Because capacity and decision-making ability may vary during the course of the study — depending on the length of the study and the progression of the disorder or disease — it is also recommended that assessments of capacity and decision-making ability be conducted periodically during an individual's participation in research, unless that participation is of very short duration.

It is critical that the conditions under which capacity is to be assessed maximize the likelihood of an accurate finding. First, the individual who is to assess capacity must be matched appropriately with the prospective research participant (Kennedy 2000). For instance, a woman with a history of sexual abuse as a child may continue to be intimidated by men in positions of authority and power and may be less forthcoming when interviewed by a male research team member than by a female member. Some commentators suggest that the assessment and monitoring of an individual's capacity to consent and to participate in a study is best done by the study's research team in collaboration with a potential participant's family members (Keyserlingk et al. 1995). Four exceptions to this basic premise have been noted: (1) when the project staff does not have the requisite skill to assess or monitor participants' capacity; (2) when there is a strong danger of conflict of interest; (3) when the individual has previously executed an advance directive for research while he or she still had capacity, but the document requires interpretation; and (4) when the protocol does not have the potential to confer a direct benefit on the participant and involves more than minimal risk.

An individual's ability to respond to questions posed or to perform well on a test of cognitive ability may also be affected by iatrogenic and institutional factors (Kennedy 2000). The individual's ability to concentrate or his or her level of awareness may be affected by medications. Older individuals are likely to be taking a greater number of medications for comorbid medical conditions. Individuals accustomed to the regimentation of life in an institutional setting may become confused or frightened with a change in routine; absent a careful assessment, signs of that confusion may be mistaken for signs of diminished capacity. Environmentally induced stress, such as sleep deprivation and recent bereavement, that results in depression and a decline in functional ability may also adversely affect the individual's decision-making ability (American Psychiatric Association 2000). Physiological causes, such as fluctuations in the blood sugar of individuals with diabetes, sodium deficiency, and electrolyte imbalances, can also affect cognition. Older individuals are more prone to medical illness and are more likely to experience adverse drug reactions or drug intolerances (Routledge et al. 2004). Because a determination of (in)capacity is so complex, it has been suggested that it should be verified through reliance on second opinions or the services of consent specialists (Bonnie 1997).

Receiving Information

Federal regulations now require that the following information be provided to all research participants during the informed consent process: (1) a statement that the study involves research, an explanation of the purposes of the research, the expected duration of the subject's participation, a description of the procedures required for participation, and the identification of any procedures that are experimental; (2) a description of any reasonably foreseeable risks or discomforts to the research participant; (3) a description of any benefits from the research that may reasonably be expected for the research participant or others; (4) a disclosure of appropriate alternative procedures or courses of treatment, if any, that might be advantageous to the research participant; (5) a statement describing the extent to which confidentiality of records identifying the research participant will be maintained; (6) for research involving more than minimal risk, an explanation as to whether any compensation or any medical treatments are available if injury occurs and, if so, what they consist of or where further information may be obtained; (7) an explanation of whom to contact for answers to pertinent questions about the research and the rights of research participants, and whom to contact in the event of a research-related injury to the research participant; and (8) a statement that participation is voluntary, that a refusal to participate will not involve any penalty or loss of benefits to which the research participant is otherwise entitled, and that the participant may discontinue participation at any time without penalty or loss of benefits to which the subject is otherwise entitled (Code of Federal Regulations 2005).

In addition to these mandated disclosures, federal regulations indicate that the following information may be provided to research participants where appropriate: (1) a statement that the particular treatment or procedure may involve risks to the research participant (or to the embryo or fetus, if the subject is or may become pregnant) that are currently unforeseeable; (2) anticipated circumstances under which the participation of a research participant may be terminated by the investigator, without the subject's consent; (3) any additional costs to the subject that may result from participation in the research; (4) the consequences of a participant's decision to withdraw from the research and procedures for orderly termination of participation; (5) a statement that significant new findings developed during the course of the research that may relate to the subject's willingness to continue participation will be provided to the subject; and (6) the approximate number of subjects involved in the study (Code of Federal Regulations 2005).

Ensuring Understanding

It is essential that individuals understand that they are participating in research and that the procedures they will undergo may not yield any direct benefit to them. Some studies have found that many research participants may not understand either that they are participating in research rather than receiving clinical care or the nature of the procedures they will undergo in conjunction with their participation (Gray 1975; Hassar and Weintraub 1976; Howard et al. 1981; McCollum and Schwartz 1969; Park et al. 1966; Riecken and Ravich 1982). Research suggests that for individuals with severe mental illness, the ability to understand is related both to the level of psychopathology and to the quality of the information presented (Benson et al. 1988).

The National Bioethics Advisory Commission (2001) recommended that the informed consent procedure be tailored to the specific abilities of each individual participant to receive and process information. For instance, in addition to bipolar disorder, some elderly participants may have hearing or vision impairments that further impede their ability to understand the information in the form in which it is presented; accommodations must be made for these limitations to ensure that potential research participants understand the substance of the information being presented. Several suggestions have been made to maximize understanding, including the use of a clear and simple presentation format for the information (Bergler et al. 1980), the provision of sufficient time to enable the individual to process the information (Morrow et al. 1978), and discussion of the information with the physician (Williams et al. 1977). Individuals may be asked to restate or summarize in their own words the information provided, to confirm that they have understood. Tailored questions, whether in multiple-choice, true-false, or essay format, may be asked of the participant following presentation of the information, to ascertain whether and how much of the information he or she understood (Bonnie 1997; Flanery et al. 1978; Hassar and Weintraub 1976; McCollum and Schwartz 1969; Roth et al. 1982; Williams et al. 1977). One commentator suggested that a family member of a person who is cognitively impaired should participate in the informed consent process to ensure understanding and provide concurrent consent (Bonnie 1997).

Voluntariness

The life situation of many individuals with bipolar disorder may affect their ability to consent or refuse consent to participate in research. One research study found that 21% of adults with serious mental illness live below the poverty threshold, compared with 9% of the general adult population (Barker et al. 1992). Many homeless individuals have a mental illness (Isaac and Armat 1990), and a lack of adequate medical care may be associated with their poverty. Consequently, the possibility of participating in research with its attendant psychiatric and medical care may represent an otherwise unavailable and unattainable resource, leading individuals to disregard the risks that may be inherent in participation and to overemphasize the likelihood that they will obtain a direct benefit from their participation (National Bioethics Advisory Commission 1998).

Some individuals may be dependent on others for their physical care, for attention to their personal needs, or for their medical care. Elderly individuals, in particular, may depend on others for assistance (Novielli and Arensen 2003). They may fear that if they refuse to participate in a particular research study, they will suffer the withdrawal or diminution of such assistance or complete abandonment. This may be of particular concern to individuals living in institutions, such as nursing homes or psychiatric hospitals (Annas and Glantz 1997). Individuals may also be concerned that they will disappoint their caregiver or care provider if they refuse to participate (Sachs and Cassel 1989). Some individuals may believe that they would not have been offered the possibility of participating in a study unless the researcher believed their participation would yield some clinical benefit to them personally. They may believe this despite all assertions by a researcher that they may not receive any personal benefit from their participation and that only future patients will derive any benefit from knowledge gained through the study. This is known as the "therapeutic misconception" (Grisso and Appelbaum 1998).

OTHER CONSIDERATIONS
Confidentiality of the Data

The protection of confidentiality of the information disclosed to the researcher may be of concern, for a number of reasons. First, confidentiality may be difficult to maintain if interviews or other procedures are conducted in the context of an institutional residence, such as a nursing home, given the physical layout of the institution, a scarcity of private space, and the possibility that the participant may have impaired hearing, requiring the researcher to speak at a level that is audible to others (Cassel 1985, 1988).

Depending on the nature of the study, attempts to access the study data could be made through the legal system. For instance, consider a study that is examining resilience and social support among the elderly. The researchers know through their interviews with a participant that he has been abusing alcohol. He is the driver in an automobile accident in which the occupants of the other car are seriously injured. The insurance company for the injured persons obtains a subpoena for the study records of this participant, claiming that the research records are relevant to the driver's negligence. This illustrates that, if researchers believe such a situation could arise, or if they are collecting data that might be of interest to law enforcement or lawyers, before collecting data they should apply for a federal certificate of confidentiality to protect the data from subpoena (National Institutes of Health 2005).

Assessing and Balancing Risks and Benefits

A decision relating to participation in a research protocol requires the decision-maker, usually the prospective participant, to balance the risks and benefits of participation. (A balancing of risks and benefits must also be done by the researcher proposing the study before its initiation and by the institutional review board [IRB] of the researcher's institution in its initial and continuing reviews of the research protocol [Code of Federal Regulations 2005].)

Commentators have identified four categories of research protocols: (1) research in which a direct therapeutic benefit to the participant is possible and minimal risk is involved; (2) research in which the participant may obtain some direct therapeutic benefit, but more than minimal risk is involved; (3) research with no expected benefit for the individual participating but with more than minimal risk; and (4) research with no expected therapeutic benefit to the participant and with more than minimal risk (Kapp 1998; LeBlang and Kirchner 1996). "Minimal risk" is often interpreted to mean that the risks of participation are no greater than those that would be experienced in the everyday course of living (Levine 1988).

The study design itself may entail significant risks. "Challenge studies" are designed "to learn more about the underlying pathophysiological mechanisms responsible for the symptomatic expression of psychiatric illnesses" (Miller and Rosenstein 1997). Such study protocols demand the intentional inducement of disease symptoms. It is not clear that the relation between the risks and potential benefits of participation can ever justify enrolling individuals in studies such as these, where under any other circumstances the instigation of symptoms would be considered harmful. Additionally, it is unclear whether informed consent is ever obtainable for studies that, by their very design, are intended to provoke symptoms of illness (National Bioethics Advisory Commission 1998).

Clinical trials and crossover trials may involve the use of "washout" periods and/or placebo controls. Washout periods, during which an individual is deprived of medication, may be used at baseline or between phases of a crossover trial to return the research participant to a medication-free baseline to facilitate evaluation of the effects of a new or different drug on symptoms or behavior. However, the sudden or rapid withdrawal of medication to accomplish this washout may result in harm to the individual, raising substantial ethical concerns. The use of placebo controls may also be ethically problematic, given individuals' possibly fluctuating ability to comprehend information and the erroneous belief that the administration of any medication must be treatment designed to benefit them (National Bioethics Advisory Commission 1998).

Direct benefits may include short- or long-term improvement in the individual's condition, an improvement in symptoms, and the slowing of a degenerative process (Keyserlingk et al. 1995). Indirect benefits may include enhanced opportunities for social interaction, increased attention from health and ancillary health professionals, and a feeling of contributing in a way that may help others. Examples of risks include the physiological effects of an experimental drug or procedure and increased levels of anxiety associated with study questions or procedures (Dresser 2001).

Research suggests that even when the risks of participation are divulged to prospective participants, individuals may have difficulty comprehending them. In one clinical trial of a drug, respondents were found to be well-informed about the study design and general risks of participation, but 39% were unable to enumerate specific minor side effects of the drug and 64% were unable to identify the serious risks of the medication that had been divulged to them (Howard et al. 1981). In yet another study, few of the respondents recognized the possibility of unknown risk, meaning risks that cannot be anticipated before initiation of the study (Gray 1975).

There is no formula to dictate how the benefits and risks of a particular individual's participation are to be weighed. In fact, there is no consensus among researchers or ethicists on the level of risk or benefit that must be present for a surrogate decision-maker to be able to consent to research participation by an individual who is cognitively impaired (Dresser 2001).

MECHANISMS FOR EXPRESSING CHOICE DURING INCAPACITY
Advance Directives for Research

Because of the intermittent nature of bipolar disorder and its potential effects on decision-making ability, it may be advisable for individuals with this illness to indicate in advance whether they wish to participate in research. For instance, an individual diagnosed with bipolar disorder may strongly desire to participate in research if the opportunity were to arise, but may fear being unable to give consent at a future date, due to an acute exacerbation of the symptoms. Accordingly, the individual might want to express this intent at a time when he or she is still able to do so, when that expression will be recognized legally as valid.

One mechanism that has been suggested is an advance directive for research. Like an advance directive for health care, such a document allows individuals to make their wishes known at a time when they retain decision-making capacity. Alternatively, individuals might execute a durable power of attorney for health care and specify that their designated agent should have the legal authority to decide for them whether participation in a particular research study would be advisable and to provide or withhold consent accordingly.

This type of advance decision-making may be an option, depending on state law; not all states provide for such a document or recognize an agent as having the authority to make research-related decisions. Even where this possibility does exist, many individuals may be unaware of the mechanism. Indeed, only a minority of elderly patients execute durable powers of attorney for health care, often because they do not know about the mechanism or erroneously assume that a relative will automatically be able to make health care decisions for them if they are unable to do so (Cohen-Mansfield et al. 1991).

There are other difficulties associated with an advance directive for research, even if a state permits this mechanism. Because the informed consent process is supposed to be ongoing throughout the course of the study, an individual who consents to participate before knowing what a study is about is not really giving *informed* consent.

Questions also arise about the current validity of a prior expression to participate in research, because the individual's situation may have changed during the intervening period of time. For instance, an individual may have indicated, while having the capacity to do so, an intent and desire to participate in research. Some ethicists, distinguishing between the "then-person," the precursor to the person who now lacks capacity, and the "now-person," have argued that, as the individual's capacity decreases, so should the weight given to his or her previously expressed wishes in an advance directive (Brock and Buchanan 1989; Dresser 1992). This perspective results in the incongruous result of the greatest weight being given to the needs of the severely demented now-self, who has the least psychological continuity with the former competent self (Klepper and Roty 1999). Others have emphasized the concept of "precedent autonomy" and have argued that past decisions of the competent then-self must be respected even if they are not consistent with the wishes of the cognitively impaired now-self (Dworkin 1994). Still others have argued for the compassionate application of the principle of precedent autonomy, which would permit the implementation of previously expressed wishes as long as doing so does not result in discomfort to the now-self (Post 1995). This discussion has occurred most frequently in the context of Alzheimer disease, where the loss of individual capacity is progressive. The relevance of concepts addressing the then-person and now-person to individuals with fluctuating capacity, such as those with bipolar disorder, has not been explored.

Surrogate Consent

Even in the absence of a legally executed document, such as an advance directive for research, some have suggested that adults who lack the capacity to consent should be able to participate in research through the consent of a surrogate. Federal regulations permit a "legally authorized representative" to provide consent in some circumstances where the prospective participant is unable to do so. The term "legally authorized representative" is defined in the regulations as "an individual or judicial or other body authorized under applicable law to consent on behalf of a prospective subject to the subject's participation in the procedure(s) involved in the research" (Code of Federal Regulations 2005).

Some states have implemented regulations or statutes that govern in addition to the federal law and may place severe restrictions on the ability of individuals who are cognitively impaired to participate in research or the ability of a legally authorized representative to consent to an individual's participation in research, or may require judicial approval for such participation. Table 13.1 provides a partial listing of the states that have such restrictions, as well as citations to the statutory provisions and relevant court decisions.

A question arises as to which individual(s) are best suited to be appointed as surrogate decision-makers. The National Alliance for the Mentally Ill has proposed family members as the most appropriate surrogates in the research context (Flynn 1997). Many IRBs allow family members or friends to give consent (LeBlang and Kirchner 1996). However, some IRBs interpret the phrase "legally authorized representative" in the federal regulations narrowly and require that the surrogate be a court-appointed guardian, a designated health care agent under a written durable power of attorney for health care, a health care surrogate as defined by the relevant state law, or a combination of these (LeBlang and Kirchner 1996). At least one commentator argued that judicial approval must be obtained any time an individual is to be involved in research if that individual is unable to provide consent (Bein 1991).

Some commentators have pointed out the dangers to an individual of having decisions made by a surrogate, whether appointed through the execution of a document or not. First, family members may be inappropriate, because of their own lack

TABLE 13.1

Examples of state law provisions restricting ability of cognitively impaired individuals and/or their surrogate decision-makers to consent to participation research

State	Limitation	Provision
California	Conservator may consent to participation "only for medical experiments related to maintaining or improving the health of the subject or related to obtaining information about the pathological condition of the subject."	California Health and Safety Code § 24175(e) (West 1992)
Connecticut	Guardian may consent to participation in any biomedical or behavioral medical procedure or participation in any behavioral experiment "if it is intended to preserve the life or prevent serious impairment of the physical health of the ward or it is intended to assist the ward to regain his abilities" and has been approved for that person by the court.	Conn. Gen. Stat. Ann. § 45a-677(e) (West Supp. 1997)
Delaware	Prohibits approaching residents of state mental hospitals for participation in pharmaceutical research if individual is "incapable of voluntary consent to care or treatment"; prohibits specified classes of state mental hospital residents from participating in pharmaceutical research, regardless of capacity.	Del. Code Ann. Tit. 16, §§ 5174, 5175 (1995)
Illinois	Parent or guardian may not consent to ward's participation in any "unusual, hazardous, or experimental services" without approval by the court and determination that such services are in the "best interests" of the ward.	§ 405 Ill. Comp. Stat. Ann. 5/2-110 (West 1993)
Massachusetts	Prohibits research on patients in mental facilities if the research will not provide direct, therapeutic benefit; prohibits research on patients with mental disabilities where the risk is greater than minimal and exceeds the benefit to the participant.	Mass. Regs. Code Tit. § 104 13.01-.05 (1995)
Michigan	Experimental psychosurgery cannot be performed on a mentally incompetent person even if the surrogate decision-maker consents.	*Kaimowitz v. Michigan Department of Mental Health*, in *Disability Law Reporter* 1:147 (1976); *U.S. Law Week* 42:2063 (Circuit Court, Wayne County, Michigan, 1973)
Minnesota	Guardian or conservator is prohibited from giving consent to experimental treatment of any kind, unless the procedure is first approved by the court, which will determine whether it is in the "best interest" of the ward.	Minn. Stat. Ann. § 524.5-313(c)(4) (2003)

continued

TABLE 13.1
Continued

State	Limitation	Provision
Missouri	Prohibits state mental health patients from being "the subject of experimental research," with stated exceptions; prohibits the conduct of biomedical or pharmacological reserach on any individual with mental disabilities, unless the research will provide direct therapeutic benefit.	Mo. Stat. Ann § 630.115(8) (West Supp. 1997)
New Hampshire	The probate court may authorize the guardian to consent to experimental treatment only after ensuring that the treatment is in the ward's "best interest."	N.H. Rev. Stat. Ann. § 464-A:25(I)(c)-(e)(1995)
New York	Residents in a facility operated by the state or licensed by the Office of Mental Health who lack decision-making capacity may not be participants in any non-federally funded nontherapeutic research that poses greater than minimal risk, unless the individual, before the onset of incapacity, gave specific consent or designated an appropriate surrogate from whom consent can be obtained.	*T.D. v. New York State Office of Mental Health*, 650 N.Y.S.2d 173 (N.Y. App. Div. 1996), appeal dismissed, 680 N.E.2d 617 (N.Y. 1997), leave to appeal granted 684 N.E.2d 281 (N.Y. 1997), appeal dismissed, 1997 WL 785461 (N.Y., Dec. 22, 1997)

of capacity, unavailability, or inattention to the needs of the individual with cognitive impairment (High et al. 1994). Second, the surrogate may act in his or her own interest, rather than that of the individual (Sachs 1994). Accordingly, it has been suggested that an appropriate surrogate is an individual who (1) is chosen, known, and trusted by the individual; (2) participates with the individual who is cognitively impaired in the informed consent process; (3) is familiar with the individual's medical and psychiatric history; (4) is familiar with the prodromal signs and symptoms indicative of a relapse; (5) is informed about and is willing to assume the responsibilities of a surrogate decision-maker; (6) is willing to overrule the individual's previously expressed desire to participate in research if the participation could adversely affect the individual; and (7) is willing and able to ensure appropriate medical and/ or psychiatric follow-up care if needed (Backlar 1998).

Assuming that a surrogate, whether legally appointed or not, is able to decide for the individual who lacks the capacity to make the decision, the question remains of how the surrogate should make that determination. Two processes have been suggested: the best-interest test and the substituted-judgment test. The best-interest test requires an assessment of what is in the individual's best interest at the time the decision by the surrogate is to be made. This perspective allows a surrogate to more easily disregard any previously expressed desire or intent of the individual with mental illness, because what was once expressed may no longer be in the individual's best interest, as determined by the surrogate. The substituted-judgment test requires that the surrogate decide the issue of research participation in a manner consistent with what the individual would have chosen if he or she had remained able to do so. This perspective allows the surrogate to preserve to a greater degree the psychological continuity between the once-capable then-person and the now-person. If an IRB permits reliance on the substituted-judgment test, the IRB may require, in addition to the surrogate's consent, the assent of the individual to participate, meaning that, to the best of the individual's ability, he or she must indicate some preference, although that indication does not rise to the level of legal consent (cf. Sachs et al. 1994).

CONCLUSIONS

The participation in research by elderly adults with bipolar disorder is essential if we are to understand the course of this disorder over the lifespan and the cumulative and interactive effects of the disease with comorbid conditions. This understanding is critical if we are to develop strategies and discover pharmaceuticals that will ameliorate the symptoms of the disease and enhance individuals' functional capacity and quality of life. However, it is mandatory that we also protect those individuals who, while assisting in this endeavor through their participation in research, are in need of additional protections.

REFERENCES

Advisory Committee on Human Radiation Experiments. 1996. *Final report*. Washington, DC: Advisory Committee on Human Radiation Experiments.

American Psychiatric Association. 2000. *Diagnostic and statistical manual of mental disorders* (4th ed., text rev.). Washington, DC: American Psychiatric Association Press.

Annas, G. J., and Glantz, L. H. 1997. Informed consent to research on institutionalized mentally disabled persons: the dual problems of incapacity and voluntariness. In Shamoo, A. E. (ed.), *Ethics in neurobiological research with human subjects: the Baltimore conference on ethics* (pp. 55–79). Amsterdam: Gordon and Breach.

Backlar, P. 1998. Anticipatory planning for research participants with psychotic disorders like schizophrenia. *Psychol Public Policy Law* 4:829–848.

Barker, P. R., Manderscheid, R. W., Hendershot, G. E., et al. 1992. Serious mental illness and disability in the adult household population: United States, 1989. In Manderscheid, R. W., and Sonnenschein, M. A. (eds.), *Advance data from vital and health statistics of the National Center for Health Statistics* (no. 218). Washington DC: Department of Health and Human Services.

Bein, P. M. 1991. Surrogate consent and the incompetent experimental subject. *Food Drug, Cosmetic Law J* 46:739–771.

Benson, P. R., Roth, L. H., Appelbaum, P. S., et al. 1988. Information disclosure, subject understanding, and informed consent in psychiatric research. *Law Hum Behav* 12:455–475.

Bergler, J. H., Pennington, A. C., Metcalfe, M., et al. 1980. Informed consent: how much does the patient understand? *Clin Pharmacol Ther* 27:435–440.

Bisbing, S., McMenamin, J., and Granville, R. 1995. Competency, capacity, and immunity. In ACLM Textbook Committee (ed.), *Legal medicine* (3rd ed., pp. 27–45). St. Louis, MO: Mosby–Year Book.

Bonnie, R. J. 1997. Research with cognitively impaired subjects: unfinished business in the regulation of human research. *Arch Gen Psychiatry* 52:105–111.

Brock, D., and Buchanan, A. 1989. *Deciding for others.* Cambridge: Cambridge University Press.

Cassel, C. 1985. Research in nursing homes: ethical issues. *J Am Geriatr Soc* 33:795–799.

Cassel, C. 1988. Ethical issues in the conduct of research in long term care. *Gerontologist* 28:90–96.

Code of Federal Regulations. 2005. Title 45, §§ 46.101, 46.102(c), 46.111(a)(4), 46.116.

Cohen-Mansfield, J., Droge, J. A., and Billing, N. 1991. The utilization of the durable power of attorney for health care among hospitalized elderly patients. *J Am Geriatr Soc* 39:1174–1178.

Dresser, R. S. 1992. Autonomy revisited: the limits of anticipatory choices. In Binstock, R. H., Post, S. G., and Whitehouse, P. J. (eds.), *Ethics, values, and policy choices* (pp. 71–85). Baltimore: Johns Hopkins University Press.

Dresser, R. 2001. Dementia research: ethics and policy for the twenty-first century. *Georgia Law Rev* 35:661–690.

Dworkin, R. 1994. *Life's dominion: an argument against abortion, euthanasia, and individual freedom.* New York: Vintage.

Faden, R., and Beauchamp, T. 1986. *A history and theory of informed consent.* New York: Oxford University Press.

Flanery, M., Gravdal, J., Hendrix, P., et al. 1978. Just sign here . . . *South Dakota J Med* 31(5):33–37.

Flynn, L. M. 1997. Issues concerning informed consent and protections of human subjects in research: hearings before the Subcommittee on Human Resources of the House Committee on Government Reform and Oversight, 105th Cong.

Garnett, R. W. 1996. Why informed consent? Human experimentation and the ethics of autonomy. *Catholic Lawyer* 36:455–511.

Gray, B. 1975. *Human subjects in medical experimentation: a sociological study of the conduct and regulation of clinical research.* New York: Wiley.

Grisso, T., and Appelbaum, P. 1998. *Assessing competence to consent to treatment: a guide for physicians and other health professionals.* New York: Oxford University Press.

Hassar, M., and Weintraub, M. 1976. "Uninformed" consent and the wealthy volunteer: an analysis of patient volunteers in a clinical trial of a new anti-inflammatory drug. *Clin Pharmacol Ther* 20:379–386.

High, D. M., Whitehouse, P. J., Post, S. G., et al. 1994. Guidelines for addressing ethical and legal issues in Alzheimer disease research: a position statement. *Alzheimer Dis Assoc Disord* 8(suppl. 4):66–74.

Howard, J. M., DeMets, D., and BHAT Research Group. 1981. How informed is informed consent? *Control Clin Trials* 2:287–303.

Isaac, R. J., and Armat, V. C. 1990. *Madness in the streets: how psychiatry and the law abandoned the mentally ill.* New York: Free Press.

Kaimowitz v. Michigan Department of Mental Health. 1973. *U.S. Law Week* 42:2063 (Circuit Court, Wayne County, Michigan).

Kapp, M. 1998. Decisional capacity, older human research subjects, and IRBs: beyond forms and guidelines. *Stanford Law Policy Rev* 9:359–365.

Kennedy, G. J. 2000. *Geriatric mental health care: a treatment guide for health professionals.* New York: Guilford Press.

Keyserlingk, E. W., Glass, K., Kogan, S., et al. 1995. Proposed guidelines for the participation of persons with dementia as research subjects. *Perspect Biol Med* 38:319–361.

Klepper, H., and Roty, M. 1999. Personal identity, advance directives, and genetic testing for Alzheimer disease. *Genet Test* 3:99–106.

LeBlang, T. R., and Kirchner, J. L. 1996. Informed consent and Alzheimer disease research: institutional review board policies and practices. In Becker, R., and Giacobini, E. (eds.), *Alzheimer's disease from molecular biology to therapy* (pp. 529–534). Boston: Birkhauser.

Levine, R. J. 1988. *Ethics and regulation of clinical research.* New Haven, CT: Yale University Press.

Loue, S. 2001. Elder abuse and neglect in medicine and law: the need for reform. *J Legal Med* 22:159–209.

Lubasch, A. H. 1982. Trial ruled in 1953 death case. *New York Times,* Sept. 14.

McCollum, A. T., and Schwartz, A. H. 1969. Pediatric research hospitalization: its meaning to parents. *Pediatr Res* 3:199–204.

Meisel, A., Roth, L. H., and Lidz, C. W. 1977. Toward a model of the legal doctrine of informed consent. *Am J Psychiatry* 134:285–289.

Miller, F. G., and Rosenstein, D. L. 1997. Psychiatric symptom-provoking studies: an ethical appraisal. *Biol Psychiatry* 42:403–409.

Morrow, G., Gootnick, J., and Schmale, A. 1978. A simple technique for increasing cancer patients' knowledge of informed consent to treatment. *Cancer* 42:793–799.

National Bioethics Advisory Commission. 1998. *Research involving persons with mental disorders that may affect decisionmaking capacity.* Rockville, MD: National Bioethics Advisory Commission.

National Institutes of Health. 2005. Certificates of confidentiality kiosk. http://grants1.nih.gov/grants/policy/coc/index.htm

Novielli, K. D., and Arensen, C. A. 2003. Overview of geriatrics. *Clin Podiatr Med Surg* 20:373–381.

Park, L. C., Slaughter, R. S., Covi, L., et al. 1966. The subjective experience of the research patient: an investigation of psychiatric outpatients' reactions to the research treatment situation. *J Nerv Ment Dis* 143:199–206.

Post, S. G. 1995. Alzheimer disease and the "then" self. *Kennedy Inst Ethics J* 4:307–321.

Riecken, H. W., and Ravich, R. 1982. Informed consent to biomedical research in Veterans Administration hospitals. *JAMA* 248:344–348.

Roth, L. H., Lidz, C. W., Meisel, A., et al. 1982. Competency to decide about treatment or research: an overview of some empirical data. *Int J Law Psychiatry* 5:29–50.

Rothman, D. J. 1991. *Strangers at the bedside: a history of how law and bioethics transformed medical decision making*. New York: Basic Books.

Routledge, P. A., O'Mahony, M. S., and Woodhouse, K. W. 2004. Adverse drug reactions in elderly patients. *Br J Clin Pharmacol* 57:121–126.

Sachs, G. A. 1994. Advance consent for dementia research. *Alzheimer Dis Assoc Disord* 8:19–27.

Sachs, G., and Cassel, C. 1989. Ethical aspects of dementia. *Neurol Clin* 7:845–858.

Sachs, G. A., Stocking, C. B., Stern, R., et al. 1994. Ethical aspects of dementia research: informed consent and proxy consent. *Clin Res* 42:403–412.

Scott v. Casey. 1983. 562 F. Supp. 475 (N.D. Ga.).

Valenti v. Prudden. 1977. 58 A.D.2d 956, 397 N.Y.S.2d 181.

Williams, R. L., Rieckmann, K. H., Trenholme, G. M., et al. 1977. The use of a test to determine that consent is informed. *Military Med* 142:542–545.

Index